Cutting-Edge Therapies for *Autism*

2010–2011

Ken Siri and Tony Lyons

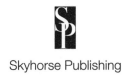

Skyhorse Publishing

Skyhorse Publishing books may be purchased in bulk at special discounts for sales promotion, corporate gifts, fund-raising, or educational purposes. Special editions can also be created to specifications. For details, contact the Special Sales Department, Skyhorse Publishing, 555 Eighth Avenue, Suite 903, New York, NY 10018 or info@ skyhorsepublishing.com.

www.skyhorsepublishing.com

10 9 8 7 6 5 4 3 2 1

Library of Congress Cataloging-in-Publication Data

Siri, Ken.
    Cutting-edge therapies for autism, 2010-2011 / Ken Siri and Tony Lyons.
        p. cm.
    ISBN 978-1-61608-025-9
1. Autism in children--Treatment--Popular works. I. Lyons, Tony. II. Title.
    RJ506.A9S57 2010
    618.92'89--dc22
                        2010003545

Printed in the United States of America

This book is for Lina, Alex, and all the kids suffering from autism, and for their parents struggling to give them the best possible life.

ACKNOWLEDGEMENTS

K en and Tony are deeply indebted to in-house Skyhorse Publishing editor Joey Sverchek, without whom we could not possibly have completed this project. We are also indebted to Teri Arranga of AutismOne who spent countless hours going over the manuscript, the jacket, and the press release and gave us excellent editorial advice.

Tony would like to thank his ex-wife Helena who has worked with Lina to the brink of insanity, utilizing many of the therapies described in this book, staying up with her when she can't sleep, calming her down when she is dis-regulated, holding, comforting, and carrying her, joining and engaging with her and giving her as much love as any human being has ever received from another human being. She is pulling Lina with both hands out of the abyss of autism.

CONTENTS

THERAPIES OF THE FUTURE

FINAL THOUGHTS

PREFACE

BY KEN SIRI AND TONY LYONS

EDITOR'S NOTE: Ken and I both have children on the autism spectrum. We don't have any financial connection to any organization, doctor or therapist included in this book. We conceived of the book as a way to learn more ourselves in order to help our children. We are happy to be able to present what we have learned regarding the resources and treatments currently available and those which are emerging. Our team of contributors is impressive. It includes leading doctors, therapists, teachers, scientists, educators, social workers and parents. **–Tony Lyons**

The central purpose of this book is to provide people interested in autism therapies—including parents, grandparents, teachers, therapists, doctors and researchers—with articles about the cutting-edge work being done in the field. This field changes rapidly and we plan to update the book annually. *Cutting-Edge Therapies for Autism* is for people who want to learn as much as they possibly can about the therapies available, and about how to do everything in their power to help the growing number of children who are suffering.

Autism is the country's fastest-growing medical emergency, affecting more children than cancer, diabetes, Down syndrome and AIDS combined. Approximately 1 million people in the United States currently suffer from some form of autism.

Autism is difficult to define. No two kids have the same exact set of symptoms or respond to the same combination of therapies. Each child's treatment plan needs to be unique, taking into consideration the specific symptoms the child exhibits, the results of tests administered, and the observations of the child's doctors, therapists, teachers and, just as importantly, parents.

Case study #1: Lina

My daughter Lina was a bright, happy, talkative, social little girl. She had some ongoing problems with eczema but, other than that, was very healthy. Just before she turned three, she was given a regimen of antibiotics for bronchitis. Shortly thereafter, she received her measles mumps and rubella (MMR) booster shot. About two weeks later, she started to drool uncontrollably. It looked like her lips and jaw muscles had gone totally numb. The pediatrician took some tests and found that she had been exposed to the Epstein Barr Virus, but couldn't tell us anything more. The drooling episode lasted a couple of weeks, during which time her speech became garbled and she began to stutter. It took an incredible effort for her to push words out of her mouth. She was like a toy running low on batteries, losing steam, losing control. As things inside of her began to disconnect, she was becoming disconnected from the world around her. A friend came over with her daughter for a play date and, after a few minutes with Lina, she asked, with real fear in her eyes: "What's going on with Lina? She seems like a different person." Lina seemed to improve after that, but then gradually deteriorated. She was first diagnosed with Sensory Processing Disorder, then Pervasive Development Disorder (PDD), and then, finally, autism. For some kids autism means screaming, biting, throwing things out the window, breaking everything in sight, even head banging. Life with them and for them can be harsh. When I look at Lina I see a peaceful, loving, gentle girl struggling to get out of a body that isn't functioning correctly. She's the victim—not me, not her mother, not her teachers, not society. The other day after slamming doors, screaming uncontrollably, and throwing things, she was able to calm down and walked over to me. I was sitting in my home office and, exhausted, she put her cheek on my arm, pulled my fingers to her back and said: "Can I please have a tickle, scratch, scratch." Lina clearly has attention deficit hyperactivity disorder (ADHD), she's obsessive compulsive (OCD), she has sensory processing disorder (SPD), is often manic, has gut and sleep issues, and her language is a constant struggle. But her mother, Helena, and I are fighting these symptoms and Lina is fighting them and we'll keep fighting them together and, God willing, we'll continue to see progress.

Case study #2: Alex

My son Alex was born in June of 1998 and developed normally, meeting or exceeding all his milestones until just after the age of 3. He attended daycare early (from age 4 months old) and was a popular and happy kid. While at daycare, Alex was able to pick up some Spanish in addition to his native English and could count to 10 in English, Spanish and Japanese by his second birthday. Medically, Alex was healthy as an infant and toddler, although he did have frequent sinus and ear infections that were treated with inhaled albuterol. He had all his vaccinations on time, the last of which followed his third birthday. By late summer folks at daycare began to comment that Alex was uncharacteristically spending more time on his own, sometimes staring out the window. A visit to his pediatrician produced an all too common "Don't worry, it's just a stage." Then Alex began to lose some speech, though he was still able to say, "Turn that off, that's scary," in response to TV coverage of 9/11. By Christmas 2001, Alex had lost a significant amount of speech, frequently stimmed by clapping his hands loudly (you never heard such a clap) and clearly had ADHD. At a holiday party that season, a person who owned a daycare center told me she thought Alex was autistic. This began our yearlong journey into the autism abyss. By the end of 2002 Alex was non-verbal and a fully diagnosed member of the autism epidemic.

There is no general consensus on what causes autism—either classic Kanner's autism or the regressive kind. Some people think it's entirely genetic, while others think it's caused by Pitocin, fluoride in tap water or tooth paste, GAMT (guanidinoacetate methyltransferase) deficiency, chemicals in foods or household products, parental age, stress, treatments for asthma given to pregnant women, vaccines and/or the preservative thimerosal in some vaccines, viruses in the stomach or perhaps a specific retrovirus known as XMRV (which is under investigation by the CDC), gastrointestinal (GI) tract problems, immune problems, impaired intestinal functioning, environmental toxins, vitamin D deficiency, seizures, mobile phone radiation, encephalitis, hypoglycemia, antibiotics, and the list goes on and on. In compiling this book we have noticed a consensus beginning to emerge that the symptoms of autism result from a perfect storm of factors that come together to create a kind of system overload, a tipping point, in a genetically predisposed child's developing immune system. Recent studies point toward this overload causing problems at the cellular level, impairing the ability of nerve cells to transmit information properly through the synapses of the brain. Furthermore, the dramatic increase in the incidence of autism spectrum disorders points toward environmental factors playing a significant role. Further supporting this is the fact that scientists have found that by introducing environmental toxins or antibiotics they can create autistic symptoms in rats.

So what happened to Lina and Alex? We believe that they were genetically predisposed to contract autism, but required a big push and that the push came from a virus and a high fever, followed by antibiotics and a barrage of vaccines, all of which occurred at a fragile developmental stage. The antibiotics disregulated the immune system and the vaccines, thrown in as an additional stressor at the worst possible time, were the final straw. We also believe that the disregulated, hyper-active immune system created an autoimmune response whereby the immune system couldn't tell the difference between healthy tissue and the antigens that it normally fights and then probably attacked the healthy tissue of both the stomach lining and the brain. We believe that this combination of factors created a gut malfunction, a kind of climate change in the stomach that made it difficult for our kids to digest certain proteins that are necessary for healthy blood-cell development and healthy nerve cell activation. The proteins in the blood cells are necessary for the healthy development of the cognitive centers of the brain and in the nerve cells they help the neurotransmitters fire up correctly, send proper messages (like pain, hot and cold, sound etc.) and connect the right and left lobes of the brain. We think that the human body can normally withstand severe complications and stressors but, for the young, predisposed child, this chain of events is just too much. While we're not scientists, like everyone reading this book, we're doing our very best to try to solve the puzzle.

As far as treatments for autism, most doctors still tell parents with absolute certainty that it is an incurable lifelong condition and that treatments simply don't work. Kim Stagliano, author of the upcoming book *All I Can Handle, I'm No Mother Teresa* about life with three autistic daughters writes:

An autism diagnosis can erase a person's ability to get solid medical care. If you brought your 6-year-old to a hospital in the throes of a seizure, the neurologists would run tests and look for the cause. When I brought my 6-year-old in, I was told, "She has autism. She has different circuitry." And then when I requested tests, I was told, "We're just not that aggressive with autism." My child has a brain and a gut and immune system just like any other child. Why does her autism negate that?

In looking at a more than 50 percent increase in the incidence of autism between 2002 to 2006, Dr. Thomas Insel director of the National Institute of Mental Health (NIMH) and chair of the Interagency Autism Coordinating Committee (IACC) the nation's top autism research coordinator, had this to say in an interview with David Kirby for the *Huffington Post*:

> This tells you that you really have to take this very seriously. From everything they are looking at, this is not something that can be explained away by methodology, by diagnosis.

He goes on to say that we should not be looking at autism as a single thing, with one cause, one treatment, one explanation. There may, in fact, be 10 or 20 or more distinct variations.

> I think this is a collection of many, many different disorders... It's quite believable to me that there are many children who develop autism in the context of having severe gut pathology, or having auto-immune problems, or having lots of other problems. And some of these kids really do recover. And this is quite different from the autism that was originally described in the 1940s and 1950s—where it looks like you have it and you are going to have it for the rest of your life.

If autism is caused by the comorbidity of the underlying medical conditions, and if there are really endless variations of autism, then why on earth wouldn't we treat these conditions, mandate that insurance companies pay for these treatments, and get on to the business of trying to heal the underlying conditions. Dr. Insel agrees and says: "We've got to be able to break apart this spectrum disorder into its component parts and identify who's going to respond to which interventions." He advocates for genetic mapping as a way to pinpoint the underlying medical conditions so that we can figure out whether an individual had been "exposed to organophosphates, or perhaps to some infection, or some autoimmune process" that interferes with the way the brain develops. Others are beginning to express similar sentiment. Dr. Christopher Walsh, Ballard Professor of Neurology and Chief of the Division of Genetics at Children's Hospital in Boston says: "I would like every kid on the spectrum to have not 'autism' but a more specific disorder. By isolating the genes involved and understanding their functions, researchers can begin to develop particular treatments aimed at particular disorders." Dr. James Gusella, Ballard Professor of Neurogenetics and director of the Center for Human Genetic Research at Massachusetts General Hospital (MGH) says: "Autism is a problem that no one person or discipline can figure out alone."

Throughout the book, we use the word "treatment" in the broadest possible sense. Nevertheless, the therapies included by no means constitute an exhaustive list. Most of the practitioners included can tell you about cases where their therapy helped decrease the symptoms of a specific child, helped the child relate better, speak better, helped minimize gut problems, or helped control behavioral problems. And they have parents to support their claims. On the other hand, most of these therapies have not undergone rigorous trials, the kind of trials that cost substantial amounts of money and often take years to complete and evaluate. As a result, there are some people who contest the claims of the practitioners or parents. In any case, by including a specific treatment, we are not endorsing that treatment or telling you that it will work for your child or patient. Nor are the 84 doctors, teachers, therapists, parents, and other experts who have contributed to this book endorsing any treatment other than the one that they are writing about. Furthermore, practically none of these therapies are endorsed by any state or the federal government or covered by health insurance.

We certainly believe that the government should mandate insurance coverage for extensive genetic, blood and spinal fluid testing before any definitive diagnosis can be given. We have heard of cases where children showed the symptoms of autism or other disorders such as cerebral palsy, multiple sclerosis, or schizophrenia, but in fact had easily treatable disorders and were fully rehabilitated. We believe these kids, like any other kids, deserve the best medical care available, including full coverage for any treatment that is recommended by a specialist in any specific underlying medical condition. Some states have already started heading in this direction. For now, the only FDA approved drugs are Abilify and Risperdal and the only therapy approved by most states is applied behavior analysis (ABA), based on the teachings of B. F. Skinner. Recently, however, practitioners and researchers have begun advocating for approaches that combine the various therapies and scientists are trying to develop ways to measure how particular therapies improve brain connections in a specific individual.

Autism costs families an incredible amount of money. Estimates range from $60,000 to $100,000 per year and that assumes that you can either find an adequate public school in your district or, more likely, a private school that your city will agree to pay for. If you can't get the school paid for, then the cost could be as high as $200,000 per year. Whoever pays, autism is a growing problem and states and the federal government need to address it. Right now, autism costs the United States an estimated 35 billion dollars per year, but that could well be the trickle that turns into a flood. We believe that by funding more research and by agreeing either to pay for a broader range of therapies or to require insurance companies to do that, states and the federal government will save money in the long run.

Dr. Insel admits that when he was in training as a psychiatrist he "never saw a child with autism." He says that he wanted to see kids with autism, but he simply couldn't find any. Now, Insel says, "I wouldn't have to go any further than the block where I live to see kids with autism." This is an epidemic. We've come from a time when 1 in 10,000 babies born in the United States exhibited symptoms of autism to a time when the statistics are roughly 1 in 100. Think about that for a moment, 1% of kids born in this country become autistic. And those statistics, which come from the Centers for Disease Control (CDC), are based on data collected four years ago, so that the current rate is estimated to be 1 in 91.

If you were to take the 57% increase in the incidence of autism between 2002 and 2006, as calculated by the CDC (which the CDC itself says cannot be explained away by a shift in diagnostic criteria) and extrapolate forward, then at least half of all children born in the United States will be autistic by 2046. And these statistics fail to differentiate between classic autism, which is characterized by a child sitting in a corner rocking back and forth with little interest in social interaction, and regressive autism, where a normally developing child suddenly loses speech, interest in social interaction with peers and develops various biomedical symptoms. Ten years ago no one talked or wrote about regressive autism and now this is the fastest growing segment of the autistic population. What if this is just a different disorder? What if it's a disorder that has gone from 1 in 200 million to 1 in 200 in a 10 year period? Then, certainly, we're looking at a medical disaster of unprecedented proportions that is here, now and warrants a response at least as dramatic as the CDCs response to swine flu or the AIDS epidemic. We could well be at the tipping point of a crisis that will soon consume our future.

We are not doctors or scientists or government officials, but dads who love our kids and want to do the very best we can for them. We don't know for sure what caused our kids' autism and maybe we never will. If it was an immune system overload, we think that in most cases the cure is going to come not from a one-off drug, but from a counterassault, an all-out systemic approach, from DIR, from ABA, from dietary interventions, from GI tract treatments, from nutritional supplements, from anti-virals, from physical therapy, from sensory integration therapy, from brain therapy, from whatever fits the individual child. The current unwillingness of insurance companies, states and the federal government to pay for therapies is typical short-term thinking. Costs will only escalate, as untreated children become adults who need to be cared for by the state. A long-term approach will ultimately save money and will undoubtedly lead to at least some children being cured. This is war and if we want these children back, if we want to stop the progress of this disorder, we are going to have to fight. There will be people, lots of people, who will keep pointing out that there is no known cure, that they believe the struggle is hopeless. They will tell you that the best thing to do is to try to protect your own sanity and save your money. Our mission is to give our children, everyone's autistic children, their lives back to the fullest extent possible. We want to be involved in finding a remedy or a series of therapies that act together to bring these kids back to themselves and to their families and to the world.

Lina and Alex may never be typical kids. But perhaps they can be in a position to make informed decisions about their own lives, to communicate with people, to experience friendship and love and passion and hope. And who knows, perhaps if we help cure them, they will be the ones who develop a cure for cancer! Whatever the outcome, until there is a cure, we will do our very best to look for promising therapies for the symptoms of autism and continue to publish *Cutting Edge Therapies for Autism* in March of every year.

—**Ken Siri and Tony Lyons**

INTRODUCTION

NAVIGATING THE AUTISM SUPERHIGHWAY: HOW TO DETERMINE IF A THERAPY IS RIGHT FOR YOUR CHILD AND FAMILY

BY DR. MARK FREILICH

If you are intently reading or just skimming through the chapters of this book, the assumption is that your child or a child you know was recently or at some time in the past diagnosed with an autism spectrum disorder.

At this point you have hopefully, to one degree or another, started to come to terms with the diagnosis and what it means for your child, for you, and for your family. You are now ready to enter the Autism Superhighway, inch by inch, or at full speed.

In either case, it is now time to gather your team of co-navigators who will assist you in putting together a GPS system with the appropriate approaches, methods, and interventions. These should all be based on your child's unique and individual profile. This profile is essential in guiding the course of treatment.

For any child with autism, determining a course of treatment using only information you have read in a book or researched on the Internet is ill-advised. One needs a qualified team of specialists to properly evaluate, diagnose, prescribe, and monitor your child's strengths and areas of need.

This book is intended to provide an overview of a variety of approaches, methods, and interventions that alone or in combination may help place a child on the road to recovery from autism. It needs to be said that at this time there is no cure for autism. There are many children, however, who have received timely and comprehensive interventions and no longer meet the diagnostic criteria for an autism spectrum diagnosis. No matter the severity of manifestations, significant benefit can be gained by the child, the family, or both, with early and intensive interventions. However, if any clinician, specialist, or intervention approach promises a cure, be very leery and scrutinize carefully the validity of these claims.

Your primary pediatric care provider should be knowledgeable about the various medical, developmental, and behavioral issues that children with autism spectrum disorders may encounter. They should be aware of the available treatment options and the specialists in your area to whom you need to be referred. They need to be open minded to ALL treatments, whether they are based on a Western medicine approach or an alternative/complementary medical philosophy. Most importantly, there needs to be close collaboration and communication between your family, your specialists/therapists, and your child's primary care pediatric physician.

Unfortunately a common etiology for autism has not been discovered. Each child may broadly share common general manifestations but the triggers and causes for these manifestations may vary greatly from one child to another. It appears that the way parents and professionals view autism today is in transition. Although many continue to view it as strictly a psychiatric or a neurologic disorder, newer viewpoints are being embraced. Autism is increasingly being viewed as a disorder with multifactorial etiologies defined by its behavioral manifestations. These include impairments in communication and social interactions, repetitive behaviors, and sensory processing and regulatory issues. Therefore, autism needs to be considered a "spectrum" disorder that not only is impacted by issues in the brain and nervous system but one that is impacted by dysfunction in the immune, gastrointestinal, and metabolic systems. Since the etiology as well as the manifestations of autism are influenced by a variety of multiple factors, a cookie-cutter or a one-size-fits-all approach to treatment and intervention programming is steering you onto the wrong road. Creating an individual profile is therefore essential to navigating the Autism Superhighway. This profile must include an assessment of the child's present developmental level. It needs to analyze the child's individual medical, genetic, behavioral, sensory processing, and regulatory profile. Consideration of parenting skills, cultural beliefs, and expectations need to be factored in.

The child's profile should and will change over time. The key to successful outcomes is establishing a cohesive team approach, with ongoing monitoring of progress to ensure treatments remain relevant and goals are always current and realistic.

One cannot promise that the Autism Superhighway your child and your family will be travelling on will offer a smooth or detour-free trip. There will be bumps, curves, and forks in the road. Remember, this is a long journey, not a short road trip. There will be many moments when you think "are we there yet?" but there will also be many scenic road stops and enjoyable attractions. Be sure to take the time to enjoy the major highlights along the way.

—MARK FREILICH, M.D.

THERAPIES

ALLERGIES, THEIR ROLE AND TREATMENT IN AUTISM

BY DR. MARVIN BORIS

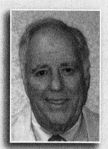

Marvin Boris, MD, FAAP, FAAAIA, FACA

Autism Associates of New York
77 Froehlich Farm Boulevard
Woodbury, NY 11797
(516) 921-3456

Associate Clinical Professor Of Pediatrics, New York University
School of Medicine
Defeat Autism Now! doctor
Fellow, American Academy of Allergy, Asthma and Immunology
Fellow, American Academy of Pediatrics
The American Academy of Environmental Medicine
Author of over fifty scientific papers
Allergy and immunology clinical practice

Autism is a complex developmental neurological disease of sensory, behavioral, communication, cognitive, and speech deficits. Many of these symptoms are mediated through inflammatory, autoimmune, and metabolic mechanisms. It has been repeatedly published that children with autism spectrum disorders (ASD) have marked alterations and elevation of cytokines, the mediators of inflammation and autoimmunity. Many factors may produce alterations in inflammation and autoimmunity, including toxins, pesticides, heavy metals, foods, chemicals, infections, drugs, vaccines, radiation, stress, and allergens.

A basic tenet of medicine is to eliminate the underlying cause of the disease, however in many instances the damage has already been done and this is not feasible. As an example, dietary manipulation of foods has, through elimination diets, benefited many children with ASD.

Avoidance of most airborne allergens is difficult. Under these circumstances allergy immunotherapy is the method of choice. Allergens affect every cell in the body, since all cells react to the allergen immunoglobulins, especially IgE and IgG. Our interest in children with ASD does not lie with the usual respiratory symptoms of allergy, but in how it affects all the other organ systems.

Our group performed and published a study, "Pollen Exposure as a Cause for the Deterioration of Neurobehavioral Function in Children with Attention Deficit Hyperactive Disorder." The effects of pollen exposure were highly significant in producing neuropsychological regression, hyperactivity, and obsessive behaviors in these groups. This illustrated well the neurogenic effects of allergen exposure and not only that the pollens produce the typical itchy eyes, runny noses, and respiratory symptoms.

Over the years, one thing I have frequently observed was that many children had behavioral problems when they returned to school in the fall. The school officials said it was psychological. However, when the child was removed from the recently painted, sprayed, or chemically cleaned environment, the symptoms and behaviors disappeared. So obviously these exposures precipitated the adverse behaviors and functioning of the children.

Allergy immunotherapy is an effective way to alleviate and prevent many of the environmentally precipitated variations in behavior in children with ASD. Several different modes of testing and treatment are currently available.

The conventional standard method utilizes prick or intradermal skin tests to determine if a person reacts to a particular antigen at a predetermined concentration. On the basis of this testing the person is administered buildup allergy injections to the positive results. The usual course requires increasing weekly injections over a period of four to six months to reach a therapeutic level.

Here I note several comments about and problems with the standard immunotherapy method. It is the effective method utilized by almost all the allergists in the United States. However this may cause several problems in the autistic population. Bringing the child to the allergist's office for these weekly injections often interferes with the child's educational and therapeutic programs. The time required to achieve an optimal dose is many months. The allergy extracts contain preservatives of phenol or glycerin, which many of the ASD children cannot tolerate.

Specific dose therapy is the allergy treatment used in our office. Physicians in the American Academy of Environmental Medicine often treat their patients through this mechanism. The extracts are made in our office from the pure basic ingredient and contain no preservatives.

In order to determine the specific antigen dose, serial endpoint testing is performed on the patient. This takes two to three hours. EMLA (Eutectic Mixture of Local Anesthetics) cream is initially applied to the child's upper arms as a local anesthetic, in order to make the treatment more comfortable for the child. A small dose of the allergy extract (e.g., dust, molds, mites, pollens, or animal extract) is injected under the skin and a wheal forms. This wheal is measured, timed for seven to ten minutes, and then measured again. It is considered positive if it grows by more than 2mm in ten minutes' time. This strongest dose that does not produce a significant increase in the size of the wheal is the treatment dose. This is the dose of that antigen that will be placed in the allergy extract. This process is repeated for all the allergens to be tested.

All the tested allergens at their specific nonreactive dosage are placed in the individual's specific extract. Since the allergy extract contains the nonreactive dose of the allergen, it is administered at home. Our policy is to give the allergy extract either as a nasal spray or an injection, whichever is easier for the family to administer to the child. The extract is administered on a daily basis. It is supplied in a thirty-dose vial, which has to be refrigerated since there are no preservatives in the vial.

Responses to the specific dose therapy are often observed in two to six weeks, not requiring the four- to six-month buildup necessary with standard immunotherapy. The most frequently observed benefits are improvement in behavior, decreased hyperactivity, improved sleeping habits, and better socialization, along with the loss of deterioration during allergy exposures.

Serial endpoint testing may be performed to help determine and possibly treat food allergies. Elimination diets are the standard and most effective process to address food sensitivities. Blood test evaluations of food allergies have inconsistent results, and I therefore do not rely on blood testing results.

Food testing is utilized on individuals who have difficulties with elimination diets and who need more information on specific foods, or to whom desensitization to foods would be beneficial. Serial endpoint testing is also a provocation test, since many people may exhibit symptoms to the food being tested, providing additional information. Unlike inhalants—where several inhalants may be tested at one time—the foods must be tested one at a time due to the possible provocation reaction. If the food shows a high sensitivity on the testing, it is recommended that it be avoided. The foods with moderate reactions can be placed in a food extract, similar to the inhalants, in order to desensitize the person to those foods. Again, the food extract may be administered using a nasal spray or injection.

Using this food desensitization treatment, I have observed over the years that many ASD children could tolerate foods which previously had adverse behavioral effects on them. This can make life more pleasant for the child and for the parent.

In summary, ASD is a biomedical disease in which both inhalant and food allergies may precipitate adverse behavioral symptoms. Testing through serial endpoints, both for inhalants and foods—with treatment based upon these results—may improve children and adults with ASD.

ANIMAL-ASSISTED INTERVENTIONS AND PERSONS WITH AUTISM SPECTRUM DISORDERS

BY DR. AUBREY FINE

Aubrey H. Fine Ed.D.

Professor
Department of Education
CA Poly University
3801 W. Temple Ave.
Pomona, CA 91768
ahfine@csupomona.edu

Psychologist Dr. Aubrey Fine has been in the field of Animal-Assisted Therapy (AAT) for over twenty-five years. He is the editor of the most widely accepted book on the subject, *The Handbook on Animal-Assisted Therapy*, has had a featured monthly column in *Dog Fancy* magazine on the human-animal bond entitled "The Loving Bond." He has also been a guest on numerous national TV and radio shows including on programs on ABC, Animal Planet, KTLA, and CNN. His newest book, *Afternoons with Puppy*, released by Purdue University in December, 2007, is a heartwarming account about the evolving relationships and outcomes among a therapist, his therapy animals, and his patients over the course of over two decades. Over this period, he has applied AAT with a variety of children with diverse forms of etiology and has witnessed many moving outcomes as a result of incorporating animals as therapeutic agents. An active faculty member at California State Polytechnic University since 1981, he was awarded the prestigious Wang Award in 2001 for exceptional commitment, dedication, and exemplary contributions within the areas of education and applied sciences.

*H*is mother always wanted him to have a dog, but wasn't quite sure how he would react. That is when I got the call. I decided that Magic—a very gentle, calm, and attentive four-year-old golden retriever who seems very comfortable working with *all children—would be his best match. She always approaches those with whom she interacts very slowly, giving them ample time to get acclimated to her presence.*

When they first met, Bob was apprehensive and used poor eye contact. He also mumbled his speech and spoke with a pedantic flair. That didn't seem to be an obstacle for Magic. She moved close to Bob, waiting for him to pet her. Their relationship was just beginning. Over the following weeks, not only did he become more comfortable with her presence, he also began to speak up and with more clarity to everybody. Puppy love and companionship may have been the initial goals, but Bob's family would quickly learn that animal-assisted interventions have much more to offer.

Introduction

The unique bond between humans and animals and its powerful impact on human well-being have been documented over hundreds of years (Wells, 2009). It is apparent that in most cases, pets fill a void in owners' lives. Instead of coming home to an empty house, people come home to the greetings of happy, loving animals, such as dogs or cats. Our pets provide companionship and unconditional love as well as providing friendship to those who may lack social contact. Within this chapter, attention will be given to explain the value of the human-animal bond, and describe how animal-assisted interventions can be a viable alternative to persons with any autism spectrum disorder (ASD). Before specifically discussing the roles that animals can have with people who have ASD, we'll first explore the value of the human-animal bond and the field of animal-assisted interventions (AAI).

Understanding the Human-Animal Bond

The American Veterinary Medical Association's Committee on the Human-Animal Bond defines the human-animal bond as, "a mutually beneficial and dynamic relationship between people and other animals that is influenced by behaviors that are essential to the health and well-being of both" (JAVMA, 1998). Data from the American Veterinary Medical Association (2007) points out that there are about seventy-two million dogs owned in the U.S. As one can imagine, many people in this country spend a great deal of their discretionary funds on their beloved pets. For example, according to American Pet Products Association (2009) $17.4 billion are spent yearly for pet food, and about $12.2 billion are spent on veterinary care.

The sense of being needed and of having a purpose in life has been researched by numerous scholars as one of the many reasons why such a bond is established. Some also believe that our relationships with animals provide social supports in vulnerable times, as well as opportunities for healthy interactions. McNicholas and Colis (2000 and 2006) suggest that animals maybe more forgiving than their human counterparts and are more accepting than fellow humans of those who may have awkward social and communication skills. Numerous research studies and papers have also been written over the past few decades that illustrate the unique physiological benefits that animals foster. The roots of these findings go back to the pioneer works of Friedmann, Katcher, and Lynch, (Friedmann et al., 1990) who demonstrated the value of caressing an animal on cardiovascular health, and decreased anxiety because of physical contact with the pet.

Since that time, there have been other researchers who have unearthed other specific physiological outcomes that are enhanced due to the bond, such as an increase in oxytocin and other healthy neurotransmitters as a consequence of gently stroking and petting dogs (Odenthal and Meintjes, 2003; and Dayton, 2010). The researchers have found that petting and interacting with the dogs also caused a decrease in cortisol levels (stress hormones). In essence, the research leaves us with an understanding that interacting with animals may be similar to a welcoming spa treatment that promotes a relaxed state. A good synthesis on this literature can be found in a paper written by Wells (2009). Finally, Dayton (2010) also reports on the research of Headey and Grabka that attempted to quantify the health correlates of pet ownership using national survey data in Australia, Germany, and China. Their results suggested that compared with those who didn't have pets, those who live with other species benefit from better overall health, get more exercise, sleep better, take fewer days off work, and see their doctors less.

Defining Animal-Assisted Interventions

The reputation of AAI has blossomed in the past several decades, ever since Boris Levinson coined the term "pet therapy" (Levinson, 1969). As a clinician, Levinson suggested that animals could provide a calming effect in therapy. Ever since that time, numerous terms have been used to explain the therapeutic use of animals. Terms such as "animal-facilitated counseling," "animal-assisted therapy and activities," "pet-mediated therapy," and "pet psychotherapy" have been used interchangeably. Nevertheless, the most widely used terms are "animal-assisted therapy" and "animal-assisted activities." Both could be classified under the rubric of animal-assisted interventions.

The Delta Society's *Standards of Practice for Animal-Assisted Activities and Therapy* defines animal-assisted therapy (AAT) as "an intervention with specified goals and objectives delivered by a health or human service professional with specialized expertise in using an animal as an integral part of treatment" (Delta Society, 1996). On the other hand, but equally valuable, animal-assisted activities (AAA) occur when specially trained professionals, paraprofessionals, or volunteers accompanied by animals interact with people in a variety of environments (Delta Society, 1996). In AAA, the same activity can be repeated for many different people or groups of people; the interventions are not part of a specific treatment plan and are not designed to address a specific emotional or medical condition; and detailed documentation does not occur.

In previous articles (Fine, 2000, 2006), the author has identified several other tenets that he believes are some of the major purposes of incorporating animals as an aspect of therapy. Briefly, two of the tenets are as follows:

Tenet 1: Animals as a social lubricant

As stated earlier, this tenet has been the primary force behind AAI. The animals act as a social lubricant and ease the stress of therapy by being comforting. The animals also act as a link in conversation between clinician and client, helping to establish trust and rapport between patient and clinician. The mere presence of an animal can also give clients a sense of comfort, which further promotes rapport in the therapeutic relationship. In regards to persons with ASD, the literature does suggest a similar outcome. For example, Martin and Farnum (2002) noted several improvements in children with ASD when they interacted with therapy dogs. It appears that including animals in therapy promoted more playful moods and better attentiveness in the youngsters who participated in the project. Martin and Farnum concluded that these changes in their behavior were a direct consequence of being around the dogs. They also explained that "animals are believed to act as transitional objects, allowing children to first establish bonds with them and then extend these bonds to humans" (Martin and Farnum, 2002).

Tenet 2: Animals as teachers

Perhaps one of the strongest outlets for applying AAI is how clinicians have often utilized animals for teaching as well as for role models. This is one of the greatest advantages of incorporating animals into therapy. Teaching animals and supporting their growth can also have therapeutic benefits for the clients. There have been many clinicians who have used the bonding relationship with the animal as a method to enhance developmental skills. For example, in a study with a child with autism, Barol (2006) used the relaxed atmosphere that the dog promoted to teach skills that were normally avoided by the young boy. Prior to the onset of her study, Barol met with the therapeutic team to discuss what sorts of activities they would offer the child, using the therapy dog as a motivational tool. For example, when asked to cut things in occupational therapy, tradition-ally the boy would often become uncooperative, squeal, and whine. However, when asked to do a similar task when cutting up bacon-like dog treats, he seemed more willing to cooperate. In addition, the speech and language therapist worked with the child to say "Here, Henry" when he gave the dog the treat. In essence, the responsibility of taking care of the animal seemed to be the impetus for his actions.

Pet Companionship and AAI: Suggestions for Applications

It is clear that there has been a recent interest in the roles that animals have in the lives of persons with ASD. In fact, in this book, there are separate chapters that highlight the value of service animals as well as that of equine therapy. Both these options also take their roots in the area of the human-animal bond, and are aspects of AAI. The author will not cover these therapies specifically, but would like to reiterate that there is some strong evidence demonstrating the value of both.

There also have been a handful of studies in the last decade demonstrating that AAI could be useful in supporting persons with ASD with many of their developmental needs. Ming-Lee Yeh (2008) suggested several interesting out-comes from her three years of research on evaluating a canine animal-assisted therapy (AAT) treatment for children with ASD in Taiwan. She reported sig-nificant improvements for the children on the social skills subscale and total score on the VABS (*Vineland Adaptive Behavior Scale*; VABS, Chinese version). She also reported that after interacting with dogs, children revealed significant improvements in various dimensions of communication and language, as well as increasing their on-task behavior.

Grandin, Fine, and Bowers (in press) have suggested several reasons why AAI may be more appropriate for some people with ASD, while others may react indifferently. One argument that was made pertains to the fact the some people may respond negatively to their interactions due to sensory oversensitivity. For example, one person with ASD may not be able to tolerate the smell of a dog, while another may have auditory oversensitivity and may not be able to tolerate the sound of a dog barking. The impact of sensory oversensitivity is extremely variable and can have a very strong effect on an interaction. For instance, when Bob first met Magic, he seemed very conscious of how she smelled. Attention was given to bathing her right before his visits with a very neutral-smelling shampoo.

On the other hand, a barking dog or a squawking bird may not bother some, while others will find it extremely aversive and offensive. Simply put, some people with various levels of ASD may avoid animals because they have extreme sensitivity to either sound or smell (it may not have anything to do with the animal specifically). One needs to carefully consider this point prior to introducing an animal.

On the other hand, some believe that persons with ASD may respond differently to animals due to their differences in cognitive problem solving. For example, Grandin and Johnson (2005) hypothesize that one of the reasons why some children and adults with ASD relate really well to animals is due to sensory-based thinking. They suggest that there may be some similarities in the way that both people with ASD and companion animals process information. In essence, animals do not think in words. They believe that dogs' cognitions are filled with detailed sensory information and their world is filled with pictures, smells, sounds, and physical sensations. Grandin et al. (in press) summarized their impressions about some of the safeguards to consider when utilizing animals in therapy, with the following conclusions. Table 1 summarizes these perceptions.

Additionally, AAI can also be applied with individuals who have a milder version of ASD. Perhaps one of the greatest benefits has been how the animals have supported companionship and friendship in the lives of people who have felt very isolated and lonely. In *Afternoons with Puppy* (2007), Fine and Eisen discussed several cases of youths with Asperger's syndrome and autism and the roles that animals had in their lives. One case that clearly stands out was that of a teenage boy diagnosed with high-functioning autism who had tremendous social skill

Table 1

	Guidelines to consider when applying AAI with persons with ASD
1.	Children and adults with ASD may relate better with companion animals because they both use sensory-based thinking.
2.	Sensory oversensitivity may have a tremendous impact on the outcome and is extremely variable. This means that some people may not be able to tolerate smells or sudden sounds from an animal. On the other hand, some will have no sensory problems with animals and will be attracted to them.
3.	Animals, specifically dogs, may communicate their behavioral intentions more easily to persons with ASD especially because their relationships are simpler.

difficulties. Unfortunately, the boy led a very isolated life until he developed an interest in the birds in my office. Eventually he adopted a bird, and it provided him with compassion and joy. He often would sit next to the bird when he was anxious and upset. The bird seemed to provide him with a blanket of warmth that helped him regulate his anxiety. He also realized the importance of handling the bird gently. They seemed to become protective of each other and enjoyed one another's company.

Concluding Remarks

George Eliot in "Mr. Gilfil's Love Story" from her book *Scenes of Clerical Life* (1857), once stated that *"Animals are such agreeable friends—they ask no questions, they pass no criticisms."* Her comments seem very apropos in our concluding remarks for this paper. The love and unconditional regard received from a pet or from a therapy animal may represent a catalyst for emotional and psychological growth. A well-trained therapy animal working alongside a seasoned therapist may be a viable team when used to promote various developmental and functional skills. On the other hand, families may want to consider adopting an animal for companionship. However, one must realize the importance of selecting a compatible pet and the need for effective training. Provisions need to be thought through to support not only the welfare of the person but also the animal. Although AAI shouldn't be unrealistically viewed as a panacea, one should not overlook the power of our connection to animals. We may find some significant benefits derived from this relationship.

ANTHROPOSOPHICAL CURATIVE EDUCATION AND SOCIAL THERAPY

BY DR. MARGA HOGENBOOM AND PAULA MORAINE

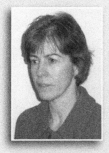

Marga G.E. Hogenboom, artsexamen Utrecht 1984, MRCGP

Camphill Medical Practice
Murtle Estate
Bieldside
Scotland
AB15 9EP
00441224868935
marga@hogenboom.co.uk
www.camphillschools.org.uk

Dr. Marga Hogenboom has worked for seventeen years as a general practitioner and school medical officer in The Camphill Medical Practice in Scotland. She specialises in Anthroposophic medicine. The Camphill School Aberdeen has ninety pupils and is accredited by the Autistic Society in the U.K. She is co-author of the books *Autism: A Holistic Approach* and *Living with Genetic Syndromes Associated with Intellectual Disability*.

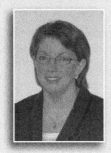

Paula Moraine, M.Ed.

pmoraine@gmail.com

Paula Moraine has been an educator for thirty-five years, working with children and adults in classrooms, residential homes, and universities. She is currently the Director of the Community Outreach Center for Literacy and Tutoring Program in Bel Air, Maryland.

History: In 1924, when attitudes toward people with special needs were radically different than they are today, Rudolf Steiner gave a seminal course of lectures to a small group of teachers and doctors, forming a fundamental basis for the Anthroposophically inspired curative work for individuals with special needs. Many decades later, the Anthroposophical curative movement has grown enormously, with more than six hundred centers and homes around the world for both children and adults. These day and residential schools practice curative education, an approach which combines education, therapy, and medicine with a strong emphasis on daily experiences of nature and the seasons of the year. In the centers for adults this curative approach is often referred to as "Social Therapy."

In these homes and schools, more than 50 percent of the children or adults will have autistim spectrum disorder (ASD), ranging from high-functioning autism to individuals who are dependent on others for their everyday care. This mix of disabilities and abilities is welcomed by the many Anthroposophical Curative Education and Social Therapy centers, and is viewed as a special strength that enhances social interaction.

Philosophy

The thought underlying Anthroposophical Curative Education and Social Therapy is that every human being has an eternal, healthy individuality. At birth, a human being incarnates into a physical body and an individual life, merging the eternal individuality with the earthly incarnation. The Anthroposophical basis of Curative Education and Social Therapy is guided by fundamental principles of Anthroposophy that includes the understanding of the human being as having a body (physical body), soul, and spirit that express through a fourfold organization of physical body, etheric body (life forces), astral body (feelings and emotional forces), and ego (the sense of "I"). As a child develops, he or she begins to feel at home in the body through a full spectrum of sense experiences that goes beyond the usual five senses, extending to twelve senses as described by Rudolf Steiner: the senses of touch, life (well-being), self-movement, balance, smell, taste, sight, warmth/temperature, hearing, language, concept, and ego.

Children with atypical development—caused by genetic factors, birth trauma, illness, neglect, or abuse—will have difficulties fully integrating in their bodies. It is not known what causes ASD, despite intensive research.

Each child on the autism spectrum will be unique and different, but may manifest similar difficulties in the twelve senses. The ASD child will often have increased sensitivity in the sense of touch, which provides us a feeling of our self or safety. They can be oversensitive to touch and even ticklish, but normal touch can be difficult for them. Curative education approaches this sensitivity thera-peutically, through massage, applying etheric oils to the children, surrounding the children with natural materials, and helping the children to experience the natural world through touch.

For children with ASD, the sense of well-being is often disturbed. The child may sleep poorly, have irregular bowel movements, strange eating habits, or can look pale and uncomfortable. Curative education emphasizes improvement in the sense of well-being through an ordered, rhythmical day, gentle sense impressions, limited exposure to media, frequent outdoor activities, and healthy natural food. Parents often notice the first area of improvement for the ASD child in a curative home is a regular sleeping rhythm.

The well-developed sense of movement and balance appears in children with Kanner's autism. These children can balance on a fence, can run, and have agility for a variety of activities. On closer observation it is clear that those are not free movements; the child cannot express his or her personality through these movements. In a curative school, there will be many opportunities throughout the day to replace these compulsive movements with outdoor play, clapping games, folk dancing, sports, horseback riding, or swimming.

We relate to the world around us through what we taste, smell, see, and through feeling warmth. All this information helps us to make sense of the world. The child with ASD often finds these normal sensory experiences overwhelming, painful, and confusing. Sounds can be distorted and too loud, visual impressions are disconnected, and taste is so acute their food intake will be limited. Those overwhelming sense impressions limit the possibility to really experience what happens in the world, and the child closes off from the world.

The child with ASD does not seem to feel well in their physical body, and indicates they are overwhelmed by sensory input. So how can curative education help these children? Through working with the twelve senses, within an organized and consistent approach, the child with ASD can gradually lean to relax, deal with their sense impressions more effectively, and eventually recognize others as separate from themselves. This is the beginning of the experience of self as a separate individuality.

The schools for Curative Education are based on the principles and practices of Waldorf Education, as established by Rudolf Steiner in 1919. Waldorf Education is based on the principle that the body, soul, and spirit of the individual child can be guided and educated through carefully balancing the education of the child's thinking, feeling, and will. This is accomplished using an articulated curriculum based on insights into the development of the child, and an evolving engagement of the developing thinking, feeling, and will of the child. The education in Anthroposophical curative schools is based on the Waldorf curriculum, adapted to support children with a variety of special educational needs.

Therapies form an integral part of daily life in the curative schools that might include play therapy, music therapy, art therapy, movement therapy, massage therapy, color/light therapy, baths and aroma therapy, and horseback riding therapy. Daily life for each child will be a mixture of educational and therapeutic activities that work together to bring about an integration of the child's physical, cognitive, and sensory capacities. Each child is allowed to develop along an individual path, so teachers and therapists are trained to be intuitive, responsive, and diagnostic with each child.

The integrated approach to education, therapy, and medicine makes Anthroposophical Curative Education and Social Therapy interdisciplinary and multimodal. Collaboration among teachers, doctors, therapists, social workers, and parents is developed to a high degree in curative homes and schools. In the curative home, the element of the family setting is added to the school day and to therapeutic hours. The child relies on consistency in all parts of their day, and the curative home is organized to provide smooth, seamless transitions between the various areas of the child's daily experience. The same is true for curative homes for adults, though the daily schedule is adapted in respect for the adults' maturity.

Best-case scenario

James, an eight-year-old boy, attends the Camphill School as a boarder. He is a very oversensitive child on the autism spectrum, he has poor sleep, no speech, and exhibits obsessive behaviour. His parents are exhausted and describe a difficult home life due to his many needs. Ten years later, he is a young man with reasonable speech, using full sentences, and engaging in simple conversations. His speech is still developing, he has learned many practical skills, remembers people, and relates to people. Although his progress is impressive, he still needs a protected environment.

Parents often note important changes in their very disabled children. Although these children may never learn to speak, and though they will need lifelong care, the parents notice that their child recognizes them and appears more peaceful in general.

Worst-case scenario

Camphill Schools integrate children of all abilities and do not have closed units. Some children with ASD can have unpredictable, or even dangerous behaviour, which can put frail children at risk despite close supervision. The Camphill Schools are not a viable option for these children.

Students with high-functioning autism often progress through the curative school acquiring adequate skills and capacities for work in other settings. These children often live at home or in groups with others, and engage in various work settings.

Training and Research

There is currently no substantive research available for the effect of the Anthroposophical Curative Education approach to children with ASD or pervasive developmental disorder (PDD). There is, however, a BA in Curative Education available through the University of Aberdeen, Scotland, offered to the teachers and therapists working in the Scottish Camphill curative schools. By paying special attention to these senses and creating specific experiences throughout the day to protect and enhance these senses, Curative Education takes on a quality of healing that supports the person with autism. There is also training in curative education available in the U.S. through the Camphill centers in Pennsylvania. Although empirical research is not available, there is a wealth of experience and practice that informs the ongoing work in curative schools, and could help form future research to reveal the effects of integrating education, therapy, and medicine in addressing the special challenges and opportunities presented by ASD.

A full description of these twelve senses and how they are incorporated into education, therapy, and medicine can be found in the book, *Autism: A Holistic Approach* (2001) by Bob Woodward and Dr. Marga Hogenboom. A full description of how these principles are implemented is given in this book. In *Holistic Special Education,* edited by Robin Jackson, the practice of creating a therapeutic education and experience for the children in curative schools and homes is described.

Camphill Communities: www.camphill.net/

Curative Education and Social Therapy International: www.ecce.eu/

Autism Spectrum Disorder and Pervasive Developmental Delay: www.nimh.nih.gov/

ANTIEPILEPTIC MEDICATIONS

BY DR. RICHARD E. FRYE

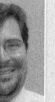

Richard E. Frye, MD, Ph.D.

Department of Pediatrics
Division of Child and Adolescent Neurology at the University
of Texas Health Science Center, and at The Children's Learning
Institute
7000 Fannin—UCT 2478,
Houston, TX 77030
Richard.E.Frye@uth.tmc.edu

Dr. Richard E. Frye received his medical degree from Georgetown University. He completed his pediatric residency training at University of Miami and child neurology residency training at Children's Hospital Boston. Following residency, Dr. Frye completed a fellowship in behavioral neurology and learning disabilities at Children's Hospital Boston. Dr. Frye completed a Ph.D. in physiology and biophysics at Georgetown University and a MS in biomedical science at Drexel University. Dr. Frye is board certified in Pediatrics and in Neurology with special competency in Child Neurology. Dr. Frye is also funded by the National Institutes of Health to study brain function in individuals with neurodevelopmental disorders. Dr. Frye is the medical director of the University of Texas medically based autism clinic. The purpose of this unique clinic is to diagnose and treat medical disorders associated with autism, such as mitochondrial disorders and subclinical electrical discharges, in order to optimize remediation and recovery.

A ntiepileptic drugs (AEDs) have many applications in autism spectrum disorder (ASD). These include the control of seizures and epilepsy; treatment of epileptic encephalopathies such as Landau-Kleffner syndrome, electrical status epilepticus during slow-wave sleep and subclinical electrical discharges; behavioral and mood regulation; migraine headaches; and periodic leg movements during sleep. When a child has more than one of these medical disorders, it is possible to select an AED that will treat several conditions simultaneously. Some of the more recently introduced AEDs such as felbamate have not gained wide enough use in ASD to determine whether they are efficacious in ASD.

Seizures Syndromes: Individuals with epilepsy related to a specific epilepsy syndrome, such as tuberous sclerosis, should be treated with AEDs that are effective for treating the specific underlying epilepsy syndrome.

Emergency Seizure Treatment: Rectal diazepam is very effective to treat prolonged seizure activity and should be prescribed to individuals with epilepsy or seizures that are at risk for such a prolonged seizure.

Epileptic Encephalopathy: AEDs have been more extensively studied for the classically recognized epileptic encephalopathies, specifically Landau-Kleffner syndrome and electrical status epilepticus during slow-wave sleep, than the less well-characterized syndromes such as subclinical electrical discharges. In general, the same medications appear to be just as effective for the all the epileptic encephalopathies. Valproate has efficacy in some cases and may be the initial treatment choice. Occasionally, oxcarbazepine may be helpful for very focal electrical discharges. Immunomodulatory treatments, specifically steroids and intravenous immunoglobulin, may also be helpful adjunctive treatments for these syndromes. For electrical status epilepticus during slow-wave sleep, diazepam prior to sleep has also been used.

Behavior and Mood Regulation: Valproate and lamotrigine are particularly effective in mood regulation, while topiramate appears to be effective for reducing impulsivity and aggressive behavior.

Migraine Headaches: Valproate, gabapentin, and topiramate have been very effective in treating migraine headaches, with topiramate being particularly effective.

Periodic Leg Movements During Sleep: Gabapentin can be useful for treating period leg movements during sleep, especially if there is trouble with sleep initiation.

AEDs were originally developed to control the abnormal electrical activity in the brain association with seizures and epilepsy. Other applications of these medications have been developed, including the use of AEDs in migraine headaches, sleep disorders, and mood stabilization and behavioral regulation in psychiatric disorders. Given their success in psychiatric and neurological disorders, they have been applied to individuals with ASD for similar indications.

Success is variable and depends on the indication for treatment. In some cases, dramatic results occur with AED treatment. It is best to select the most likely medication for the indication that will produce minimal side effects based on the profile of the patient. Poor results with AED treatment should lead to the consideration of alternative therapies, or to prompt the investigation of underlying medical disorders that have not been investigated. For example, poor success for behavioral control with an AED might prompt the investigation of gastrointestinal symptoms that are not obvious, or a trial of psychoactive medications. Seizures-like events that do not respond to AEDs should be reviewed carefully. If a video electroencephalograph has confirmed an electrographic correlate to the clinical behavior, more extensive metabolic or neuroimaging investigations might be indicated.

Side effects of AEDs highly depend on the medication. In general, newer AEDs (lamotrigine, oxcarbazepine, topiramate, levetiracetam) have fewer serious side effects than the older AEDs (phenobarbitol, phenytoin, primidone, carbamazepine). The exception to this is valproate, which appears to have good efficacy for many indications that affect children with ASD. The side effects profiles have not been studied in ASD specifically, so it is not known whether children with ASD have a higher incidence of side effects than other populations of children. In general, almost all AEDs can cause neurological side effects (ataxia, tremor, nystagmus), behavioral side effects (hyperactivity, agitation, aggressiveness), gastrointestinal side effects (abdominal pain, nausea), and an allergic reaction which can be severe in some cases. As discussed below, the incidence of side effects varies with the specific AED used, and the more serious side effects can be avoided with careful monitoring. Thus, it is best to have a practitioner with experience in these medications prescribe the AED and monitor the patient. In general, it is best to avoid older AEDs (phenobarbitol, phenytoin, primidone) that have a high incidence of cognitive and neurological side effects, as such side effects can exacerbate behavioral and cognitive abnormalities associated with ASD. Care should also be taken when using multiple AEDs. Since almost all AEDs elevate the rate of birth defects, it is important to carefully consider the choice of AEDs in potentially sexually active females.

There are specific side effects that every practitioner should be aware of and should communicate to the patient when prescribing AED medication:

Valproate: Valproate can result in serious side effects. However, valproate has remained one of the most widely used AEDs for ASD due to its efficacy, the relatively low incidence of serious side effects, and the ability to detect serious side effects with careful monitoring. The most serious side effects are hepatotoxicity, hyperammonemia, and pancreatitis. Several precautions can be taken to prevent these side effects from occurring. In general, a complete blood count, liver function tests, and amylase and lipase should be monitored during the initial period of starting the medication, and if the patient experiences gastrointestinal symptoms. Once a stable dose has been selected, the patient can be monitored approximately every three months. Hepatotoxicity is believe to be more prevalent in children under two years of age, so it is best to avoid prescribing valproate to very young children. Carnitine can help with the metabolism of valproate and may mitigate hepatotoxicity. Thus, cotreatment with carnitine is recommended. Common side effects of valproate include weight gain and thinning of the hair. The latter is believed to respond to selenium (10–20 mcg per day) and zinc (25–50 mg per day). Long-term use of valproate has been linked to bone loss, irregular menstruation, and polycystic ovary syndrome.

Lamotrigine: Lamotrigine has a low incidence of serious side effects and is generally well-tolerated. The most serious side effect of lamotrigine is a life-threatening rash known as Stevens-Johnson syndrome. Increasing the lamotrigine dose slowly toward the target dose can reduce the risk of this reaction occurring. Any parent or patient should be alerted to look for this adverse reaction.

Steroids: Common side effects include weight gain, edema, mood instability, and insomnia. Serious side effects include hypertension, immunosuppression, gastrointestinal ulceration, and glucose instability. Anyone on steroids should be closely monitored, especially if steroids are used for an extended period of time.

Intravenous Immunoglobulin: Common reactions include rash, headache, and fever, requiring prophylactic pretreatment for these side effects in some patients. This treatment is contraindicated in individuals with kidney or heart problems and should be administered by a practitioner familiar with the treatment.

Oxcarbazepine: Hyponatremia can develop in some individuals.

Topiramate: Common side effects include weight loss and cognitive and psychomotor slowing. Topiramate is minimally metabolized by the liver and is excreted mostly unchanged by the kidneys. Topiramate can cause a metabolic acidosis, nephrolithiasis, and oligohidrosis. Thus, this medicine should be avoided in individuals with kidney disorders, and parents and patients should be careful in hot weather. Glaucoma has occurred in rare cases, so any vision symptoms should be considered carefully.

Levetiracetam: Overall, levetiracetam has a low incidence of serious side effects and has minimal effects on liver metabolism. The most prevalent side effects are behavioral, and include agitation, aggressive behavior, and mood instability. Levetiracetam has been linked to suicide in a few individuals without

ASD. Preliminary reports suggest that cotreatment with pyridoxine helps mitigate behavioral side effects.

Diazepam: The most common reaction is drowsiness. Respiratory depression can occur if given at high doses.

Vigabatrin: Vigabatrin is associated with a progressive and permanent visual loss. Thus, its use is usually restricted to control of seizures in tuberous sclerosis.

Children with ASD have a high incidence of medical disorders that may guide the practitioner to choose a particular AED.

ASD Symptoms	Avoid	Possible Alternative
Gastrointestinal disorders	Valproate	Lamotrigine
Poor growth	Topiramate	Lamotrigine
Overweight	Valproate	Topiramate, Lamotrigine, Levetiracetam
Behavioral problems	Levetiracetam	Lamotrigine, Valproate, Topiramate

ANTIFUNGAL TREATMENT

BY DR. LEWIS MEHL-MADRONA

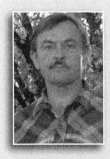

Lewis Mehl-Madrona, MD, Ph.D., MPhil

Education and Training Director
Coyote Institute for Studies of Change and Transformation
Burlington, VT and Honolulu, HI
Department of Family Medicine
University of Hawaii School of Medicine
Honolulu, HI
PO Box 9309
South Burlington, VT 05407
mehlmadrona@gmail.com
(808) 772-1099

Dr. Lewis Mehl-Madrona graduated from Stanford University School of Medicine and completed his family medicine and his psychiatry training at the University of Vermont College of Medicine. He earned a Ph.D. in clinical psychology at the Psychological Studies Institute in Palo Alto and also became a licensed psychologist in California. He took a Master's in Philosophy degree from Massey University in New Zealand in Narrative Studies in Psychology. He is American Board certified in family medicine, geriatric medicine, and psychiatry. He is the author of *Coyote Medicine*, *Coyote Healing*, *Coyote Wisdom*, *Narrative Medicine*, and, most recently, *Healing the Mind through the Power of Story: The Promise of Narrative Psychiatry*. He is the Education and Training Director for Coyote Institute for Studies of Change and Transformation, based in Burlington, Vermont and in Honolulu, Hawaii and is Clinical Assistant Professor of Family Medicine at the University of Hawaii in Honolulu.

O verview. The reduction in amount of fungi in the digestive tract is part of a larger group of interventions commonly called biological therapies. In this review, we will focus on the evidence for fungal involvement in the symptoms of autistic children, discuss the ways in which the amount of fungi in the gut can be reduced, and review the evidence that exists to support these practices.

Autism and Digestive Difficulties

Children diagnosed with autism do have considerable digestive difficulties. In 2003, Rosseneu studied eighty children diagnosed with autism who also had digestive symptoms, finding that 61 percent had abnormal gram negative endo-toxin-producing bacteria, 55 percent had overgrowth of *Staphylococcus aureus* and 95 percent had an overgrowth of *Escherichia coli*. He did not find abnormal amounts of fungus.

Candida Overgrowth

The main fungal culprit implicated in autism is *Candida albicans* (Edelson, 2006). Generally this fungus is kept under control by the bacteria that live within the gut. However, exposure to antibiotics can kill these bacteria resulting in a proliferation of *Candida*. It lives on the moist dark mucous membranes which line the mouth, vagina, and intestinal tract. Ordinarily it exists only in small colonies, prevented from growing too rapidly by the human host's immune system, and by competition from other microorganisms in and on the body's mucous membranes. When something happens to upset this delicate natural balance, *Candida* can grow rapidly and aggressively, causing many unpleasant symptoms to the host. Vaginal yeast infections present the most common case in point.

High levels of *Candida* are thought to release toxins which are absorbed into the bloodstream through the blood, thereby causing difficulties. Edelson links an overgrowth of *Candida* to confusion, hyperactivity, short attention span, lethargy, irritability, and aggression. He further cites headaches, abdominal pain, consti-pation, excess gas, fatigue, and depression as linked to *Candida* overgrowth. Sup-port for the *Candida* overgrowth theory is often sought in the observation that people treated for *Candida* become worse for two to three days before becoming better. This worsening is supposed to relate to "die-off" of the yeast. As the fungi die, their cell walls open, releasing the intracellular contents into the gut. Some components of this intracellular material are thought to be cause symptoms in humans. Further proof is offered in the form of organic acid analysis of the urine. When organic acids are found in the urine that are only produced by yeast, presumably the yeast are releasing these acids into the gut to pass through the gut wall into the bloodstream to be removed by the kidneys. Popular books on *Candida* include William Crook's *The Yeast Connection Handbook*. Organic acid urine testing is performed at The Great Plains Laboratory in Overland Park, Kansas.

Many children afflicted with autism have had frequent ear infections as young children and have taken large amounts of antibiotics. These are thought to exaggerate the yeast problem. Other possible contributors to *Candida* overgrowth are hormonal treatments; immunosuppressant drug therapy; exposure to herpes, chicken pox, or other "chronic" viruses; or exposure to chemicals that might upset the immune system.

Another reported reason for fungal overgrowth is a faulty immune system. A relationship between autism and immunity was proposed over forty years ago based on the detection of autoimmune conditions in family members of children diagnosed with autism (Money et al., 1971; Ashwood et al., 2004. Pardo and Eberhart, 2007). Numerous scientific reports of immune abnormalities in people with autism have been published (Ashwood and Van de Water, 2004, Hornig and Lipkin, 2001). These include defects in antibody production, imbalances between the different parts of the immune system, and higher rates of infections in children diagnosed with autism. The production of lymphocytes has been found to be decreased (Stubbs & Crawford, 1976).

A year later, Stubbs (1977) supported an altered immune response among "five of thirteen autistic children who had undetectable titers despite previous rubella vaccine, while all control children had detectable titers. This finding of undetectable titers in autistic children suggests these children may have an altered immune response." Children diagnosed with autism do not always respond to vaccination, having no evidence of being immunized a year after a rubella vaccine was given.

In one study, 46 percent of families of children diagnosed with autism have two or more members with autoimmune disorders such as type I diabetes, rheumatoid arthritis, hypothyroidism, and lupus (Pardo & Eberhart, 2007). Antibodies have been found in children diagnosed with autism against their own nerves and their myelin covering, nerve receptors, and even brain parts (Jepson, 2007). The commonly recognized clumsiness of many autistic children has been linked to antibodies attacking the Purkinje cells in the cerebellum (Rout and Dhossche, 2008) which are the cells that control coordinated movements. Inflammation has been found in the brains of children with autism (Vargas et al, 2005).

Once we eliminated barley malt and all other malted products (maltodextrin, malted barley flour, and so on), vinegar, and yeast, the improvement was dramatic. We began to see the light at the end of the tunnel, but little did we know how long that tunnel was. Reaching the end of the tunnel is still a goal, although after more than eight years, we are much closer. Eight years ago, simply decreasing Avi's headaches to once a week or once every two weeks, and seeing his behavior improve and his autistic symptoms decrease, were major victories. We had turned the tide before we lost Avi altogether. He was coming back to us, very, very slowly. It took two more years, and much more experimentation, to completely eliminate Avi's debilitating headaches. Another two years of experimentation eliminated Avi's eczema and itching.

Oxalic Acid and Yeast

Oxalate and its acid form oxalic acid are organic acids that are primarily from three sources: the diet, from fungus such as *Aspergillus* and *Penicillium* and *Candida* (Fomina et al, 2005, Ruijter et al, 1999; Takeuchi et al, 1987), and from human metabolism (Ghio et al, 2000).

Researcher Susan Owens discovered that the use of a diet low in oxalates markedly reduced symptoms in children with autism and PDD. For example, a mother with a son with autism reported that he became more focused and calm, that he played better, that he walked better, and had a reduction in leg and feet pain after being on a low-oxalate diet. Prior to the low-oxalate diet, her child could hardly walk up the stairs. After the diet, he walked up the stairs easier (Great Plains, 2008).

Oxalates in the urine are much higher in individuals with autism than in normal children. In one study, 36 percent of the children with a diagnosis of autism had values higher than 90 mmol/mol creatinine, the value consistent with a diagnosis of genetic hyperoxalurias, while none of the normal children had values this high.

Supplements can also reduce oxalates. Calcium citrate can be used to reduce oxalate absorption from the intestine. Citrate is the preferred calcium form to reduce oxalate because citrate also inhibits oxalate absorption from the intestinal tract. Children over the age of 2 need about 1000 mg of calcium per day (Great Plains, 2008). N-Acetyl glucosamine is used to stimulate the production of the intercellular cement hyaluronic acid to reduce pain caused by oxalates (Vulvar Pain Foundation, 2008). Chondroitin sulfate is used to prevent the formation of calcium oxalate crystals (Shirane et al, 1988). Vitamin B6 is a cofactor for one of the enzymes that degrades oxalate in the body and has been shown to reduce oxalate production (Chetyrkin et al, 2005). Increased water intake also helps to eliminate oxalates (Great Plains, 2008). Probiotics may be very helpful in degrading oxalates in the intestine. Individuals with low amounts of oxalate-degrading bacteria are much more susceptible to kidney stones (Kumar et al, 2002). Both *Lactobacillus acidophilus* and *Bifidobacterium lactis* have enzymes that degrade oxalates (Azcarate-Pearil et al, 2006). Increased intake of essential omega-3 fatty acids, commonly found in fish oil and cod liver oil, reduces oxalate (Baggio et al, 1996).

Non-pharmacological Therapies

The most common means of restoring *Candida* populations to desirable levels is through ingesting healthy bacteria, generally species of *Lactobacillus*. These potions of bacteria are generally called probiotics, and are safe and effective. Reduction of dietary sugar and carbohydrates is also advocated, along with a yeast-free diet.

Saturated Fatty Acids

Undecylenic and caprylic acids are common medium-chain saturated fatty acids used to treat fungal infections. Common sources of caprylic acid are palm and coconut oils, whereas undecylenic acid is extracted from castor bean oil. Palm and coconut oil and castor bean oil are also used. Both have been shown to be comparable to a number of common antifungal drugs. A typical dosage for caprylic acid would be up to 3600 mg per day in divided doses with meals. Undecylenic acid is commonly taken in dosages of up to 1000 mg per day in divided doses.

Useful herbs include berberine, an alkaloid found in an herb called barberry *(Berberis vulgaris)* and related plants as well as in goldenseal, Oregon grape root and Chinese goldthread. This herb is commonly used in Chinese and ayurvedic medicines for its antifungal. *Oregano vulgare* is an effective antifungal. Carvacrol, one of its components, was found to inhibit *Candida* growth. Garlic *(Allium sativum)* contains a large number of sulphur containing compounds with anti-fungal properties. Because of the many different compounds with anti-fungal properties in garlic, yeast and fungi are less likely to become resistant. Fresh garlic was significantly more potent against *Candida albicans* than other preparations. Colloidal silver is a suspension of silver particles in water. Colloidal silver is said to be effective against yeast and fungi species including *Candida*. It works by targeting the enzyme involved with supplying the fungus with oxygen. Cellulase is the enzyme that breaks down cellulose, the main component of the yeast cell wall. When it comes into contact with yeast cells, the cell wall is damaged and the organism dies. Plant tannins are natural substances found in black walnut and other plants. They are found in red wines and redwood trees. They have an antifungal effect.

Antifungal medications. Antifungal medications include fluconazole, ketoconazole, itraconazole, or terbinafine and are used, sometimes for as long as one to two months. Antifungals are usually monitored with liver function tests every one to three months, since these drugs can cause liver damage. Sometimes Amphotericin B is used as an oral liquid because it is not absorbed by the intestines into the blood stream but will still kill intestinal yeast. Nystatin is another oral medication that is not absorbed by the intestines and is relatively safe to use over long periods of time.

Outcomes

No systematic studies have been conducted of antifungal regiments for children diagnosed with autism. Difficulties exist in making such studies. Autism is most likely what is called a polymorphic condition. Many pathways lead to the same symptoms. Some of these pathways could involve *Candida*; others, not. Finding the children who would respond could be a challenge. Many case reports exist of children who have improved with antifungal treatment. Case reports, however, cannot rule out the possibility of the treatment working because of what I call the "Pygmalion effect"—that people become what we expect them to become. It's a kind of social placebo effect. When we believe in a treatment, we can make it powerfully effective, even though it may have no intrinsic biological efficacy

In general, candidal overgrowth in the intestines of children diagnosed with autism has not been documented (Wakefield et al., 2000) by endoscopy. In 1995, two brothers were reported whose symptoms were associated with *Candida* overgrowth. Both improved following *Candida* elimination (Shaw, 1995).

One example of a common kind of story comes from the book, *Feast Without Yeast: 4 Stages to Better Health*: The authors' 4½-year-old son was writhing on the floor screaming. "He had been behaving this way on and off for six months. . . . At age two he had been fine. From two-and-a-half to age four, his development had slowed down, but had not stopped. Starting a few days after his fourth birthday, he began to lose his speech . . .

"He lost his toilet training, stopped eating and lost . . . weight. . . . [He] could not use his hands. He sat in a swing spinning much of the day. He had lost all emotional contact except with his mother, and that was fleeting . . .

"We took away chocolate, peanut butter, orange juice, aged cheeses, and some other foods. The improvement was immediate. Avi looked and acted as if a weight had been lifted from his head. Only then could we see the onset of separate headaches, when we would make a mistake and give him foods we weren't supposed to, or when he would eat something that we learned later caused problems. We saw the headaches set in about three times a week instead of being chronic.

His symptoms . . . began to diminish. He no longer screamed all the time. His behavior improved. He seemed more with us, more engageable. If he accidentally ate the wrong foods, the screaming began again . . . "

"We got our next break about eight weeks later with the Jewish holiday of Passover. For this holiday, all foods containing yeast, leavening and fermented foods are eliminated. This holiday lasts eight days. Three days into Passover, our son was clearly improving again. He appeared much more comfortable. . . . His behavior had improved to the point that he was accepted into a special education speech and language summer program.

"After that first Passover holiday, one of the many health care professionals we were seeing suggested we look at an outstanding book called *The Yeast Connection* by Dr. William Crook. Dr. Crook compiled treatment histories of people who have problems with something called *Candida albicans*, a type of fungus which at times resembles yeast. We found that Dr. Crook recommended eliminating many of the foods we had found to be problematic for Avi, although there were some very significant differences at that time. . . . Within a few days of starting on the nystatin, Avi made a year's growth in playground development. He got off the swings, where he usually spent his hours of playground time. He began climbing jungle gyms, sliding down slides, and beginning to look like a four year old kid again. Avi still did not get his speech back, but he was beginning to be able to function.

"Many people ask us whether this treatment has been a cure; for our son. We cannot say that it has been, but we cannot say that it has not been. Avi still does not talk fluently, but he has words, and can communicate. He types independently, too.

"Talking is not the only important part of life. Avi now is able to relate to people emotionally. He is out of pain.

Avi has now started his fourth year of high school, and is doing great.

"Before we began treating Avi with dietary intervention, Avi could not tolerate the presence of other children before starting on this diet. He could not tolerate being touched. Now Avi loves tickles, hugs, and touches, even from strangers."

Another famous case occurred in 1981, when Duffy, the 3½-year-old son of Gianna and Gus Mayo of San Francisco began to developmentally regress. The Mayos were lucky enough to take Duffy to allergist Alan Levin who found that Duffy's immune system was severely impaired. Duffy had been given a number of treatments with antibiotics, which were intended to control his ear infections. Levin tried Nystatin, an antifungal drug which is toxic to *Candida* but not to humans. Duffy at first got worse (a common reaction, caused by the toxins released by the dying *Candida* cells). Then he began to improve. Since Duffy was sensitive to molds, the Mayos moved inland to a dryer climate. Since *Candida* thrives on certain foods (especially sugars and refined carbohydrates) Duffy's diet required extensive modification. Duffy became active, greatly improved child with few remaining signs of autism. The Los Angeles Times published a long, syndicated article about Duffy in 1983, which resulted in letters and phone calls from parents of autistic children throughout the country. There were many autistic children whose problems started soon after long-term antibiotic therapy, or whose mothers had chronic yeast infections, which they had passed along to the infants.

I have similar cases to report. I can say that the process of eradicating *Candida* has benefited many children in my practice. What I cannot say is that the problems were caused by the *Candida*. Healing is a process. When we believe in a process, then healing happens. David Peat in *Blackfoot Physics,* discusses the embeddedness of the English language in nouns and in a linear, mechanical, "thing" view of the world. We want things to work. Instead, it is more common that processes work. The process of eliminating *Candida* has helped many children, which is different from saying that eliminating *Candida* helped them. I don't know how many "things" are interchangeable in a process of healing. I don't know how much any individual "thing" matters. Double-blind, randomized, controlled trials are ideal for comparing to things. They are poor for determining if a process of healing can help a particular condition. Within a process of healing, these trials help us to compare two "things". We have yet to accomplish a clinical trial on eliminating yeast, but, for now, I continue to enthusiastically pursue the process of healing through eliminating yeast. This process I know to work.

APPLIED BEHAVIOR ANALYSIS

BY JENIFER CLARK

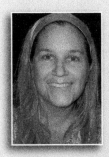

Jenifer Clark, MA, Ph.D. (c)

New York, NY
212-222-9818
clarkjenif@aol.com
MERIT-consulting.org
JeniferClark.com

Jenifer Clark has been working with children and families for over fifteen years. She received her master's in psychology from NYU and is completing her Ph.D. in clinical psychology at CUNY. She has worked as an ABA therapist and consultant since 1992. She specializes in working with children with autism and has taught atypical development at Hunter College. Currently, she is the director of Boost!, an afterschool program for children with autism. This program focuses on teaching socialization and leisure skills to children on the spectrum, incorporating typical children as peers and social models. Ms. Clark is the co-founder and therapist for Sibfun, a support group for siblings of children with special-needs. She consults at special needs and typical schools and continues to consult with children and families.

Applied Behavior Analysis (ABA) is a treatment model that is extremely effective in remediating many of the cognitive, attention, and language based areas of deficit typical to autism. ABA is currently one of the most common interventions and the core of many educational programs for treating children on the autistism spectrum.

ABA is very methodical and scientific. Programs rely on data to demonstrate measurable gains and it should be evident that the procedures employed were responsible for the improvement in behavior. Goals are written up as programs, which are broken down into small, more easily mastered steps. The procedures for how each step will be taught is described in minute detail. Included in each treatment goal is specific mention of what the instructor will do or say to elicit a specific response and what specific response is expected from the child. Additionally the "error correction" is outlined. Error correction is the steps that will be taken if the desired response is not elicited.

Empirical research has played a pivotal role in the widespread acceptance and use of ABA. The controlled studies performed by Lovaas and his colleagues in the 1980s were some of the first empirically based examinations of treatment methodology and outcome to be conducted in the field of autism. Lovaas was able to demonstrate the effectiveness of ABA on the development of receptive and expressive communication, daily living skills, fine and gross motor skills, socialization, and daily living tasks. Importantly, the studies that were done by Lovaas and his colleagues found that a program should be between 30 to 40 hours per week to optimal in terms of efficacy. He was also able to identify that only 2 percent of his control group (receiving only ten hours of intervention each week) was able to mainstream in what was identified as "spontaneous recovery." This was in contrast to the approximately 50 percent of children who were treated with a more intensive program (30 to 40 hours) and were able to attend school in typical educational settings with typical peers (Lovaas). This research led to the conclusion that the more intensive the ABA program is, the better the outcome. The ABA philosophy is that children with autism should be appropriately engaged most of their waking hours.

The most important aspects of ABA stem from the concept of operant conditioning, the idea that one can use external reinforcement to increase the likelihood that a particular behavior will occur. Operant conditioning is considered to be a critical concept in the treatment of autistic children because they frequently lack the capacity to learn from their environment and appear to be less motivated to do so. It seems to evade the child with autism that it is in their best interest to learn to speak. External rewards can function as motivators and increase the autistic child's capacity to learn and to attend.

In operant conditioning, it is understood that there is a relationship between a verbal request or visual presentation (the stimulus) and a desired behavior that can be developed through reinforcing individual trials. Eventually, the discriminative stimulus (Sd) comes to indicate that a particular behavior is expected. If the subject engages in the expected behavior, then reinforcement is provided. The delivery of this reinforcement increases the chance that this sought after behavior would be emitted again in response to the Sd. So for example, one Sd might be "stand up." If the child stands up then a reinforcer would be delivered, thus increasing the likelihood in the future that when the child hears someone ask him to "stand up" he will oblige.

These principles are present and influential in the lives of typical children and adults as well. We are all encouraged to repeat experiences that are reinforcing. Similarly, it is second nature for most parents to praise and reinforce the behavior that they want their child to engage in more frequently. As infants and toddlers begin to achieve milestones such as walking and talking, parents tend to be very encouraging and attentive. First words and approximations are highly reinforced through the praise, excitement, and attention of parents. These reinforcers encourage the neurotypical child to practice and expand their communicative attempts. In many ways, ABA merely takes this naturally occurring phenomenon and formalizes it. By having the child sit at a table to practice this work, distractions can be minimized. For children who need to be taught to attend to and understand spoken language, verbal praise may not be reinforcing yet. Other reinforcers that have been established as desirable can be substituted while these areas are remediated. Many children with autism quickly come to appreciate social interactions as powerful reinforcers but it may take some specific interventions early on in the treatment to allow them to benefit from these more typical interactions.

Starting Treatment

In the initial phases of treatment, the most critical goals are helping the child to regulate and establishing trust in the relationship. Most children with autism tend to be poorly regulated. This may be indicated by rapid and unpredictable shifts in mood, frequent tantrums, aggressive acts, and even self-injurious behaviors. Many autistic children in the initial stages of treatment are internally driven and are resistant to having external demands placed on them. They have their own agenda that they are rigidly adhering to and resist disruptions in their routine.

The remediation-based aspect of ABA sets out to put structure in place and begin working on the areas of core deficit which leave these children so reliant on their maladaptive coping strategies. The child with autism may be very resistant to this change. This is when it is critical that the therapist be both thoughtful about the experience of the child but clear about the expectations. The therapist is setting boundaries which are a part of typical development. Children with autism may express anxiety about beginning the structured work of remediation but I have never met a child who wasn't glad to have learned to speak or communicate with others. These interventions are in their best interests but they can be put forth in such a way that the therapist remains connected to the child but is firm about expectations.

In order to communicate with the child in the early stages of treatment, these communications may have to be modified. For instance, if the child has a language processing issue, it is necessary that communication be conveyed visually. Token systems can be very effective in allowing children to understand the expectation and extend beyond a 1:1 reinforcement ratio (being reinforced for each trial). The expectation may be that the child imitates a gross motor movement (a precursor to being able to imitate those around him). For example, in a three-token system, the instructor can show the child that if they imitate three times, they can engage in a preferred activity or, in other words, be reinforced. This message can be conveyed with three stickers or three tokens. Each time the child successfully performs the activity they will receive a token or sticker to reward a successful response as well as to indicate that they are getting closer to completion and being tangibly reinforced. The first attempt to use a token system may be very difficult but each successive attempt will be easier than the one that preceded it. The child will begin to develop trust in the therapist that their communication or promise (we will do this three times and you can engage in your preferred activity) will be upheld.

Such systems are not unique to children with autism. There are many situations in life which provide us with an indication of when something will be complete. We may look ahead when reading something less interesting to see how many more pages are left. We might look at the time left on the treadmill when we set out to run for a designated period of time. Many school children look at the clock near the end of the day to see how much time is left before dismissal. In essence, a token system is a similar indication. We are acknowledging that children with autism are doing hard work and we are simply trying to increase motivation but at the same time make it clear when they will have completed a task.

There is a trust that begins to evolve through the work and this occurs in part as the child begins to realize that the instructor will not ask the child to do something that they are incapable of doing. In behavioral terms, there is a concept known as "prompt fading." This implies that the instructor may initially provide a very high level of prompt or support to ensure success. Returning to the example of clapping hands, as the child begins to understand what is expected of him and what the motor pattern feels like when you attempt to imitate that particular action, the therapist can fade back their level of prompt. So initially, she may clap the child's hands for him, and as he begins to understand what is expected of him and how to accomplish that, the level of prompt will be reduced. The next step may be setting the child's hands up in a clapping position and later just touching the child's elbows.

To fade out prompts effectively, the therapist must be skilled at intuiting the needs of the child. Some children may require no assistance at all to be successful in such an activity while others require assistance that is quickly faded, and still others will require assistance for some time. The therapist can also assess the type of intervention or prompt that would be most helpful to a particular child. Some children might find imitating actions challenging because of their difficulty attending to the visual information being presented. A child with these particular issues would be best served by an intervention which drew their attention to the visual demonstration (perhaps waiting until the child is looking or attracting their visual attention prior to engaging in the action). Other children may have difficulty translating what they have observed into a message that allows them to imitate the movement.

One such child had a very poor capacity to imitate gross motor activities. I observed as he watched me carefully but repeatedly engaged in a different motor response than the one I had done. This three year old was particularly attracted to language and words, and so I put in an intermediate step of asking him what I was doing. He responded "clapping hands." I encouraged him, "so you do it." He quickly began clapping. He was then able to imitate five different actions without pause. Helping him to translate the visual into verbal and to use self talk to help him know what to tell his body to do helped him significantly. Although this additional step helped the boy mentioned, such an intervention would be an unnecessary obstacle for many other children with autism. This illustrates the importance of designing interventions that are specific to the strengths and challenges of the particular child.

Parents are often trained by ABA therapists to incorporate behavioral strategies and philosophies into their parenting techniques. Behaviorists recognize that negative behaviors are often unknowingly reinforced by parents, meaning that although they might ignore their child's inappropriate behavior some of the time, they occasionally attend to it. That occasional or intermittent reinforcement is in fact the most powerful way to assure that the child will continue the behavior. The child, unsure when the parent will respond, but confident that they will respond at some point, continues to emit the problematic behavior.

Many parents of a child with autism are taught about a concept known as extinction. This concept implies that in order to extinguish an undesirable behavior, the behavior should never be reinforced. If the behavior is occasionally reinforced, that is the equivalent of an intermittent reinforcement schedule and the behavior will continue to occur. Extinction requires that a behavior be consistently ignored.

Parents who are dealing with their autistic child's problematic behaviors are encouraged to examine how they might be reinforcing them. For instance, the parents of an autistic child who tends to throw screaming tantrums throughout the day, might be trying to put his tantrums on extinction. The parents might be successfully ignoring the tantrums while at home but when he throws a tantrum at the playground, his parents might pick him up and bring him home to avoid creating a scene. Being picked up and carried home from the playground may in fact be reinforcing to the child and therefore increase the likelihood that the tantrum behavior will continue.

Behavioral therapists typically conduct a functional analysis to determine the antecedents and potential reinforcers for a particular problematic behavior. Such analyses demonstrate that negative attention is sometimes reinforcing to a child and even more so to a child with autism. Parents are taught to carefully evaluate their response patterns and to be consistent with regard to problematic behavior.

The more that parents of children with autism can incorporate sound behavioral practices in a natural way with their autistic child, the better that child's prognosis will be. All parents use behavioral practices in their interactions with their children and in the case of ABA, this approach has been made more methodical and exact. ABA is an extremely effective methodology for remediating the core deficits of autism and this empirically supported fact makes it a leading intervention for children on the spectrum. The brain-based nature of autism requires that children with autism receive remediation. The plasticity of the human brain implies that neurological change can occur and ABA has proven success in this domain.

AQUATIC THERAPY

BY ANDREA SALZMAN

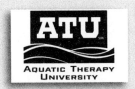

Andrea L. Salzman, MS, PT

Aquatic Therapy University
3500 Vicksburg Lane #250
Plymouth, MN 55447
(800) 680-8624
info@aquatic-university.com
www.aquatic-university.com (Aquatic Therapy University)
www.aquatic-sensory-integration.com (Aquatic Sensory Integration)

Ms. Salzman is the Director of Practice for Aquatic Therapy University (ATU) which provides curriculum-based studies in aquatic therapy. Salzman has served as:
• Editor-in-Chief, Journal of Aquatic Physical Therapy;
• Seminar Instructor, two hundred-plus aquatic therapy seminars;
• Founder, Aquatic Resources Network, clearinghouse of information on aquatic therapy and related topics;
• Creator, Aquatic Health Research Database (AHRD);
• Author, five textbooks and over three hundred magazine articles;
• Manager, Regions Hospital Therapy Pool;
• Adjunct Faculty, College of St. Catherine's PT program.
In 2010, Salzman was honored with the highest award given to aquatic physical therapists, the Judy Cirullo Leadership Award, from the American Physical Therapy Association. Salzman has also received the Aquatic Therapy Professional of the Year and Tsunami Aquatic Awards from the Aquatic Therapy and Rehabilitation Institute (ATRI). Special thanks to Jennifer Tvrdy, OTDR/L for her assistance in making Aquatic Sensory Integration techniques accessible to parents and therapists everywhere.

Parents have a powerful weapon in their fight against autism: water. The bathtub, shower, or public pool can offer countless opportunities to tame transitional stresses, promote social encounters, correct out-of-kilter motor systems, and promote sensory integration.

In water, parents have the power to harness buoyancy, viscosity, turbulence, surface tension, refraction, and thermal shifts. [1] Aquatic therapy offers so much promise for this population that entire therapy pools have been designed with these children in mind. [2-3] Additionally, training seminars, textbooks, and DVDs have been developed to teach therapists and parents to perform sensory integration in water. [4-5] Even Internet-based social networking sites have gotten into the act by devoting entire discussion groups to aquatic therapy for the sensory-challenged child. [6]

As always in the field of physical medicine, research lags behind anecdotal evidence. Intuitively, many pediatric clinicians believe in the power of the pool. In the literature, clinicians have reported a substantial increase in swim skills, attention, muscle strength, balance, tolerating touch, initiating/maintaining eye contact, and water safety during their sessions with young children with autism. [7-10] Parents who require assistance creating aquatic treatment ideas and skill-specific challenges can benefit from reading their findings.

To date, there are no gold-standard clinical trials which support aquatic therapy for the treatment of autism. This is interpreted—in all probability, pre-maturely—by some as a reason to deny aquatic therapy for this diagnosis.

As one example, Aetna Insurance has made a special notation of the fact that they will not reimburse for aquatic therapy services for autism or asthma (strangely specific rulings), while they will reimburse for water-based treatment of the musculoskeletal patient. [11] In this author's opinion, this represents a fun-damental misunderstanding of what aquatic therapy is.

Insurers who deny aquatic therapy, yet readily approve of their land-based counterparts, do not understand that the pool is just another tool. Much like a therapeutic ball, a bolster, a mat or a swing, the pool is a means to an end, not a treatment in and of itself.

Truly, there is no such procedure as aquatic therapy. Instead, there is neu-romuscular re-education, trained in the water. Or therapeutic exercise per-formed in a space dominated by buoyancy. Or sensory training practiced in a room overloaded with warm, viscous molecules. Insurers who would never consider denying therapists the right to use a splash-table or bucket in the clinic have little leg to stand on when denying those same clinicians the right to a *really big* pail. [12]

So what special opportunities can the pool provide? In addition to the normal therapy pursuits of strengthening, balance training, and range of motion (ROM), the pool is an excellent location to work on:

- Transitional stress
- Social interactions

- Body awareness and kinesthesia
- Tactile processing
- Vestibular processing
- Visual processing

Transitional Stress

According to Laurie Jake CTRS, CEDS, children with autism have difficulty with change because they are unable to distinguish relevant from irrelevant information, resulting in huge difficulties with decision-making. Such kids often cannot "make up their minds" or make a simple A-versus-B choice.

These kids have a need for sameness and have a strong need for rituals and routine. Free time is very difficult for them to manage. Additionally, children with autism have organizational and sequencing problems. These children don't know where to start, what comes next, or when a task is finished. The child's life can become one long series of tragic interruptions. [13]

Water activities can provide autistic children with the opportunity to embrace change. Even the act of entering the pool from the deck is a massive leap into uncertainty, and parents looking for ways to promote acceptance of change can use the pool for this end.

For instance, parents who are greeted with unceasing crying jags every evening at bath time can try this trick for co-bathing. Take a towel, swaddle the child, offer the child the bottle, and then lower the child into a warm bath cradled in your arms. This works best if the child can be handed to an already-positioned parent ready in the tub. The transition is smoothed by the act of swaddling, immersion in skin-temperature water, and positioning in the cradling/nursing position. Yet, the child is successfully making a transition. Over time, the props can be removed and the transition can become more dramatic.

Even more than the bathtub, a therapy or community pool can be a daunting place for children with sensory integration issues. As a shield, children often seek out a comfort place in the pool—a place where they feel the safest. Parents or therapists who choose to work in the water should work from the child's chosen safe spot, leave for a little bit, and return again and again.

In addition to aiding with transitional skills, water activities can also provide autistic children with the opportunity to socialize and form attachments. It helps that pool-time seems less like therapy and more like fun. For many children on the spectrum, abnormal or absent social interactions are the painful realities of life with a disability. [13]

Social Interactions

Children with autism often choose to work in solitude even when surrounded by others. In water, parents can encourage their children to work with others. A parent could divide a pair of water crutches between two children and then challenge both to work together for a common goal, such as picking up a ball, lifting it out of the water, and carrying it to a target site, suggests Kari Valentine, OTR/L. Since neither child can achieve this with only one crutch, they will have to work together.

Some therapists who work in water have found role-playing scenes from books or a beloved movie a natural way to encourage interaction. As an example, it is possible to tap into the Harry Potter phenomenon by acting out the "best Potter moments" in the pool. Use a large dumbbell as a pogo stick and have races to outrun dragons and Death Eaters and the like. The rewards? Enhanced body awareness, balance, and the ability to adapt to changes in the plot of a verbal story—as well as to engage in creative play.

Once childhood morphs into adolescence, friendships, friendly competition, and a healthy interest in the opposite sex can become powerful motivators. The pool is a natural environment for these normal social interactions to take place. Oftentimes the pool is such a natural place for play, that children can exceed their parents' socialization expectations. [14]

Body Awareness and Kinesthesia

Many children with autism are afraid of movement, afraid of water splashing their face, and unable to use equilibrium reactions in an effective way. And while the pool may be the perfect place to work on these deficits, there is also a potential risk that the weightlessness which occurs in water will disrupt already atypical feedback loops. Additionally, the refraction of light on the water's surface can limit a child's ability to self-monitor limb placement, and visual cues are untrustworthy. So, does it even make sense to work on body awareness and kinesthesia in the pool?

Although it is true that quiet, full-body immersion can dampen proprioceptive input, the wise therapist or parent knows how to harness the effects of turbulence and momentum for enhancing body awareness and kinesthesia. Simple childhood games like whirlpool (running in one direction in a circle and then quickly reversing direction to move against the "current") can create opportunities for feedback loops which are unachievable on land.

Shay Vanderloo, COTA suggests that parents get creative to help facilitate a child's interest in water. Vanderloo believes in the power of role-playing. For instance, the parent can create a make-believe Egyptian adventure. Wrap the child in different textured wet towels and then challenge him to break through the towels to get free to save the "ruby"—a toy jewel floating on a mat—by jumping into the pool. The goal? To increase kinesthetic input, and diminish hypersensitivity. [15]

Kary Valentine, OTR/L suggests positioning flotation mats shaped like animals so the child can crawl, walk, or slide on his belly with weight on his back. After navigating the animal train, send the child to the water gun area where his hands, feet, legs, and arms re squirted with water to help with desensitization and body awareness.

Therapists or parents who want to jack up the mental intensity during water-gun time can have their patients call out the names of the body part hit by the stream of water. Or, better yet, both parent and child can take turns. The parent begins the game by "hitting" the child's right hand with a stream of water. The child then tries to replicate this effort by using his gun to return the favor. [15]

If a child is having difficulty with weightlessness, it is possible to achieve proprioceptive input by having him scrunch his body into a ball while hanging onto the wall and then push backwards, shooting into the middle of the pool.

The game "Simon says" can be used to both assess and encourage proprioceptive awareness. Make use of this kid's game to teach better body control. Or make use of wet, clingy items such as towels, fabric shower curtains, and even discarded clothing to morph a dress-up game into a therapeutic session designed to enhance proprioception. [15]

Tactile Processing

The water in a pool provides a singular opportunity to alter tactile input. During water activities, the hairs on the body "catch" water molecules as the molecules whisk by, creating a mild shearing effect on the limb. Additionally, the deeper the limb is immersed beneath the surface, the greater the hydrostatic pressure. Initially, this pressure can cause the tactile receptors to fire, but over time, the constant pressure can result in a shut-down effect.

Thus, it is possible to increase—or decrease—the amount of tactile input the child receives by putting him into the pool. But what if the child is so averse to noxious stimulation that he won't even place his face near the water's surface? Stock up a therapeutic toolbox with everyday items easily purchased such as car wash mitts, sponges, and window clings. In the water, it becomes possible to stroke cheeks with cheap paint rollers and drape soaking-wet bath towels over heads to increase tolerance for abrasive touch and pressure. [16]

Vestibular Processing

In the water, the therapist or parent has the ability to challenge the vestibular system in ways unachievable on land. In fact, in some ways, the water offers the perfect environment to enhance vestibular input

An inexpensive way to convert your therapy pool into a vestibular challenge is to perform hammock swings. Purchase a child's parachute or a net hammock. Spread out the parachute or hammock and have the child climb aboard. Swing the fabric through the water: up, down, side to side, tilted, and rotated. Move the child rapidly, then slowly, then rapidly again. The child can sit, kneel, lie supine, or even stand in the hammock during this task. To make this task more interactive, ask the child to sing in time to movements and to anticipate movements before they happen. [17]

Another option? The floatation mat. Rolling is always a strong vestibular task, and one of the best ways to perform this in the pool is on a floatation mat.

Visual Processing

In the pool, the therapist or parent has the ability to challenge the visual system in ways unachievable on land. Because light refracts when traveling from air to water (making it difficult to track what the body is doing underneath the surface), the pool can create a nice training ground for children who rely too heavily on visual cues.

Additionally, there are certain elements intrinsic to a swimming pool (turbulence, airborne splashing, flowing current from jets) which create a visual, tactile, and proprioceptive feast. This makes it possible for children to "feel" what they see. Sight becomes palpable. And this amplifies the therapeutic possibilities. [18]

Parents and therapists who choose to take their children to the water's edge will find a host of opportunity within. It becomes immediately possible to challenge or protect, to stimulate or soothe—all with little effort and much satisfaction. In the water, parents will find a weapon in their arsenal, and a companion for their journey along the spectrum.

For More Information

Aquatic Sensory Integration. Training opportunities for parents and therapists of children with sensory issues. Books, DVDs and hands-on educational seminars. Aquatic Therapy University. Plymouth, MN. Ph: (800) 680-8624. Web: www.aquatic-sensory-integration.com.

AquaticNet Social. Networking Site for Aquatic Therapists & Parents. Aquatic Resources Network. Plymouth, MN. Web: www.aquatictherapist.ning.com.

Aquatic Health Research Database. Over eight thousand aquatic therapy-related research abstracts, including research on the benefits of aquatic therapy for children. Aquatic Resources Network. Plymouth, MN. Ph: (800) 680-8624. Web: www.aquaticnet.com.

ART THERAPY APPROACHES TO TREATING AUTISM

BY NICOLE MARTIN AND DR. DONNA BETTS

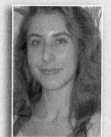

Nicole Martin, MAAT, LPC, ATR

Sky's The Limit Studio, LLC
Lawrence, KS 66044
(785) 424-0739
arttherapyandautism@yahoo.com
arttherapyandautism.com

Sky's The Limit was founded in 2007 by Nicole Martin, a registered art therapist, licensed professional counselor, and artist living in Lawrence, Kansas. As the big sister of a brother with autism, she is dedicated to improving public access to creative arts therapy services tailored specifically to the needs of people on the spectrum. STL's treatment model is a synthesis of her many years of experience working in developmental/behavioral art therapy, applied behavior analysis, and recreational arts and disabilities programs. She is the author of *Art as an Early Intervention Tool for Children with Autism* (2009) and various articles, and received her training at the School of the Art Institute of Chicago.

Donna Betts, Ph.D., ATR-BC

Art Therapy Program
The George Washington University
1925 Ballenger Avenue, Suite 250
Alexandria, VA 22314
dbetts@gwu.edu
www.art-therapy.us
www.gwu.edu/~artx/

Dr. Betts is a registered and board-certified art therapist and assistant professor in the George Washington University graduate art therapy program. Dr. Betts serves on GW's Autism Initiative Committee, which is working toward the establishment of the GW Autism Research, Treatment & Policy Institute. Her own research addresses the clinical utility of art therapy approaches with individuals on the autism spectrum. Dr. Betts is also the author of the Face Stimulus Assessment (FSA), (Betts, 2003, 2009) a performance-based, nonverbal drawing instrument used primarily to identify strengths of people with autism and related disabilities, establish treatment goals, and determine progress in therapy. Ongoing research related to the reliability and validity of the FSA is another focus of Dr. Betts's work.

Art therapy is a mental health profession that uses the creative process of art-making to improve and enhance the physical, mental, and emotional well-being of individuals of all ages (AATA, 2009a). Art therapy is based on the belief that the creative process involved in artistic self-expression helps people to increase self-esteem and self-awareness, achieve insight, develop interpersonal skills, resolve conflicts and problems, manage behavior, and reduce stress.

Creative expression has been used for healing throughout history (AATA, 2009b). In the early 20th century, psychiatrists became interested in the artwork created by their patients with mental illness. Educators simultaneously discovered that children's art expressions reflected emotional, developmental, and cognitive growth. By midcentury, hospitals, clinics, and rehabilitation centers increasingly incorporated art therapy programs along with traditional therapies.

Today, art therapy integrates the fields of human development, visual art (drawing, painting, sculpture, and other art forms), and the creative process with models of counseling and psychotherapy (AATA, 2009a). Art therapy is used in a number of settings with individuals of all ages, and with a variety of mental and emotional problems and disorders, and physical, cognitive, and neurological problems.

Art therapy is an effective approach when working with individuals with autism spectrum disorder (ASD). Art therapy involves the application of techniques specifically designed to reduce the symptoms of autism and promote healthy self-expression. A number of clinical reports support the use of art therapy with ASD, as well as with individuals with developmental disabilities in general (Gilroy, 2006).

The art therapist is adept at facilitating therapeutic processes with the use of visual art media and modalities such as painting and drawing, sculpture, cartooning, clay modeling, animation, and puppetry. The sensory appeal of the art materials makes them desirable tools for self-regulation and self-soothing. Projects designed to tackle specific treatment goals are limitless and may include group murals (to work on collaboration, reciprocity, and flexibility skills), portrait drawing (to work on face processing and relationship skills), friendship boxes (to work on memory and relationship skills), and many more (Martin, 2009a).

Art therapy differs from art education due to the therapist's expertise in the psychological application of art techniques, master's-level training in child development, knowledge of autism spectrum disorders, and how to tailor projects accordingly. An art therapist working in this specialty should be fluent in developmental/behavioral art therapy approaches, have a solid understanding of early childhood artistic development, have experience in the use of current best practices in behavioral and communication supports for individuals with autism, and be a patient and enthusiastic coach. Improving artistic skills and striving for aesthetic beauty are desirable qualities and will help maintain the client's enthusiasm, but remain secondary to the focus on personal growth and reduction of symptoms.

No possible risks or side effects from art therapy with this population have been published to date; however, the risks that can arise from poorly selected art materials and their poorly supervised use must be carefully considered. Art therapists should know the toxicity level and ingredients of all their art supplies as well as the allergies, diet restrictions, and behavioral patterns of their clients, and pair them wisely. For example, a child on a gluten-free diet should avoid traditional playdough since it contains wheat flour, and a child who tends to throw objects should not use sharp tools without close supervision. Art therapists can start by offering a sensible variety of nontoxic materials and then increasing the variety, number, and quality as the child matures. Art materials should also be carefully matched to the child's symptoms and energy level; a poor match can aggravate or encourage symptomatic behavior, while a good match can soothe and create an appropriate outlet for symptoms (Martin, 2009a).

The wide range of symptoms experienced by people with ASD makes them very unique in presentation, so treatments must be tailored to a range of varying needs (Evans & Dubowski, 2001). It is especially important to offer a safe, predictable, and stable environment by providing therapy at the same time every week and setting up materials in an orderly fashion. By doing so, the art therapist establishes psychological continuity and a stable environment for the client (Stack, 1998). Treatment takes place within the professional therapeutic relationship between the art therapist and the client, in either private sessions or a group setting. Additionally, an art therapist can train the client's caregivers and teachers in the use of art therapy techniques in order to help generalize progress to the client's natural environment, such as home or school.

To begin, the art therapist assesses the individual's skills and interests in order to formulate individualized treatment goals. Using a combination of formal and informal assessment, the art therapist determines the client's capacity for imagination and socialization, artistic developmental level, the impact of different art materials on the client's senses and behavior, and the client's initial interests and personality, before developing appropriate treatment goals. Assessment tools such as the Face Stimulus Assessment (Betts, 2003, 2009) and the Portrait

Drawing Assessment (Martin, 2008) can provide insight into the skills of clients with autism.

Art therapy helps clients with autism on many different levels. Major treatment goal areas include socialization, communication, and sensory regulation (Martin, 2009b). Martin (2009a) highlights six treatment goal areas that distinguish art therapy from other therapies used to treat autism: imagination/abstract thinking skills, sensory regulation and integration, emotional understanding and self-expression, artistic developmental growth, visual-spatial skills, and appropriate recreation/leisure skills.

Early intervention is crucial. Goals that a child with ASD might accomplish in art therapy include age-appropriate drawing or modeling skills, improved self-expression and reduced anxiety or frustration, independent or semi-independent use of art making as a coping skill or self-soothing tool, improved social skills such as project collaboration and flexibility, and age-appropriate imagination and ideation skills.

The art therapist's ability to troubleshoot possible hindrances to the client's interest in art—such as sensory discomfort, perfectionism, anxiety, difficulty translating or generating ideas, compulsive/impulsive behaviors, lack of personal relevancy, or past punitive experiences associated with art materials—and take corrective action, means that art therapy has the potential to benefit the majority of individuals with autism, not just those who demonstrate a precocious talent.

To illustrate with a case example, an individual with autism who is withdrawn may be approached through the objects and activities that he or she prefers (Kramer, 1979). By beginning with the familiar and progressively introducing the new, clients with ASD are more willing to accept the unfamiliar. For instance, Dr. Betts once worked with a student who was obsessed with his own wet saliva. The boy was fascinated with the patterns of movement he created with his spit, and this is what kept him engaged in the kinesthetic activity. Thus, Dr. Betts came up with a way to divert the boy away from his excessive interest in saliva by introducing a dry substance—sand. In his art therapy sessions, the boy was encouraged to play with sand and its containers in a tabletop box. As he learned about how to manipulate his environment through sand play, his obsession with the spit eventually disappeared. With Dr. Betts's continuous encouragement and praise for using the sand, contained within the boundaries of a box, the client progressed toward a more flexible and mature ego functioning. He therefore made gains that addressed his Individualized Education Program (IEP) goals related to cognitive, behavioral, and emotional growth.

Including art therapy as a component of early intervention treatment helps individuals with autism form good habits for a lifetime of using art as a vital means of expression. Appropriate art therapy goals and projects can be created for a person with ASD at any age, level of functioning, or initial interest level. All individuals with autism can benefit from learning how to express their thoughts, feelings, and interests in a creative, hands-on way, whether to ease and enhance communication, externalize feelings of anxiety, or simply realize their potential as imaginative, productive human beings.

9

BIOFILM PROTOCOL

by Ken Siri

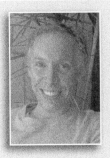

Kenneth J. Siri

Ken Siri, a former Wall Street analyst who covered the healthcare industry, is the single father of an autistic boy. Now a freelance writer, he is working on a title for the fall, *1001 Tips for the Parents of Autistic Boys*. Ken has become active in the autism community in New York City where he and his son reside, most prominently as a member of the Rebecca School PTA.

Introduction

Doctors now know that autism is not only a neurological condition but also an immune inflammatory condition, impacting the gut along with the brain. In fact, many of the symptoms associated with autism (stimming, hyperactivity, self-injurious behaviors, aggression) are related to the gut. Doctors on the cutting edge of autism research, such as Dr. Anju Usman, have had success treating autistic children by addressing persistent gut dysbiosis. A highly promising cutting-edge therapy in this realm is known as the biofilm protocol.

What is a biofilm:

- A biofilm is a collection of microbes growing as a community, forming a matrix of extracellular polymeric substance (EPS) separated by a network of open water channels.
- The architecture is an optimal environment for cell-cell interactions, including the intercellular exchange of genetic material, communication sig-

nals, and metabolites, which enables diffusion of necessary nutrients to the biofilm community.

- The matrix is composed of a negatively charged polysaccharide substance, held together with positively charged metal ions (calcium, magnesium, and iron).
- The matrix in which the microbes are embedded protects them from UV exposure, metal toxicity, acid exposure, dehydration salinity, phagocytosis, antibiotics, antimicrobial agents and the immune system.
  (Usman DAN! Presentation, October 9, 2009)

Treatment Development

The gastrointestinal (GI) tract or gut contains the largest collection of microorganisms in the body (over a trillion bugs) and is the first line of defense in the body's immune system (the gut accounts for about 70 percent of the body's immune system). A healthy gut contains "good" bacteria; symbiotic flora growing in the GI tract, known as microbiota. These good bugs fight off pathogens and allergens.

This complex ecosystem of organisms needs to be in balance; stresses including a history of excessive antibiotics can unbalance the gut, killing off healthy flora and microbes (good bugs), allowing clostridia and yeast (bad bugs) to overgrow.

When the balance of good and bad bugs is disrupted, the immune system becomes weakened, leading to chronic infections, inflammation, and autoimmunity. This condition, of gut bugs out of balance, is known as dysbiosis.

Once bad bugs take over the GI tract, they are notoriously difficult to eliminate. Frontline treatment typically involves changing the diet and adding probiotics. If the patient has a serious dysbiosis problem (yeast), then antifungals (typically nystatin and Diflucan) are used. For many of our autistic kids the results from this standard therapy are fleeting or nonexistent, as they have had undiagnosed or improperly diagnosed GI issues for significant periods of time (often years). When these typical treatments do not work, it may be that the bad bugs have become protected by a pathogenic biofilm, which was produced over time by the dysbiosis.

Pathogenic Biofilm Indicators—a stool test ordered by a doctor can help confirm

- History of frequent antibiotics usage, and or usage at a young age (typically for ear infections) while the immune system was developing
- Dairy intolerance

- Poorly formed stools (color, consistency, undigested food)
- Chronic constipation and or diarrhea
- Aggression, self-injurious behavior, irritability, mood swings
- Poor sleeping behaviors
- Colic or reflux
- Thrush and history of diaper rash—skin problems, eczema, acne, rash
- Abdominal distention, bloating
- Initial response to antifungals, but relapse after discontinuation

How does this happen? Well, in order to hide from the body's immune system, bad bugs (when untreated) cause a chronic infection in the child, generating the pathogenic biofilm, which acts as a protective matrix, cloaking the same bad bugs from the immune system. This allows the bad bugs to thrive and produce toxic byproducts, leading to food sensitivities, GI dysfunction, and autoimmunity. This protective matrix makes pathogenic biofilm difficult to diagnose and treat.

GI (Gastrointestinal) Dysfunction

Maldigestion—Food sensitivities (dairy, gluten, soy, etc), poor weight gain, low essential amino acids, low stomach acid/bloating

Malabsorption—vitamin deficiencies, fatty acid deficiencies, dry skin, irregular stool

Immune Dysregulation/Inflammation—stims, sleep disorders, aggression, and self-injurious behaviors.

Treatment of pathogenic biofilm can help the immune system restore normal gut flora and improve symptoms associated with autism. Unfortunately, pathogenic biofilms are resistant to many antimicrobials and antibiotics in standalone therapy.

> **Note:** There are two types of biofilm communities, symbiotic, and pathogenic. Symbiotic are produced by good gut bugs and protect the gut lining. Symbiotic biofilms occur normally in the body around mouth, teeth, lungs, sinuses, and other areas. Pathogenic biofilm are those that can cause a disease.

Practitioners use a biofilm protocol to deal with the most persistent GI issues. The goal of the protocol is to sterilize the organisms in the gut which are creating the pathogenic biofilm and leading to abdominal illness and digestive problems as evidenced by poor stool quality (infrequent, discolored, poor consistency). The following is the latest iteration of the protocol.

The protocol

A biofilm approach follows four steps:

1. Lysis/Detachment
    a. Oral Na (sodium) EDTA, ethylenediaminetetraacetic acid (an iron chelating compound), and enzymes (nattokinase, lumbrokinase, chitosan) are given on an empty stomach.

    Note: EDTA works as an antifungal enhancing agent, lactoferrin acts to block further biofilm development, and the enzymes help to break down or degrade the biofilm.

    i. Patients with dairy allergies should not take lactoferrin
    ii. Patients with shellfish allergy should not take chitosan
    iii. If severe GI issues are present, enzymes should not be give on an empty stomach
    iv. Avoid iron, calcium, or magnesium supplements within two hours of administration.

2. Microbial killing
    a. Natural antimicrobials or pharmaceutical agents given one hour after lysis/detachment. Agents will depend upon testing
    b. Start with natural antimicrobials; pharmaceuticals later, if organisms remain
    c. Killing bugs is secondary to creating a hostile environment for them

3. Cleanup
    a. Activated charcoal to help prevent symptoms of die-off and aid in removal of toxins, such as ammonia
        i. Remember to give activated charcoal space, at least two hours from step two and any other supplements/meds (they get absorbed by the charcoal).

4. Rebuild/Nourish the gut lining
    a. An hour plus outside microbial killing
    b. Utilize probiotics, prebiotics
    c. Probiotic- and prebiotic-rich foods
    d. Nutritious, nontoxic foods; think organic, hormone-free, antibiotic-free. Consider Specific Carbohydrate Diet (SCD). Use digestive enzymes with meals

e. Supportive nutrients

   i.   Probiotics are live organisms which confer a health benefit. You want a good quantity and quality of organisms

   ii. Prebiotics are nondigestible food ingredients that benefit the patient, stimulating the growth of beneficial bacteria. Can be given as supplement and/or in foods—legumes, peas, soybeans, fruit, garlic, onions, leeks, and chives. Act as a food source for good bacteria. Also act to inhibit pathogens and reduce clostridia toxins

   iii. Give away from microbial killing phase (two plus hours)

Layman translation is as follows:

Step 1 Lysis/Detachment

Break open the biofilm protecting the bad gut bugs utilizing the combination of Na EDTA and the enzymes mentioned above. To make life easier, there are now a couple of products on the market that combine these. InterFase by Klaire Labs and Biofilm Defense by Kirkman Labs are now available. Either, or the combination above, are given on an empty stomach.

Step 2 Antimicrobial killing

An hour after completing the lysis/detachment step is the optimal time to give the antimicrobials. Your doctor can suggest a cocktail, but they typically include Diflucan, neomycin, and other antifungals/antimicrobials. Your doctor will also devise the dosage of each drug given the patient's size and specific gut issues.

Note: The antifungals will require a prescription, and the enzymes are typically only available to physicians, so working closely with a doctor trained in biofilm will be necessary. Easiest formulation is capsules/pills, some are available in suspension but it is worth it to transition a child to capsules if they are not already familiar. We have had success using applesauce on a spoon with a single pill/capsule each time, working from the smallest to largest each session.

Step 3 Cleanup

The body, properly fortified with nutritious food, will perform this task on its own in most cases. If experiencing a die-off reaction (increased negative behaviors) use of activated charcoal (from you local health food store) will assist in the cleanup. It may also be useful to give the activated charcoal anyway, during the initial week or so, to capture the ammonia and other byproducts generated from the lysis/detachment step. Remember, with activated charcoal, give two hours outside any supplement or medication, as the charcoal will not discriminate what is absorbs.

Step 4 Rebuild the gut

Here, probiotics are given following a meal (dinner works best) to help grow the good gut bug colonies. Again, this should be at least two hours after or before activated charcoal is given. After a meal is ideal, as a full stomach is occupied and less likely to have digestive juices available to destroy the probiotics (i.e., acid in the stomach is occupied). Note that if enzymes are given to help the patient digest certain proteins, notably dipeptidyl peptidase-IV (DPP-IV) or other proteases to help digest gluten and casein, their use may need to be suspended during the bio-film treatment, as these enzymes could inflame a seriously stressed GI tract.

Ideally this treatment is continued until stools normalize and the gut returns to normal. Enzymes may then be reintroduced.

Results

Parents should expect a die-off reaction with increased gas and loose, bro-ken-up stools, and potentially increased negative behaviors (stimming, upset, aggression) for a short period of time. The duration of treatment is based on how quickly stools and bloating normalize, typically reported to be weeks to months. Do not get discouraged—the treatment takes time, as pathogenic biofilm has taken time to be created, and will likewise require time to be removed. As stools and bloating normalize, expect to see improved overall behaviors, better sleep, disappearing rash, and markedly improved mood, allowing for increased regula-tion and attention and focus.

Potential side effects include irritability, aggression, stimming, hyperactivity, sleep disturbances, and rash. These could be the due to yeast or bacteria flare-up, detox reaction (too rapid a removal of heavy metals leading to vitamin and min-eral deficiency), and stress on liver or kidney. Die-offs usually create an excess release of toxins, including ammonia, which is why activated charcoal should be used at the start of the treatment.

10

BIOMOLECULAR NUTRIGENOMICS: NUTRIGENOMIC DNA TESTING AND RNA-BASED NUTRITION

BY DR. AMY YASKO

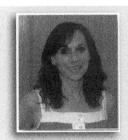

Dr. Amy Yasko, Ph.D., NHD, AMD, HHP, FAAIM

Neurological Research Institute, LLC
279 Walkers Mills Road
Bethel, ME 04217
207.824.8501
www.DrAmyYasko.com

Amy Yasko received her undergraduate degree in chemistry and fine arts from Colgate University and her PhD in the department of Microbiology, Immunology, Virology from Albany Medical College. Her postdoctoral work included fellowships in the Department of Pediatric Immunology and the Cancer Center at Strong Memorial Hospital, as well as the Department of Hematology at Yale Medical Center. Dr. Yasko was Director of Research at Kodak IBI as well as a principle/owner of several biotechnology companies including Biotix DNA and Oligos Etc., Inc. After receiving additional degrees as a traditional Naturopath and becoming a Fellow in Integrative Medicine, Dr. Yasko shifted her focus from biotechnology to natural medicine. With her knowledge in these various fields she developed a protocol including a nutrigenomic test used to aid in addressing such complex conditions as autism, chronic fatigue syndrome, and other chronic neurological issues. Through the use of herbs and supplements and biochemistry testing to chart client progress, many who follow her protocol have improved and have even recovered. Dr. Yasko has spoken at conferences hosted by the NY Academy of Science, is listed in Who's Who in Women, has received the CASD Award for RNA research in autism and has published numerous articles as well as chapters in books related to her more conventional work in biotechnology. At present she donates much of her time on her discussion group www.ch3nutrigenomics.com and offers advice and suggestions to the many who seek her help on their path to recovery.

Multifactorial diseases are caused by infections and environmental events occurring in *genetically susceptible individuals*. Basic parameters like age and gender, along with other genetic and environmental factors, play a role in the onset of these diseases. Infections combined with excessive environmental burdens only lead to disease if they occur in individuals with the *appropriate genetic susceptibility*.

One clear, definitive way to evaluate the genetic contribution of multifactorial disease is to take advantage of new methodologies that allow for personalized genetic screening. Currently, tests are available to identify a number of underlying genetic susceptibilities based on allelic variations that are found in the DNA. Unfortunately, the use of this testing has fallen short of expectations. Perceived impediments to the use of genetic screening to identify underlying susceptibilities to disease include fear of job discrimination, loss of insurance coverage, and the inability to address diagnosed disease states. The lack of use of this powerful diagnostic technology highlights the need for adequate means to address the results of personalized genetic testing. It is a travesty to have the ability to specifically identify genetic weaknesses, yet have this technology underutilized out of fear. It points to a dire need for therapeutic technologies that take advantage of this same genetic information with an eye toward personalized treatment or nutritional supplementation, rather than simply personalized diagnosis.

The field of nutrigenomics is the study of how different foods can interact with particular genes to decrease the risk of diseases. Biomolecular nutrigenomics takes this concept a step further, analyzing the molecular signaling pathways that are affected by specific single-site base changes, and then utilizes combinations of nutrients, foods, and natural ribonucleic acids to bypass mutations and restore proper pathway function.

A central pathway in the body that is particularly amenable to biomolecular nutrigenomic screening for genetic weaknesses is the methionine/folate pathway. As a result of this decreased activity in the methylation pathway, there is a shortage of methyl groups in the body which would otherwise serve a variety of important functions.

Methyl groups are CH3 groups that are moved around in the body to turn on or off genes. There are several particular sites in this pathway where blocks can occur as a result of genetic weaknesses. Supplementation with appropriate foods and nutrients will bypass these mutations to allow for restored function of the pathway.

The methylation cycle is the ideal pathway to focus on for nutrigenomic analysis and supplementation. The function of this pathway is essential for a number of critical reactions in the body. A consequence of genetic weaknesses (mutations) in this pathway is increased risk factors leading to a number of serious health conditions. Defects in methylation lay the appropriate groundwork for the further assault of environmental and infectious agents resulting, in a wide range of conditions including diabetes, cardiovascular disease, thyroid dysfunction, neurological inflammation, diabetes, chronic viral infection, neurotransmitter imbalances, atherosclerosis, cancer, aging, schizophrenia, decreased repair of tissue damage, improper immune function, neural tube defects, Down's syndrome, multiple sclerosis (MS), Huntington's disease, Parkinson's disease, and Alzheimer's disease, as well as autism.

Methylation is also directly related to neurotransmitter levels; methylation of intermediates in tryptophan metabolism can affect the levels of serotonin, and intermediates of the methylation pathway are also shared with the pathway involved in the actual synthesis of serotonin and dopamine. In addition to its direct role as a neurotransmitter, dopamine is involved in methylating phospholipids in the cell membranes to increase membrane fluidity. Membrane fluidity is important for a variety of functions, including proper signaling of the immune system as well as protecting nerves from damage. A number of serious neurological conditions site reduced membrane fluidity as part of the disease process, including MS, amyotrophic lateral sclerosis (ALS), and Alzheimer's disease. In addition, phospholipid methylation may be involved in modulation of NMDA (glutamate) receptors, acting to control excitotoxin damage.

Increases in certain inflammatory mediators of the immune system such as IL-6 and TNF-α lead to decreases in methylation. Chronic inflammation would therefore exacerbate an existing genetic condition of undermethylation. The inability to progress normally through the methylation pathway as a result of methylation cycle mutations could lead to a buildup of precursors of the methylation pathway, including the excitotoxin glutamate.

The building blocks for DNA and RNA require the methylation pathway. Without adequate DNA and RNA, it is difficult for the body to synthesize new cells. This would result in a decreased level of new cells, including critical cells of the immune system, the T cells. De novo T cell synthesis is necessary to respond to bacterial, parasitic, and viral infection, as well as for other aspects of the proper functioning of the immune system. T cells are necessary for antibody-producing cells in the body (B cells), as both T helpers and T suppressors are needed to appropriately regulate the antibody response.

In addition, decreased levels of methylation can result in improper DNA regulation. DNA methylation is necessary to prevent the expression of viral genes that have been inserted into the body's DNA. Loss of methylation can lead to the expression of inserted viral genes.

Proper levels of methylation are also directly related to the body's ability to both myelinate nerves and to prune nerves. Myelin is a sheath that wraps around the neuronal wiring to insulate and facilitate faster transmission of electrical potentials. Without adequate methylation, the nerves cannot myelinate in the first place, or cannot remyelinate after insults, such as viral infection or heavy metal toxicity.

A secondary effect of a lack of methylation and hence decreased myelination is inadequate pruning of nerves. Pruning helps to prevent excessive wiring of unused neural connections and reduces the synaptic density. Without adequate pruning, the brain cell connections are misdirected and proliferate into dense, bunched thickets. These metabolically caused changes in brain function can be mitigated if the underlying genetic weaknesses that are causing these changes are identified and supplemented nutritionally using biomolecular nutrigenomic analysis.

In general, single biomarkers are identified as indicators for specific disease states. However, it is possible that for a number of health conditions, including autism, it may be necessary to look at the entire methylation pathway as a "biomarker" for underlying genetic susceptibility for a disease state. It may require expanding the view of a "biomarker" beyond the restriction of a mutation in a single gene, to a mutation somewhere in an entire pathway of interconnected function.

This does not mean that every individual with mutations in this pathway will be autistic or will have one of the health conditions listed above. It may be a necessary but not a sufficient condition. Most health conditions in society today are multifactorial in nature. There are genetic components, infectious components, and environmental components. A certain threshold or body burden needs to be met for each of these factors in order for multifactorial disease to occur. However, part of what makes the methylation cycle so unique and so critical for our health is that mutations in this pathway have the capability to impair all three of these factors. This would suggest that if an individual has enough mutations or weaknesses in this pathway, it may be sufficient to cause mutlifactorial disease, as methylation cycle mutations can lead to chronic infectious diseases and increased environmental toxin burdens, and have secondary effects on genetic expression.

By looking at diagrammatic representations of the methylation pathway and relating the effects of genetic polymorphisms to biochemical pathways, it is possible to draw a personalized map for each individual's imbalances, which may impact upon their health. By identifying the precise areas of genetic fragility, it is then possible to target appropriate nutritional supplementation of these pathways to optimize the functioning of these crucial biochemical processes. Key nutrients or foods that can aid in helping to bypass methylation cycle mutations are ribonucleic acids, or RNA.

The methylation pathway is particularly amenable to RNA-based supplementation, as these pathways are not only necessary to convert homocysteine to methionine, but are also needed for the synthesis of pyrimidines and purines for new DNA and RNA synthesis. By supplementing these pathways with appropriate nutrients, it is possible to optimize the functioning of these crucial biochemical processes.

CENTER FOR AUTISM AND RELATED DISORDERS, INC. (CARD)

BY DR. DOREEN GRANPEESHEH, DR. JONATHAN TARBOX, AND DR. MICHELE BISHOP.

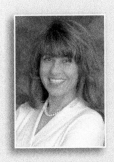

Doreen Granpeesheh, Ph.D., BCBA-D
Jonathan Tarbox, Ph.D., BCBA-D
Michele Bishop, Ph.D., BCBA-D

19019 Ventura Boulevard, 3rd Floor
Tarzana, CA 91356
http://centerforautism.com/
(818) 345-2345

Dr. Doreen Granpeesheh is the Founder and Executive Director of the Center for Autism and Related Disorders (CARD) and the Founder and President of the Board of Autism Care and Treatment Today (ACT Today!). Dr. Granpeesheh received her Ph.D. in Psychology from UCLA and is licensed by the Medical Board of California and the Texas and Arizona State Boards of Psychologists. Dr. Granpeesheh holds a Certificate of Professional Qualification in Psychology from the Association of State and Provincial Psychology Boards, is a board-certified Behavior Analyst, and has been providing behavioral therapy for children with autism since 1979. She is a member of numerous scientific and advisory boards, including the U.S. Autism and Asperger's Association, *The Autism File* magazine, Autism 360/ Medigenesis and the 4-A Healing Foundation. Dr. Granpeesheh is also an active member of the Autism Human Rights and Discrimination Initiative Steering Committee, and sits on the Oversight Committee of the Department of Developmental Disabilities for the State of Arizona. In addition, Dr. Granpeesheh currently serves as first Vice Chair of the National Board of Directors of the Autism Society of America. Dr. Granpeesheh has had numerous publications on issues concerning the diagnosis and treatment of autism and currently oversees the behavioral treatment of over a thousand patients through CARD's twenty clinic sites across the globe.

The Center for Autism and Related Disorders (CARD) was founded in Los Angeles, California in 1990 by Dr. Doreen Granpeesheh. Currently, CARD has seventeen office locations in the United States, across six states, two international sites in Australia and New Zealand, two affiliate sites in the United

Arab Emirates and South Africa, and reaches out through consultation to families affected by autism on every continent.

CARD provides a wide range of services for children and adults with autism, pervasive developmental disorder not otherwise specified (PDD-NOS), and Asperger's disorder. These services include behavioral, diagnostic, and psychometric evaluations and assessments, specialized services such as feeding, medical treatment facilitation, and short-term challenging behavior interventions, as well as our core model of early intensive behavioral intervention (EIBI) in the client's home, school, and community. In addition, CARD is heavily invested in the training of parents and other professionals through the provision of continuing education classes and online trainings, while CARD's research and development department is engaged in numerous areas of research, including evaluation of medical interventions, to further delineate the subtypes of autism spectrum disorder (ASD). CARD researchers have published over fifty research articles in peer-reviewed scientific journals and have contributed over twenty chapters to edited scientific texts. CARD's mission is to provide the highest-quality behavioral intervention to the maximum number of children with autism possible, around the globe.

Assumptions at the Heart of CARD Therapy

CARD believes that all people with ASDs are capable of learning. Although there is currently no way to predict the outcome of treatment for any individual, we strongly believe that all children with ASD have a right to the most effective treatment available in the world.

CARD's philosophy is behavioral. CARD believes that everything a person says or does is behavior, and that all behavior can be improved or enhanced via learning opportunities in the environment. The belief that all human beings, with or without disabilities, have the capacity to learn, prevents blaming the child's disability when a teaching procedure fails. Instead, it leads to an understanding and respect for personal dignity, individuality, and self-determination of people with ASD, and encourages the expression of personal beliefs, feelings, interests, and preferences.

While our intervention follows the principles of learning and behavior, at the core of our philosophy is also the belief that learning occurs best under conditions of stable health, adequate sleep, and functional regulation of sensory input. As such, in our application of behavioral treatment, we recognize and identify these factors in our clients and adjust our interventions so as to maximize our outcomes.

CARD believes that recovery from autism exists. We have observed recovery in a significant percentage of the children we have served (see Granpeesheh, 2008; and Granpeesheh, Tarbox, Dixon, Carr, & Herbert, 2009 for discussions of recovery). However, while recovery becomes possible for a group of children with particular characteristics, it is not the single goal of intervention. Our goal is to help each child achieve the most they can, and in doing so, live a more fulfilling and independent life.

The CARD Model of Treatment for Children with ASD

The first controlled study on a comprehensive ABA program for children with autism was by Ivar Lovaas in 1987. Subsequent studies replicated the general findings of Lovaas (1987) and have provided more detail (see Granpeesheh, et al., 2009 for a more thorough review). Some of these findings indicate that ABA treatment should begin as early as possible (Fenske et al., 1985; Harris & Handleman, 2000), that children who receive more treatment hours per week (i.e., thirty or more) have better outcomes than those who receive fewer (e.g., fifteen or less) (Lovaas, 1987; Granpeesheh et al., 2009), and that continuing ABA treatment for two or more years (Eikeseth, 2002; 2007; Howard et al., 2005; Sallows & Graupner, 2005) will lead to optimal outcome.

This form of ABA is commonly referred to as early intensive behavioral intervention (EIBI). The CARD model of intervention builds upon the core principles of EIBI while providing a more holistic approach to treating autism.

The primary goal of treatment at CARD is to develop unique and individualized programs based on the individual's particular strengths and weaknesses. As such, our treatment begins with a comprehensive evaluation and assessment. Our assessments include all areas of functioning, such as speech and language, cognition, adaptive, play, social, motor, academic, and executive functioning skills, and are conducted via psychometric assessments, questionnaires completed by caregivers, and through direct observation. In addition, various instruments are administered for diagnostic purposes, to determine frequencies of challenging behaviors, and to determine sensory dysregulation in the visual, auditory, tactile, and proprioceptive modalities. Finally, where possible, full medical and health evaluations are requested, thereby enabling us to develop a full profile of the client and to design an individualized treatment program that meets each client's unique needs.

After determination of a client's skills and needs, all underlying or comorbid medical issues and dietary needs are dealt with so as to stabilize the client's health, sleep, and resulting ability to attend. Sensory dysregulation of any type is noted, and adjustments are made to the client's program, stimuli used, and modality of treatment delivery so as to maximize the client's ability to receive the instruction provided, and the program of behavior intervention is initiated.

Most of the clients treated at CARD enter the program at the age of two and receive intensive services over the course of four years, with the ultimate goal of recovery at the age of six. For these children, the first year of treatment consists of intensive work on language and behavior with progression into social skills in the second year, more abstract cognitive and executive functioning skills in the third, and a gradual fade-out of services in the final year. The intensive services are usually provided initially in the child's home, with a transition to the child's school and community as the child's age allows.

The procedures used in our program are based on the principals of behavior analysis. With our younger clients (ages one to three), our delivery involves more social and play-based interventions, while our toddlers (ages three to five) mostly receive therapy through a combined discrete trial and natural environment modality. The discrete trial method is a highly structured behavioral protocol that involves concise instructions, clearly defined behavioral responses, and immediate delivery of rewards, while the natural environment training model allows the client to practice the skills he has learned in his various unstructured daily life settings.

The progression of a client's program depends on his or her incoming skills. While most clients begin with minimal language and severely deficient social skills, the range of clients we treat mandates a broad variety of instructional content areas within our curriculum. Individuals with the less severe diagnoses of PDD-NOS or Asperger's syndrome often require instruction only in the social, cognitive, and executive functioning areas, and these areas of instruction are delivered through a more cognitive behavioral format.

Over the course of CARD's twenty-year history, we have treated thousands of individuals with ASD. Our clients have taught us that any skill can be learned when provided at the right time and within the right order of instruction. The content of the CARD curriculum addresses all areas of functioning, providing over three thousand lessons across the following eight domains: 1) language, 2) play, 3) social skills, 4) motor, 5) academics, 6) adaptive skills, 7) cognition, and 8) executive function. The curriculum programs are based on age-appropriate norms following the development of skills in typically developing children.

For our older clients (ages ten to twenty-one), our CARD II program focuses on independent living skills, successful employment, development of leisure activities, building friendships, and attending college, trade, or vocational school.

Since all of our clients have unique needs and strengths, there is no "typical" client at CARD and the particular regimen of treatment, including delivery protocol, number of hours, and specific content, are all determined individually.

Outcome of CARD Clients

Several current studies and recent publications speak to the outcome of CARD clients. In a study on the effects of CARD treatment, we found that greater intensity of treatment and beginning treatment at a younger age both contribute to faster learning rates during CARD therapy (Granpeesheh, Dixon, Tarbox, Wilke, & Kaplan, 2009). In a study currently underway, we have found that children who received twenty-five or more hours of therapy per week made significant gains in all areas of functioning. Of particular note is the finding that 96 percent of the group studied met criteria for an ASD according to the Autism Diagnostic Observation Schedule (ADOS) at intake, while only 64 percent of that group still met criteria for an ASD according to the ADOS after two years of treatment. In a recent study, we reported the results of a retrospective evaluation of CARD clients who had recovered from autism, and described the course and outcome of treatment for thirty-eight recovered children (Granpeesheh, Tarbox, Dixon, Carr, & Herbert, 2009). Our studies on the outcome of CARD treatment have replicated the general findings in the published literature. That is, an intensity of twenty-five or more hours per week of treatment, beginning at a young age, optimizes positive outcome, even resulting in recovery for some children.

In conclusion, CARD is among the largest autism treatment organizations in the world. CARD's state-of-the-art services, global reach, and comprehensiveness of scope are matched by none. What sets the CARD model apart from others is our open-minded and holistic approach to autism treatment and our insistence on a comprehensive application of ABA treatment to every imaginable skill a person with ASD may need to learn. Over the course of the last two decades, with the rising incidence of ASD, we have experienced a tremendous increase in the demand for CARD treatment services. This has led to the opening of our Specialized Outpatient Services clinic, where we provide feeding intervention services and short-term intervention for severely challenging behaviors, as well as the development of an online web-based system of training, assessment, and behavioral programming, based on the CARD Curriculum, called SKILLS

(Shaping Knowledge through Individualized Life Learning Systems). SKILLS consists of online delivery of the CARD curriculum, the CARD SKILLS Index (a comprehensive assessment of child functioning linked directly to the curriculum), as well as electronic training resources and a globally accessible repository for data storage and analysis. The last two decades have been very productive for CARD and the next twenty years promise to be even better, as we expand our suite of services and our capacity for disseminating effective autism treatment around the globe.

CENTER FOR AUTISM SPECTRUM DISORDERS, MUNROE-MEYER INSTITUTE

BY DR. TIFFANY KODAK AND DR. ALISON BETZ

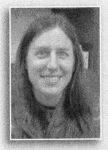

Tiffany Kodak, Ph.D.

Dr. Tiffany Kodak is an Assistant Professor in the Department of Pediatrics at the University of Nebraska Medical Center and Assistant Director of the Early Intervention Program in the Center for autism spectrum disorders at the Munroe-Meyer Institute. She graduated from Louisiana State University in 2006 with a Ph.D. in School Psychology. Dr. Kodak completed her graduate internship at The Marcus Institute in Atlanta, Georgia under the supervision of Drs. Wayne Fisher, Henry Roane, and Michael Kelley. Her post-doctoral fellowship was completed in 2006 under the supervision of Dr. Wayne Fisher. Her research has focused on several general topics, including the assessment and treatment of problem behavior, choice, behavioral economics, and skill acquisition with individuals diagnosed with autism and severe behavior disorders. She has published sixteen peer-reviewed research studies, and worked directly with individuals with developmental disabilities for fifteen years. Dr. Kodak is on the editorial board and served as the editorial assistant for the *Journal of Applied Behavior Analysis*, is a Board Certified Behavior Analyst (BCBA), and the recipient of the APA (Division 25) Applied Behavior Analysis dissertation award in 2006.

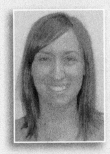

Alison Betz, Ph.D.

Dr. Alison Betz received a Master of Arts in Behavior Analysis from Western Michigan University, and her Ph.D. in Disability Disciplines with a specialization in Applied Behavior Analysis from Utah State University. She is currently completing a post-doctoral internship at the University of Nebraska Medical Center's Munroe-Meyer Institute. Her research interests and publications have focused increasing communication and social skills of young children with autism. She is currently focusing her research efforts on the assessment and treatment of severe problem behavior with individuals with disabilities. Other research interests include increasing the response variability of individuals with autism, the effects of token reinforcement, and schedules of reinforcement.

For more information about the programs in the Center for Autism Spectrum Disorders contact cawilli1@unmc.edu. To refer a child for services in the CASD, please fax (402) 559-5004 or email cawilli1@unmc.edu referrals, including child's name, date of birth, reason for referral, and contact information.

Munroe-Meyer Institute, University of Nebraska Medical Center

The Center for Autism Spectrum Disorders opened at the Munroe-Meyer Institute opened in 2006 as part of the University of Nebraska Medical Center. The center focuses on using the principles of behavior analysis to assess and treat child with autism and other developmental disabilities. The primary goal of the center is to improve the lives of children with autism spectrum disorders (ASD) and their families by: (a) providing comprehensive, state-of-the-art clinical services; (b) advancing knowledge about the causes of and treatments for ASD through systematic research; and (c) disseminating information about effective assessment and treatment through education, professional training, and consultation. There are three departments included in the Center for Autism Spectrum Disorders: Early Intervention Program, Severe Behavior Program, and the Pediatric Feeding Disorder Program. This chapter will focus on the Early Intervention and the Severe Behavior Programs.

Early Intervention Program

The emphasis of the Early Intervention Program within the Center for Autism Spectrum Disorders is to provide highly specialized services to children diagnosed with an autism spectrum disorder (ASD) between the ages of two and nine. The program utilizes assessment and treatment procedures based on the principles of Applied Behavior Analysis (ABA). Our program focuses on teaching (a) language, (b) academic and pre-academic skills, (c) appropriate social behavior, and (d) daily living skills (e.g., potty training).

In order to teach a variety of skills that are individualized to the specific needs of each child, it is the mission of the program to improve the quality of life for children with ASD and their families by providing empirically supported and comprehensive treatment services, developing and refining assessment and treatment procedures through systematic research, and promoting generalization and maintenance of acquired skills.

Program Description

The Early Intervention Program at the Munroe-Meyer Institute offers a continuum of services including evaluation, school consultation, clinic-based intervention, and home-based program development. Each child receives services based on his or her individual needs.

During therapy sessions, highly specialized techniques are used to teach children a variety of skills. Trained therapists conduct instructional procedures across settings ranging from individualized seat work, to naturalistic play interactions with adults and/or peers. A psychologist with specialty training in applied behavior analysis oversees all therapy sessions. Therapists record each occurrence of targeted skills, and the accuracy of the data is checked frequently. Session-by-session data are graphed, reviewed, and analyzed each day by therapists and supervising psychologists. Data are used to guide program development and refine the academic interventions.

Like many of their typically developing peers, children with ASD may not acquire skills through daily interactions in their home or school environment. To effectively teach children with ASD, tasks are broken down into small, measurable units, and each skill is practiced repeatedly until the child masters the skill. Some skills may serve as building blocks for other more complex skills (e.g., imitation, attending). Thus, we may begin working on more basic skills that allow children to acquire building blocks that prepare the child to learn more advanced skills and learn in a number of different environments. Once a skill is mastered, it is practiced periodically to make sure the child continues to maintain previously mastered skills over time. Parents are also provided with information and materials to work on mastered skills in the home environment. It is our goal for children to exhibit all newly learned skills in a variety of environments and with a variety of people.

If a child in the Early Intervention Program displays problem behavior that is of concern to the parents or school personnel, assessment and treatment procedures will be utilized to reduce the occurrence of the challenging behaviors.

Initial Evaluation. Children will be seen by a team of specialists with training and expertise in educational interventions. Some children may benefit from highly intensive early intervention, while other children may only require limited visits to our clinic or consultation between our staff members and school personnel. Our evaluation process may require an extended period of time because children respond differently to different academic instructional procedures. Our goal is to identify a number of instructional procedures that will result in the most rapid acquisition of targeted skills.

Treatment. Based on the needs of each individual child, a curriculum of academic, pre-academic, social, and language skills are developed. Targeted skills are worked on each day until the child reaches mastery criterion for the skill. Our model of intervention combines aspects of Discrete Trial Training, Natural Environmental Training, and Verbal Behavior. Treatment procedures may include Discrete Trial Instruction, Natural Language Paradigm, Incidental Teaching, Peer Mediated Strategies for social skills development, as well as a number of other empirically-validated procedures based on the principles of ABA.

Parent Training. Once an effective treatment is developed and the child has mastered some of the targeted skills, we train parents and other care providers to use the teaching strategies in other environments. The long-term success of the treatment depends on how accurately the program is carried out by parents, teachers, in-home aids, and other care providers. We encourage school personnel to participate in training as well. Our goal is to teach everyone who interacts with the child to use the instructional procedures that result in learning new skills and maintaining previously learned skills.

Severe Behavior Program

Approximately 10–15 percent of children with autism, developmental disabilities, and traumatic brain injuries engage in some form of destructive behavior such as aggression, self-injury, pica, or property destruction. The purpose of the severe behavior program within the Center for Autism Spectrum Disorders is to provide specialized services to individuals with autism and other developmental disabilities who display these destructive behaviors. It is often the case that children who do display these problematic behaviors pose a health risk for the child or to others, limit their learning and development, cause stress and hardship on their families, and may be at risk for long-term institutional care. Thus it is the mission of this program to improve the quality of life of the children who display destructive behaviors, and their families, by (a) providing the most advanced treatment services; (b) perpetuating the development and refinement of effective treatments of severe behavior through systematic clinical research; and (c) promoting the widespread dissemination of effective treatment technologies through highly specialized training and consultation.

Program Description

The severe behavior program provide specialized treatment to school-aged children (three to twenty-one years old) that display such severe destructive behavior that it poses a risk to self, others, or to the environment, and who cannot be safely managed or treated in a less-structured and intensive program. The program offers a continuum of services, including initial evaluation, outpatient services, day treatment, and parent/caregiver training. An individualized program is created for each child, and that child moves through the program based on his or her personal needs.

Following the initial evaluation, during which the child and family meet with a team highly experienced in the assessment of severe problem behaviors and recommendations are given, the child may be referred to one of the following programs:

Day Treatment or Outpatient Services. Children with less severe behaviors are typically referred to outpatient therapy. With outpatient services, children are typically seen from one or two hours per day, one to five days per week. Children displaying more severe problem behaviors are typically seen in our day treatment program, in which the child is seen five or six hours, five days per week. Regardless of whether the child is referred to outpatient services or day treatment, the assessment and treatment of the problem behaviors are conducted in a similar manner.

All sessions are conducted in a specialized therapeutic environment that allows us to safely evaluate potentially dangerous behaviors. For each child, we begin therapy by conducting analog sessions that directly test the effects of specific environmental antecedent and consequences on the problem behavior. Data are collected on the targeted behaviors on computers by the therapists are reviewed by a licensed psychologists on a daily basis. The session data are then analyzed to develop and refine an individualized treatment for the child. Furthermore, all assessments and treatment components are evaluated systematically by using single-case research designs. This allows us to identify, refine, and replace ineffective components of the treatment plan.

Parent Training. The long-term success of the recommended treatment plan developed during therapy sessions is dependent on the accuracy of implementation by parents and caregivers. Thus, parent and caregiver training is a critical component of our program. Parent and caregiver training typically involves written and spoken instruction, modeling, behavioral rehearsal or role play, and systematic feedback during therapy sessions. Once the parents or caregivers demonstrate competency in implementing the treatment at the clinic, therapists then observe parents implementing the treatment in the home and other naturalistic settings. Furthermore, we provide treatment recommendations and training for the child's school or other caregivers.

CHELATION: REMOVAL OF TOXIC METALS

BY DR. JAMES B. ADAMS

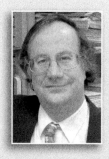

James B. Adams, Ph.D.

Professor
School of Mechanical, Aerospace, Chemical, and Materials
Engineering
Arizona State University
PO Box 876106
Tempe, AZ 85287-6106
(480) 965-3316
(480) 727-9321 (fax)
http://autism.asu.edu

James B. Adams is a President's Professor at Arizona State University, where his research is focused on the causes of autism and how to treat it. He is also President of the Autism Society of Greater Phoenix, and is co-leader of the Autism Research Institute/Defeat Autism Now! Think Tank. His research includes toxic metals/chelation, nutrition (vitamin/minerals, essential fatty acids, amino acids), neurotransmitters, and GI issues. He is the proud father of a daughter with autism.

Rationale: Many children with autism have a low amount of active glutathione, and a higher fraction of their glutathione is oxidized (inactive). Glutathione is the body's primary defense against mercury, toxic metals, and many toxic chemicals, so a low level of glutathione results in a higher body burden of toxins. Also, many children with autism had increased use of oral antibiotics in infancy, which alter gut flora and thereby almost completely stop the body's ability to excrete mercury. Normalizing glutathione, restoring gut flora, and removing toxic metals often results in reduction of the symptoms of autism.

Also, a major study by our group found that much of the variation in the severity of autism was associated with the level of toxic metals in the urine.

Preparation for Treatment: Prior to beginning chelation, it is important to first prepare the body for it. This includes:
1) Reducing exposure to toxins (by using organic food and reverse osmosis water, no mercury fillings, avoiding pesticides, etc.).
2) Improving levels of essential vitamins and minerals—see section on vitamins and minerals.
3) Improving glutathione levels—see section on glutathione.
4) Treating gut dysbiosis—see sections on gut treatments.

Testing:

It is difficult to assess toxic metal body burden. The best approach is to use a challenge dose of the relevant chelator (DMSA, DMPS, or possibly EDTA), and measure the level of toxic metals in the urine before and after taking it. A large increase indicates that the metals are present, and that the medication is helpful in removing them.

Hair, blood, and unprovoked urine testing only indicate recent exposure to toxic metals, and are *not* useful in determining past exposure. Children may have a high body burden but a low level in their current hair, blood, or urine.

The urinary porphyrins profile is a test of porphyrin production in the kidneys. Abnormal porphyrins may indicate an increased body burden of mercury, lead, or other toxic metals, but other factors such as oxidative stress might instead account for abnormal porphyrins, so the test results can be difficult to interpret.

Treatment: The chelation treatments I recommended include DMSA and DMPS, and possibly TTFD. These treatments should only be done under physician supervision, with regular evaluation of kidney and liver function and white blood cell count. All of the treatments except IV-DMPS can be done at home. DMSA is best for removing lead, and DMPS is best for removing mercury.

Length of Treatment: It is recommended to measure the amount of toxic metals in urine (preferably in a first-morning urine sample) before starting treatment. Then, every month or so, collect urine for about 8 hours after DMSA or DMPS treatment, and measure levels of toxic metals again. When the levels are within the lab's reference range (which is for people NOT undergoing chelation), then the chelator has probably removed most of the metals that it is able to. Since DMSA and DMPS bind to different metal differently, it is probably useful to use one until it urinary excretion is low, and then switch to the other. It may be useful to do a challenge dose every six months or so, as lower, maintenance doses may be helpful.

DMSA (dimercaptosuccinic acid): Oral DMSA is approved by the FDA for treating lead poisoning in children. Some of the compounded rectal suppositories also appear to increase excretion of toxic metals, but the transdermal forms do not measurably increase excretion of toxic metals.

Safety: DMSA only slightly affects excretion of most essential minerals, so a basic mineral supplement can compensate for this. The exception is that the first dose of DMSA removes a significant amount of potassium (equivalent to that in a banana), and that is not included in mineral supplements, so one or two servings of fresh fruit or vegetables should be consumed to restore potassium levels. DMSA also significantly increases excretion of cysteine, so that should be supplemented before and/or during therapy.

DMSA has a small chance of increasing liver enzymes or decreasing blood cell count, so those should be monitored during treatment. A major research study published by our group found that DMSA was generally very safe, and was highly effective in removing toxic metals, improving glutathione, normalizing platelets (a marker of inflammation), and possibly beneficial in reducing the symptoms of autism.

DMPS (2,3-dimercapto-1-propanesulfonic acid): DMPS is not approved by the FDA, but a physician may have it legally compounded for IV, oral, and rectal use, all of which increase excretion of toxic metals. The transdermal form does *not* appear to increase excretion of toxic metals.

Safety: DMPS slightly increases the excretion of some essential minerals, so a basic mineral supplement is recommended to compensate for this loss. It is unknown if it causes a loss of potassium. DMPS has a small chance of increasing liver enzymes or decreasing blood cell count, so those should be monitored during treatment.

TTFD (thiamine tetrahydrofurfuryl disulfide): A small pilot study of TTFD (used as a rectal suppository) resulted in some increase in excretion of arsenic and possibly other metals, and also significant reduction of autistic symptoms. The transdermal form may also work, although more study is needed.

Safety: TTFD appears to be very safe, with animal studies at high doses finding no evidence of toxicity.

More info: Anyone considering chelation therapy is urged to read the Defeat Autism Now! Consensus Report on Treating Mercury Toxicity in Children with Autism, available at www.autismresearchinstitute.com. This report provides more detailed advice on pretreatments, treatments, dosages, and safety.

ARI Survey of Parent Ratings of Treatment Efficacy:

	% Worse	% No Change	% Better	Number of Reports
Chelation	2%	22%	76%	324

Research:

There is substantial evidence to suggest that many children with autism suffer from exposure to mercury, and probably other toxic metals and toxic chemicals. The data includes:

1) A literature review by Bernard S et al. showing that the symptoms of autism were very similar to those of people suffering from infantile exposure to mercury poisoning.

2) A study by James et al. found that children with autism had low levels of glutathione, which is the body's primary defense against mercury.

3) A large study by Nataf et al. found that over half of children with autism had abnormal levels of a porphyrin in their urine that highly correlates with a high body burden of mercury.

4) A study by Bradstreet et al. found that children with autism excreted three to six times as much mercury as did typical children when both were given DMSA.

5) A baby hair study by Holmes et al. found that children with autism had unusually low levels of mercury in their baby hair ($\frac{1}{8}$normal), suggesting a decreased ability to excrete mercury. A replication study by Adams et al. found similar, although less dramatic, differences. The Adams et al. study also found that children with autism had much higher usage of oral antibiotics than did typical children, which is important because usage of oral antibiotics almost completely stops the body's ability to excrete mercury.

6) A small pilot study by Adams et al. found that children with autism had twice as much mercury in their baby teeth than did typical children, suggesting that they had a higher body burden of mercury during their infancy, when the teeth formed. That study also found that children with autism had a much higher usage of oral antibiotics during their infancy, similar to their baby hair study.

7) Two studies of airborne mercury, in Texas and in the San Francisco Bay Area, found that the amount of mercury in the air correlated with the incidence of autism.

8)   There have been nine epidemiological studies of the link between thimerosal in vaccines and autism. Four published studies by the Geiers have consistently found that children who received thimerosal in their vaccines had a two to six times higher chance of developing autism than those who received thimerosal-free vaccines. Four published studies by groups affiliated with vaccine manufacturers have failed to find a link, and one was inconclusive. Three of the studies were conducted in other countries where the usage of thimerosal is much less and the incidence of autism is much lower, so those results have limited relevance to the U.S.

COMPUTER-BASED INTERVENTION—WHAT'S IT ALL ABOUT?

BY VALERIE HERSKOWITZ

Excerpt from the book, *Autism & Computers: Maximizing Independence Through Technology.*

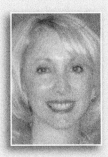

Valerie Herskowitz, MA, CCC-SLP

info@valerieherskowitz.com
www.valerieherskowitz.com

One of the world's foremost speakers on the subject of computer-based intervention (CBI) with autism, Valerie Herskowitz was the founder of Dimensions Therapy Center. She has expanded her computer-based intervention for families on an international scale by establishing a "global autism support village" through podcasts, webcasts, and other cyber tools. Ms. Herskowitz's career as a speech pathologist spans the past thirty-two years, and she was the recipient of the Stevie Lifetime Achievement Award in 2004 for her work with individuals with autism. Her youngest son, Blake, was diagnosed in 1993 with autism. Her professional journey as a therapist and as a parent of a child with autism have combined to give Ms. Herskowitz the unique insights to help families cope with problems they face in parenting a child with autism. She is the author of the book, *Autism & Computers: Maximizing Independence Through Technology* (2009). For more information about computers and autism, or to buy her book, log onto: www.valerieherskowitz.com.

It is important to start on the road to technology literacy early. The reason is based on the science and research that supports early training of any sort. It deals with early intervention and neuroplasticity, which revolves around the brain's ability to reorganize itself by forming new neural connections throughout life (Medicine.net). The brain is an organ that changes from response to experience.

There are several studies that support early intensive behavioral intervention (e.g., Anderson et al., 1987; Fenske et al., 1985; Lovaas, 1987; Smith et al., 2000)

Though the types of therapy models have varied in the studies, they have certain things in common. They all incorporated curriculums in the areas of attention and focusing, language, and social skills, and they all used a behavioral approach. Each model utilized twenty-five hours per week of structured stimulation, and they promoted the inclusion of parents and families into the intervention process. When these factors occur together, there is evidence that many children show significant increases in communication, IQ, and educational placement.

Computer-based intervention or CBI incorporates all of the above features. There are software programs that teach skills in the areas of attention, language, and social interaction, and they are taught using effective behavioral methods. I don't recommend that CBI be implemented twenty-five hours a week, but I do feel that it needs to be an integral part of a home-based intervention program. And I highly recommend that family members become active in the process.

From a physiological perspective, let's look at the reasons why early intervention is successful in utilizing the concept of neuroplasticity. According to the website Neuroscience for Kids, neuroplasticity consists of several different processes that occur throughout a person's life. There are certain periods of one's life, however, where plasticity occurs more frequently. During the first two years of life, the synaptic connections of each neuron increase until there are twice as many synaptic connections as in an adult's brain. As time continues, there is a degenerative process called pruning which continues until the cell dies. This pruning process can be affected by the activity of cell interaction, however. Therefore, cells that are activated are strengthened, and those that are not activated are pruned. The pruning process continues until approximately age sixteen, so as you can see, early stimulation has a huge impact on brain development.

From a cellular and molecular level, researchers have demonstrated how sensory, perceptual, and language functions are influenced by our experiences. They have surmised that the brain is most susceptible to modifications for language acquisition within the first six years of life. The brain still retains the ability to acquire language skills in a slower manner up until the age of twelve. After that, there is a significant slowdown. It doesn't come to a complete halt by any means, but it may be more difficult to accomplish.

Jason's Success Story

Jason had been diagnosed with autism approximately a year before his mother brought him into my office for a consultation. He was 3½ years old and had received speech therapy services through the state-funded early intervention program. For six months, Jason's therapist focused on developing his speech skills, which were nonexistent at the time. She also worked with Jason's mother to incorporate techniques in the home. After the six months, the early intervention services ended, and Jason had not made significant progress in his ability to communicate his wants and needs. Needless to say, he was becoming increasingly more frustrated.

In order to get what he wanted, he pulled his caretaker to the area where his desired item was located, and he sort of flipped the caretaker's arm up toward the item. If what he wanted wasn't in plain sight, it usually took several attempts before the caretaker (usually his mother) figured out what he wanted. Sometimes, the failed attempts resulted in huge outbursts from Jason. What worried his mother even more was the fact that Jason was becoming more and more remote as his inability to communicate increased.

I asked Jason's mother if he had been exposed to any other communication techniques such as picture systems, sign language, or electronic devices. His mother said that toward the end of the early intervention services, the therapist had started some sign language, but he hadn't caught on to it yet. I also asked whether he had been exposed to technology in any way. His mother revealed that Jason did like to randomly push the keys on the computer keyboard, but there hadn't been any attempts to formally teach him computer usage.

I spent some time working with Jason to see what he was able to do and what he seemed to be interested in. He didn't show any interest in verbal speech, and he wasn't able to repeat the sounds or words that I demonstrated. I also tried to get him to imitate some gross motor movements, like touching his head or clapping his hands. He was unable to accomplish this successfully, which led me to believe that he wasn't ready for sign language training since it requires the ability to imitate motor movements. His attention was very short, and he had difficulty focusing on these tasks.

Using toys, I tried to determine if Jason had the ability to cause things to happen. This skill, which we call "cause and effect," is very important. If a child doesn't understand that he has the ability to make something happen, he won't understand the point of using communication, which is a cause-and-effect activity. Jason was able to demonstrate his ability to control in a very rudimentary way. Though he hadn't been exposed to computers formally, I took him to the computer to see what kind of interest I could muster from him. His focusing wasn't great, but I was able to grab his interest when I used entertaining and lively introductory programs.

Jason began to work with us in the office and with his mother at home. We began training him to use the Picture Exchange Communication System (PECS) system using photos and also introduced him to a program I designed called Pre-Sign, which develops the prerequisite skills needed to learn sign language. To increase his cause-and-effect skills, we introduced Jason to a wonderful series of animated programs that are used for young children with special needs. In addition to increasing this skill, we were able to improve his attention and focusing. We also used other software for developing his understanding of language skills. These programs, again developed for those with beginning language skills, helped him to comprehend the meaning of words.

After six months, Jason was able to communicate his wants and needs using the PECS system. He had finished the Pre-Sign program, and we moved him into our sequel program, Sequenced Sign. He was using the computer via a touchscreen very well at this point. His cause-and-effect and attention skills had increased so significantly on the computer that we decided it was time to begin work on verbal speech. Instead of using traditional verbal behavior methods, however, which try to stimulate speech by having the child imitate the therapist, we used a computer program which has voice recognition skills. The child is asked to repeat different sounds into a microphone, and that action causes an animated character to perform. This activity proved to be quite successful, resulting in Jason attempting verbal imitation.

Jason continued to make great strides from there. After one year, he was verbalizing while using the PECS pictures and signs. He was quite communicative, which caused his behavior to improve. Eventually, we moved out of PECS into a dedicated voice output system. His experience in computer usage proved to be a tremendous asset as he learned to use the touchscreen communication device with ease. Through the device and computer-based intervention, he learned how to string words together to make short sentences. Ultimately, we were able to discontinue the voice output system because Jason developed the ability to speak on his own.

By the time Jason was in the first grade, he had been included in regular education with supports. He continued with his computer-based intervention program, in which the areas of advanced language and social pragmatics were stressed. As the years progressed, reading skills programming, especially in the areas of comprehension, were included in his training.

Jason is now eleven years old and in middle school. Though he still has challenges, he's living a life that includes the prospects of going to college. What is possible for him is beyond anything his parents could have dreamed for him just eight years ago. Technology continues to have a huge influence on his life: He e-mails his friends regularly and loves his iPod. He now wants a cell phone, which his mom has been thinking about getting for him.

Jason is a huge success story. The early influence of computer-based intervention proved to be the catalyst that helped him to become quite productive in his life. Not all individuals reach this level of functioning, but many do increase their abilities significantly through early technology training.

Helping Older Children and Adults

What if your child or student is older? Is all hope lost? Certainly not! As previously mentioned, brain plasticity does not stop for the entire lifetime of a person. Dr. Merzenich, the neuroscientist often referred to as the "father of neuroplasticity," has been involved in some interesting work regarding older individuals. He and his colleagues have recently created a computer-based program called Brain Fitness, which is designed to strengthen the brain in order to increase speech and agility. Dr. Merzenich's early work involved the research design of a similar computer-based training program called Fast ForWord. This program was designed for children and adolescents who demonstrate significant language impairments.

Think about the last time you tried to learn a new skill. Perhaps you and your spouse decided to take dance lessons, you decided to try to learn a little Italian before your trip to Italy, or you needed to learn a new computer application at work. There may have been a little bit of a learning curve, but you probably were able to gain some skill in these areas. Granted, it wasn't easy, and you probably won't be on *Dancing With the Stars* in the near future. But I'm sure you were able to learn enough to add enjoyment to your life.

Taking on technology in later years is much the same way, even for a person with developmental disabilities. I have a student that is actually my age. (If you have done the math, you may have figured out that I'm in my early fifties.) We started working together approximately seven years ago. Bobby lives with his brother, who referred Bobby to me. At the time, Bobby's language consisted of one- to two-word sentences, and he was difficult to understand. He had no reading skills and was unable to tell time. He was high functioning in other areas and held a job in the food court at the local mall, but he had virtually no experience using computers or any other technological application.

Initially, I felt that Bobby should focus on developing his language skills. I wanted to increase his ability to produce longer sentences, so I introduced him to a program called Sentence Developer, which I created for the students in my office. It's a visual system designed to teach sentence structure. From a technological prospective, it's fairly easy to use. Bobby was able to learn how to use a mouse very quickly, so the touchscreen wasn't necessary.

This program was Bobby's first introduction into the world of computers. Though the technological learning curve was short, the impact of these exercises on his language development was significant. This experience also gave him the confidence to move on to more sophisticated computer usage.

We moved on to programs designed to improve his speech production. These applications, which are a little bit more involved from a technological perspective, allowed Bobby to record his own voice. We also incorporated a reading program, as well as an application to teach Bobby some time-telling skills. Through the last few years, Bobby has become quite skilled in computer technology. Aside from the skills he has acquired through the training, he feels that he's part of the world that he lives in and feels pride in his accomplishments.

Bobby loves the fact that he is computer literate at this time of his life. His brother purchased the reading program, and Bobby enjoys practicing the exercises at home. Bobby's story shows that we are never too old to acquire computer or technology skills.

Had Bobby been given the opportunity to obtain computer training when he was young, would he have been more able to utilize technology than he is today? My experience tells me that the answer to this question is yes, but this type of instruction simply wasn't available to him until seven years ago. Still, what he has accomplished in that span of time is quite remarkable and compelling. So, if anyone ever tries to convince you of the old adage, "You can't teach an old dog new tricks," please disregard it as an untruth.

Why CBI is Successful

I have identified several factors that CBI offers which explain its success with individuals on the autism spectrum.

Predictability. Every parent, teacher, or therapist of a child with autism will agree that, for the most part, our children have issues with new people, new foods, and new experiences—just about "new" anything. Conversely, they seem to handle familiar situations well. They thrive in a ritualistic environment and deteriorate when something is strange to them. Computer-based intervention offers a mode of treatment that can provide familiarity and predictability. Certainly, this isn't the case the first time the individual begins the process, but as time goes on, the training takes on a *sameness* even when the actual exercise changes. The program starts up the same each time, and/or the animation is the same. The format of the exercises is the same, and if you use multiple programs from a particular software manufacturer, the format of other programs is similar, if not identical, to the programs the child is already using.

As therapists, teachers, or parents, we will have a shorter learning curve as well, since the software designers often create a series of programs that present different exercises in the same format.

Animation. I feel that animation is a make-it or break-it situation. Some children need the animation that is provided by many of these programs, and others find it a major distraction, may be afraid of it, or become overstimulated by it. This is why many of the manufacturers of these programs have included the ability to turn the animation feature on or off. You don't have this ability, however, with off-the-shelf software or programs that you purchase in a store rather than from a vendor who sells software specifically for the special needs population.

The animation can be used for several purposes: First, it's used as a reinforcer, so that when the child performs the task correctly, an animated character comes out and congratulates the child for a job well done. Another function of the characters is as a prompt device. Often, they will appear above the correct answer when the child has demonstrated the need for cuing. Then, as the child progresses, the animation will not appear. Lastly, there are several programs that utilize animation as the actual characters in the program. In this case, the intention is to increase attention and focus on the task.

If you take a look at off-the-shelf software, you often find that animation is used for other purposes as well as the above. There may be several animations on the screen at a time, and this can be quite distracting to many of the kids. The last thing we need is for our children to be *more* distracted than they already are.

Looking forward instead of down. When I started working with children on the computer, there was one thing that I noticed immediately. It seemed that they had a much easier time focusing on what they saw on the computer versus what I presented on a table when I worked with them off the computer. I initially concluded that it was the computer program alone that caused them to be more focused and attentive. But after awhile, I began to realize that it was because they looked forward when working on a computer rather than down. When they looked straight ahead, I was able to maintain their attention for a much longer period of time.

I have done my own quasi-experiment and have often utilized this vertical plane presentation when working off the computer with the children as well. Sure enough, I have found that children do seem to be able to sustain attention more appropriately this way. It makes sense. It's more natural if you think about it. When you watch TV or talk to someone, what direction are your eyes looking? You may sometimes look slightly down or slightly up if you're talking to someone who is shorter or taller. But most often, we are looking forward. It's not only a better way to teach our kids, but it's also more pragmatically appropriate. Do we really want to teach our children to focus down? No, we want them to focus forward as they will need to do when conversing with another person or watching the teacher at school.

From a therapeutic and educational sense, it's important to always try to maximize learning for all students. One way that therapists and teachers accomplish this is by recognizing different learning styles in their students. Some obvious ones are auditory learners versus visual learners. Delving into the entire subject of various learning styles is beyond the scope of this book, but software manufacturers of these types of programs have taken into account that individuals will vary greatly in terms of which sense they learn from. Therefore, they have made considerable efforts to include a great deal of auditory and visual approaches. For example, pictures are one stimulus, as well as the voice of the narrator who gives the directive. The only time that this varies is when the task requires the individual to just respond to a visual *or* auditory directive. Then, of course, both the visual and the auditory are not given. We call this a multimodality approach.

The term "modalities" refers to the way information is processed. If it is processed by seeing the information, it's obviously visual. If it's processed by hearing the information, it's auditory. Even though every individual learns through one channel better than the other, in most cases, presenting information in both an auditory and visual format is the best way to maximize learning. So, the child sees the picture, hears the words, maybe sees the written words, and sometimes gets visual cuing, etc. This multi-stimulation is often how we can make sure that the student has had the best opportunity for learning.

CRANIOSACRAL AND CHIROPRACTIC THERAPY: A NEW BIOMEDICAL APPROACH TO ASD

BY Dr. Charles Chapple

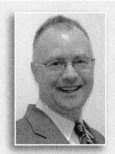

Charles W. Chapple, D.C., F.I.C.P.A.

Advanced Chiropractic Health Center
360 E Irving Park
Roselle, IL 60172
(630) 894-8778
www.drchapple.com

Dr. Charles W. Chapple completed his undergraduate studies at Nazareth College of Rochester, New York, receiving a bachelor's degree in biology before earning his doctorate degree in chiropractic from the National College of Chiropractic in 1991. Dr. Chapple holds many post-graduate certifications in areas such as chiropractic pediatrics (Fellowship in International Chiropractic Pediatric Association), acupuncture, applied kinesiology, and spinal rehabilitation. Dr. Chapple's studies have also encompassed treating neurological challenges involving children with developmental and learning delays, such as Sensory processing disorders: ADHD to Autism. A portion of his Roselle, Illinois practice focuses on the noninvasive benefits of chiropractic and craniosacral therapy to address retained primitive reflexes and sensory processing disorders. Dr. Chapple has a son on the spectrum, and thus finding solutions for individuals diagnosed with ASD is both a professional focus and a personal passion.

One has only to imagine themselves in the uncharted surroundings, where their frame of reference is skewed not only for all that they hear, see, touch, taste, and smell (the far senses) but also for their body awareness, movement, and balance (the near senses). These are challenges common to sensory processing disorders, which encompass a continuum of conditions ranging from attention

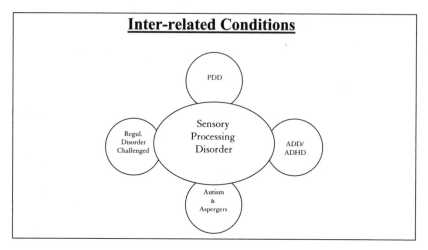

Figure 1.

deficit hyperactivity disorder (ADHD) to autism spectrum disorder (ASD) (See Figure 1).

Although the extent of these challenges can vary within the spectrum of disorders, their expressions can also provide many indicators for productive therapy, particularly when applied to the relationship between the nervous system and biomechanics. Individuals on the spectrum often give indications of areas

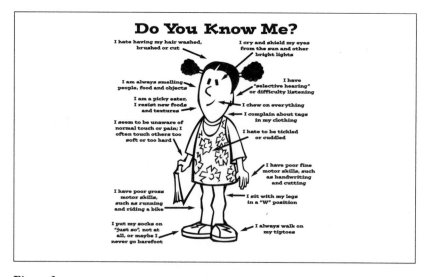

Figure 2.

Primitive-Postural Reflexes

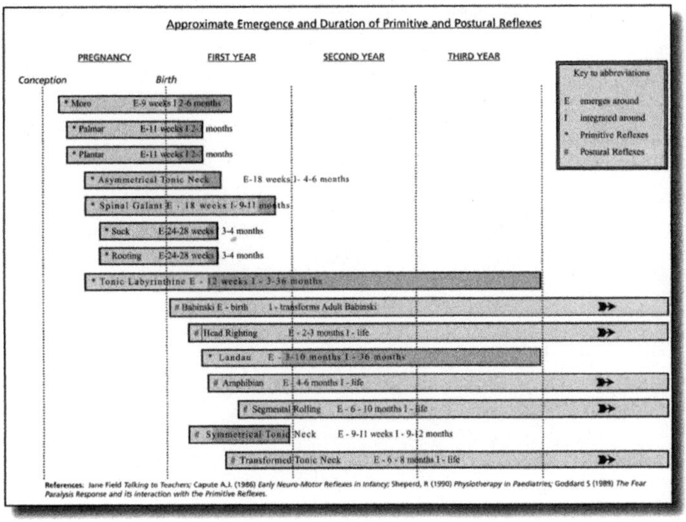

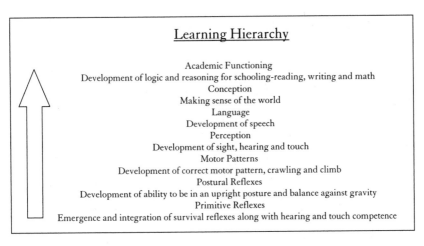

Figure 3.

within their nervous system in need of attention, through biomechanical manifestations (See Figure 2).

The central nervous system (CNS) and the facilitation of the biomechanics of its intimately related boney and membranous protective network (i.e. the cranium, the spine, and their attachments) through chiropractic, and craniosacral therapy (CST) enable a profound link through improved motor input to sensory system

Learning Hierarchy

Academic Functioning
Development of logic and reasoning for schooling-reading, writing and math
Conception
Making sense of the world
Language
Development of speech
Perception
Development of sight, hearing and touch
Motor Patterns
Development of correct motor pattern, crawling and climb
Postural Reflexes
Development of ability to be in an upright posture and balance against gravity
Primitive Reflexes
Emergence and integration of survival reflexes along with hearing and touch competence

Figure 4.

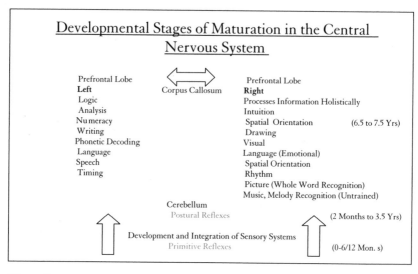

Figure 5.

regulation necessary for brain communication and development. This motor to sensory to brain connection works towards benefiting the functional interaction between an individual's internal and external environments. More simply, movement grows the brain, and chiropractic and CST fine tune movement. The CNS is the circuitry that—along with many other amazing functions—connects an individual to their senses, and the senses to their reflexes.

The recognition that reflexes and sensory processing cannot be separated is significant in benefiting individuals with diagnoses on the spectrum, especially when considering the *primitive reflexes*. Often these individuals on the spectrum are caught in a "sensoreflexive no-man's-land", where they remain under the involuntary control of the *retained primitive reflexes* instead of the voluntary control of their *postural reflexes* (See figure 3). Further correlations have been drawn between motor development and academics (See Figure 4), as well as the necessity of first fostering the integration of primitive to postural reflexes in order for subsequent appropriate right- and left-brain communication and their relevant developmental stages (See Figure 5). Authorities in this field state that reflex profiles which are moderately to severely imbalanced would require specialized teaching and attention to motor imbalances, as well as a reflex stimulation/inhibition program in order to achieve sustained long-term improvements in development. Facilitating these functions of the CNS is critical to enabling *brain* to *body* interactions.

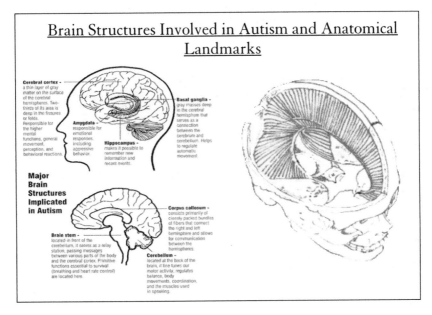

Brain Structures Involved in Autism and Anatomical Landmarks

Cerebral cortex -
a thin layer of gray matter on the surface of the cerebral hemispheres. Two-thirds of its area is deep in the fissures or folds. Responsible for the higher mental functions, general movement, perception, and behavioral reactions.

Amygdala -
responsible for emotional responses, including aggressive behavior.

Hippocampus -
makes it possible to remember new information and recent events.

Basal ganglia -
gray masses deep in the cerebral hemisphere that serves as a connection between the cerebrum and cerebellum. Helps to regulate automatic movement.

Major Brain Structures Implicated in Autism

Brain stem -
located in front of the cerebellum, it serves as a relay station, passing messages between various parts of the body and the cerebral cortex. Primitive functions essential to survival (breathing and heart rate control) are located here.

Corpus callosum -
consists primarily of closely packed bundles of fibers that connect the right and left hemisphere and allows for communication between the hemispheres.

Cerebellum -
located at the back of the brain, it fine tunes our motor activity, regulates balance, body movements, coordination, and the muscles used in speaking.

Figure 6.

Recognizing how our sensory system gathers information to regulate sensory input and knowing how an individual responds to particular sensory stimuli, can suggest a biomechanical approach to improve communication between the body's structure and function. For example, if an individual self-stimulates by rocking their head from side to side, particularly when stimulated by sound, this could indicate an improper regulation of the cranial nerve responsible in part for perception of sound and balance. So, this individual's rocking could be an attempt to self-regulate the sensory system as a result of difficulty with sound or balance, or both. Therefore, treatment would be intended to address the biomechanics in common to this cranial nerve and brain stem, such as the areas including but not limited to the temporal and adjacent cranial bones, cervical spine, and sacrum. Also the familiarization of the brain structures involved in ASD and their relation to the protective boney and membranous network which surrounds them is of great utility in treatment (See Figure 6).

Chiropractic and CST are gentle and noninvasive, hands-on approaches that assist the communication of the CNS, which is essential to both an individual's interaction with the surroundings and quite possibly to appropriate behavior. Benefits are intended through both these approaches' ability to access the body's circuitry in order to reduce or remove the interference upon it. The stimulation

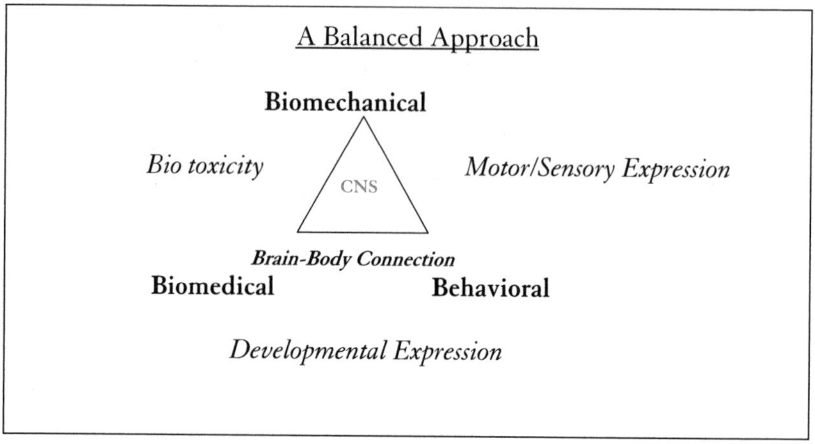

A Balanced Approach

Biomechanical

Bio toxicity   CNS   *Motor/Sensory Expression*

Brain-Body Connection
Biomedical   **Behavioral**

Developmental Expression

Figure 7.

of motor input through chiropractic and CST facilitates sensory input, which drives brain function and development. Therefore, both chiropractic and CST should be considered as an integral part of a balanced approach for treatment (See Figure 7).

Chiropractors identify a biomechanical complex of functional and/or structural and/or pathological articular changes that compromise neural integrity and

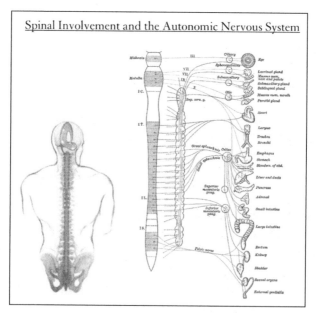

Spinal Involvement and the Autonomic Nervous System

Figure 8.

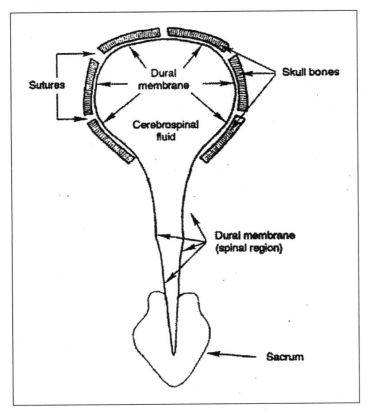

Figure 9.

may influence organ system function and general health (See Figure 8) (called *subluxations* as an academic term), and utilize gentle spinal pressure techniques called *adjustments* to reduce or rid this complex. This biomechanical complex is characterized by:

- Irregular boney mechanics or spinal misalignment
- Nerves imbalances
- Muscle irritations
- Tissue inflammation
- Degenerative wear

CST focuses on relieving pressure on the brain and spinal cord through manual pressure techniques used at the cranium and sacrum. The CST system

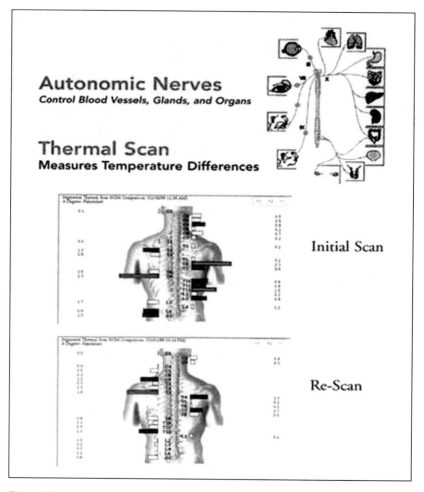

Figure 10.

consists of membranes and cerebral spinal fluid, which protect the CNS (See Figure 9). Restrictions in this system are detected, and corrections are identified through manual monitoring of the craniosacral rhythm (CSR). Subluxations, as well as variations in the CSR (6–12 bpm), could indicate any number of motor, sensory, reflex, or neurological impairments, as well as causes of pain.

Healthcare practitioners are challenged to quantify variations of CNS communication within SPD conditions.

Frequently conventional tests appear unremarkable. Noninvasive tests such as infrared thermography (IF) and surface EMG (sEMG) can accompany a thorough history, exam, and other clinically relevant testing in order to illustrate altered CNS demands.

Infrared thermography measures temperature variations along the spine as indications of imbalances in the autonomic nervous system, which can result from altered biomechanical complexes within the CNS (See Figure 10).

Chiropractic adjustments and CST work to restore more appropriate motor, sensory, reflex, and neurological input and improve motor to sensory to brain communication, therefore working within the body and not outside it.

Although there is no health care that is guaranteed or without risk, chiropractic and CST are among the safest and most effective approaches in benefiting the CNS, and therefore hold great potential as an integral part of a balanced approach in benefiting individuals challenged with SPD: ADHD to autism.

DANCE/MOVEMENT THERAPY

BY MARIAH MEYER LEFEBER

Mariah Meyer LeFeber, MA, LPC, R-DMT, DTRL

Hancock Center for Dance/Movement Therapy
16 N. Hancock St.
Madison, WI 53703
(608) 251-0908
www.hancockcenter.net
mariah@hancockcenter.net
info@hancockcenter.net

Mrs. LeFeber is a dance/movement therapist and licensed professional counselor living in Madison, Wisconsin. She embodies her love of movement in both individual and group treatment for children affected by autism and mental illness. Beyond her passion for the healing power inherent in dance/movement therapy, Mrs. LeFeber further pursues her love of dance by teaching yoga for children and performing with a modern dance company.

Movement is a language. For children affected by autism, movement may be the only language they can rely on. Children with autism often have limited verbal abilities, making it extremely difficult for them to reach out to others (Hartshorn et al., 2001). When words fail, dance/movement therapy fosters a child's ability to relate, communicate, and connect on a nonverbal level.

Dance/movement therapy (DMT), which uses movement as a "universal means of communication," is a valuable form of communication for children with autism, especially those with underdeveloped speech skills (Erfer, 2005, p. 196). Dance/movement therapy provides the space for these children to explore and discover their bodies, while unlocking their potential for creativity. Children are encouraged to find themselves in a supportive environment where there is no "right" way to express or create (Canner, 1968).

As defined by the American Dance Therapy Association (ADTA), dance/movement therapy is "the psychotherapeutic use of movement as a process which furthers the emotional, social, cognitive, and physical integration of the individual" (American Dance Therapy Association, 2008). Dance/movement therapy is an effective form of treatment for people with developmental, medical, social, physical, and psychological impairments (Levy, 2005). This expressive therapy is a bridge, linking creative expression through movement with psychological theory (Kestenberg et al., 1999).

Dance/movement therapy emerged in the 1940s in the United States. Marian Chace, also known as "The Grand Dame" of dance/movement therapy, led the emerging field. Through her work teaching dance to people with varied abilities, Chace recognized the profound impact of the movement on various facets of her student's lives, and began to bridge her work in dance to the world of Western medicine. In 1942, Chace was asked to bring this work to St. Elizabeth's Hospital in Washington, D.C. Here, psychiatrists also realized the benefits of this expressive and healing movement. In 1966, the American Dance Therapy Association formed, with Chace as the first president (Levy, 2005).

A second wave of dance/movement therapists emerged in the 1970s and 1980s. During this period, dance/movement therapy sparked the interest of many professionals, and therapists began experimenting with the use of the form with a variety of populations—including autism. In the midst of this, dance/movement therapy was also officially categorized as a form of psychotherapy.

In application, dance/movement therapy fosters socialization and communication in clients who otherwise might find it difficult to relate. The ability to engage fully through nonverbal activity sets dance/movement therapy apart from other forms of therapy. It creates an affirming environment for clients, where they are able to experience the value of belonging. Ultimately, dance/movement therapy provides both a bridge for contact and a medium for reciprocal communication for children with autism (ADTA, 2008).

A few basic principles form the guiding theory of dance/movement therapy. These overarching tenets of the field include the belief that: behavior is communicative, personality is reflected through movement, changes in movement will eventually lead to changes in personality, and the larger an individual's movement repertoire, the more options individuals have when it comes time for them to cope with the environment (Kestenberg et al., 1999; Meekums, 2002). The actual practice of dance/movement therapy relies on the observation of movement behavior as it emerges in relationship, more specifically the therapeutic relationship between client and therapist. Dance/movement therapists are trained to understand, reflect, and eventually expand on the nonverbal expression of their clients (Adler, 2003). A consistent, supportive and accepting atmosphere is used to begin the process of relationship formation, along with the following: mirroring (reflecting rhythms, patterns, and vocalizations expressed by the client), eye contact, touch, vocalizations, props, and rhythmic body action (ADTA, 2008; Erfer, 1995). In particular, props can be helpful with this population because they are very concrete and tangible, thus serving as a connecting medium between client and therapist.

In addition to the mirroring technique mentioned above, the approaches of both attunement and shape-flow adjustment (from the Kestenberg Movement Profile, one of many movement-analysis systems utilized by dance/movement therapists) help build the therapeutic relationship and augment the therapist's ability to make clinical choices. As described by Loman (1995), "attunement is based on sharing qualities of muscle tension, and Shape-Flow Adjustment is based on a similarity of breathing patterns and shape of the body between individuals" (p. 222). Within the therapeutic relationship, attunement builds a sense of empathy between therapist and client, while shape-flow adjustment builds trust in the relationship (Loman, 1995).

A constant priority, the initial and overarching goal for dance/movement therapists working with autism (or with any population) is to reach out and meet a client at his or her functioning level. Once this relationship has been established, it serves as a consistent guiding principle behind the work and emerges in the balance between the physical and relational. In the dance/movement therapy setting, relationships occur as a byproduct of the body in action and physical movement flourishes because of the trust built within the therapeutic relationship. When the physical and relational aspects of the work are in balance, movement truly can serve as a language for universal communication.

When building treatment goals, each child with autism presents with specific needs and challenges, yet a handful of goals are generally applicable. The first of these goals is increasing sensory motor and perceptual motor development, directly targeting the motor deficits often faced by children with autism spectrum disorder (ADTA, 2008; Erfer, 1995). By working from both a functional and expressive standpoint, dance/movement therapists can use simple vocabulary and movement to stimulate perceptual, gross, and fine motor skills. An example of this is teaching children the perceptual concept of "in and out" by having them physically step inside of a space (i.e., a hula hoop) and then outside of that same space. Through the gross motor movement, the children experientially learn the concept, which can then be generalized to other areas.

The second goal for dance/movement therapists is to help clients improve their socialization and communication skills. As the therapeutic relationship builds, clients increase their ability to interact as part of a group and communicate (verbally or nonverbally) within that group. Steps toward these goals include: increasing eye contact, participating in shared rhythmic activities with engagement (and independently whenever possible), recognizing and responding to group members, increasing proximity to the group, decreasing a need for interpersonal distance, developing trust, and forming an understanding of "self" as opposed to the "others" outside of the self (ADTA, 2008).

Although these social and communication goals can be met through several modalities, dance/movement therapy is unique because the steps towards these goals can all be experienced on a kinesthetic level. For example, in group rhythmic activity, group members move together with similar rhythms, intensities, and physical tensions. This extension of movement throughout the body helps a client to integrate what may be a fragmented sense of self (Levy, 2005). Moving small movements into total body activity helps build cohesiveness and a sense of grounding, not only for the person as an individual, but also for their identity as a group member. The similar rhythmic and movement patterns allow each client to feel that they belong on a nonverbal level.

Thirdly, building off of the growing understanding of self vs. others, dance/movement therapy works to foster body awareness and nurture a client's personal self-concept. By reflecting a child's movement nonverbally and then translating what is seen into simple language (i.e., mirroring the child in moving their head side to side, while verbalizing "I see you moving your head"), the dance/movement therapist positively verbalizes how the child appears, inherently improving his/her body awareness or body image. The simple verbalizations, or the "noticing" of what is going on, also help to structure the experience for the participant (Loman, 1995). As an added benefit, this verbalization of action naturally increases the movement repertoire of the client (applicable to goal one), as he/she is exposed to not only the conscious experience of his/her own movement but also that of the others in the room.

"Body image is one of the most fundamental concepts in human growth and development and one that appears to be lacking in children who are autistic" (Erfer, 1995, p. 197). Standing behind this concept, body awareness and a positive body image are imperative as the two combined form a foundation for a basic understanding of the self. Not only does the development of body awareness parallel sensorimotor development, the movement experience also helps children to orient to their space, their own bodies, and the others in the room. This orientation occurs on both an internal (self to self) and external (self and others) level. Because body image is formed from input from the vestibular, kinesthetic, proprioceptive, visual, and tactile systems, movement is an all-encompassing medium for the development of an individual's self-concept (Erfer, 1995).

A 1985 research study conducted by Enid Wolf-Schein, Gene Fisch, and Ira Cohen studied the use of nonverbal systems in children with autism and mental retardation. The study came to the conclusion that "dance/movement therapy should be considered an intervention for persons with both autism and mental retardation since there are indications that deviations in nonverbal behaviors do contribute to the overall pathology of the individuals" (Wolf-Schein, Fisch & Cohen, 1985, p. 78). This serves as an example of one of many studies indicating the potential for healing when combining dance/movement therapy and autism.

In more recent years, neuroscientists have been increasingly interested in the presence and impact of mirror neurons on mental health and relationships. Regarding this research, Cynthia Berrol notes, "a keystone of the therapeutic process of dance/movement therapy, the concept of mirroring is now the subject of neuroscience. The domains of mirror neurons currently under investigation span motoric, psychosocial and cognitive functions, including specific psychological issues . . . " (Berrol, 2006, p. 303). Dance/movement therapy inherently engages this mirror neuron system in the brain, for both those moving and those witnessing the movement of others. Since autism possibly relates to deficiencies in the mirror neuron system of the brain, dance/movement therapy has the potential to unlock and develop some of these deficient areas through the process of movement.

Risks and side effects related to dance/movement therapy are minimal. Movement may not be the preferred modality for expressing or relating for all individuals, although many who are open to trying the format find that it is a truly accessible approach to therapy. Like with any kind of movement, a person must be cautious and only do what is safely within their physical means in order to avoid any physical harm to self or others, within the process.

The American Dance Therapy Association (ADTA) is the professional organization for dance/movement therapists in the U.S. and beyond. To learn more about the field or find a dance/movement therapist in your area, visit the website at www.adta.org or contact the national office by phone at (410) 997-4040.

THE DEVELOPMENTAL, INDIVIDUAL DIFFERENCE, RELATIONSHIP-BASED (DIR) MODEL

BY DR. GIL TIPPY

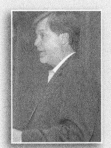

Gil Tippy, Psy.D.

DrGilTippy.Wordpress.com

Dr. Gil Tippy is the Clinical Director and one of the founders of the Rebecca School in Manhattan, a school for children with neurodevelopmental disorders of relating and communicating. Here he has been directly supervised by Stanley Greenspan, MD for the last four years. He is he Executive Director of the Center for Parents and Children in Sea Cliff, New York, a not-for-profit community center for children, both typically developing and those with neurodevelopmental disorders. He is the founder of Higher Standard Spectrum Services in Oyster Bay, New York, and has been a teacher, a supervisor of teachers, a psychologist, or all three at once, for the last thirty years. In every setting, and across the neurodevelopmental spectrum, Dr. Tippy works in the DIR model.

In this chapter I am going to talk about the Developmental, Individual difference, Relationship-based (DIR) model of intervention in ASD. You may find it a little bit easier to read than other chapters, maybe a little more friendly and personal, and that is deliberate. You should feel that I am in the room talking to you, trying to build a relationship, because, after all, this is a model that depends on the relationship between two people. So, let's start right here, in the relationship between you, the reader, and me, the writer of this chapter.

If I were going to design an intervention for autism spectrum disorders, or for anything else really, I would want to know what the core deficits of the disorder were. Seems sensible to me that you would want to attack the core deficits as directly as possible. You wouldn't address skin paleness for congestive heart failure, you would hope that paleness would take care of itself when you address the failing ability of the heart to pump the blood around the body. So, before I pick an intervention for ASD, I want to know what the core deficits are. Since I'm a Psychologist, I look to the Diagnostic and Statistical Manual of Psychiatric Disorders, the DSM-IV-TR. This is a big thick book that has every psychiatric condition listed in it, and the diagnostic criteria for each of these disorders. Psychologists use it to diagnose, and insurance companies use these criteria to pay, so it seems like a pretty solid authority.

The way the DSM works is that you have to have some symptoms from group one, some from group two, and some from group three, and so forth. If you have the right combo, then you get the diagnosis. I have picked the diagnostic criteria for autistic disorder, but I could just have easily picked the criteria for pervasive developmental disorder—NOS, or Asperger's disorder. Let's take a look at the criteria for autism.

You need, "A total of six (or more) items from (1), (2), and (3), with at least two from (1), and one each from (2) and (3)." The very first criteria listed is a "qualitative impairment in social interaction, as manifested by at least two of the following symptoms. The first symptom listed is, "(a) marked impairment in the use of multiple nonverbal behaviors such as eye-to-eye gaze, facial expression, body postures, and gestures to regulate *social interaction*." (Italics mine.) So, the very first criteria in the diagnostic manual is about social interaction. It's not about flapping or other stereotypic behaviors—it is about social interaction. Notice that they mention "eye-to-eye gaze" as a nonverbal behavior that may be missing in autism, but they put it in the context that the eye-gaze is not being used to regulate social interaction. Typically, human beings use their eyes to regulate the social space between them and the other person. If I were standing in front of you now, I could make eye contact with you, you would look back at me, and we would begin to have a social interaction. Nowhere does the DSM imply that kids with autism won't look at you, it says they don't use the eye-gaze to mediate the social space. So, the intervention you want is not to tell the kids, "Look at me. Good! Look at me!" and then reinforce it. The intervention you want should address the core deficit, the social interaction. By the way, you often see studies that say they prove some behavioral intervention works because they have improved eye-gaze. This is nonsense, because you can make anyone look at you, but it is an entirely different thing to help someone with ASD to use eye-gaze the way it is used typically between two people, to mediate the social interaction.

The next criteria is, "(b) failure to develop peer relationships appropriate to developmental level." So, the second symptom listed under part one is also about relationships. In this case the relationship is not adult to child, but peer relationships. If you want to address the core deficits, you want to address relationship and interaction.

The next symptom mentioned is "(c) a lack of spontaneous seeking to share enjoyment, interests, or achievements with other people (e.g., by a lack of showing, bringing, or pointing out objects of interest)." Kid, and adults typically do this. They say, "Hey, I have this cool thing that I'm interested in. Look. Do you see how cool this is? Do you like it too?" This is how kids typically interact, and this is how we all interact. "Did you see the game last night? What did you think?" Typical kids get there between two and six months of age, but kids on the spectrum may not be there yet, regardless of age. While other interventions may be able to get kids to look at things by pointing at them and then directing their eyes to them, it is quite a different thing to get them to share an interest with another, and consider the other's opinion. If your intervention does not address this, it is not attacking the core deficits of the spectrum disorders.

I could go on and on with the diagnostic criteria, but there isn't room in this chapter, and you would get bored. Let me just say that as you go deeper into the diagnostic criteria for autistic disorder in the DSM you want to make sure that your intervention addresses, " social interaction, peer relationships, seeking to share enjoyment, interests, or achievements with other people, social or emotional reciprocity, the ability to initiate or sustain a conversation with others," and a "lack of varied, spontaneous make-believe play or social imitative play appropriate to developmental level." All of these things are the core deficits of autism, and if your intervention does not take them as the direct target of your work, then you are not doing the most appropriate intervention. You may have evidence that your intervention correlates with some external behavior, but your evidence is not relevant. We, in the autism treatment community, would be better served if we changed the emphasis from "evidence-based practice," to "*relevant* evidence-based practice."

The "D" in DIR

DIR is a developmental model like all the developmental models you have studied in your high school, undergraduate, and graduate classes. Like Piaget or Gesell, it comes from the well-established tradition in psychology of looking at how humans develop, and how that development can go wrong. It is a stage model, like most developmental models, and while it allows for some movement up and down the developmental milestones, for the most part, one milestone builds on the one before it. So the "D" in DIR is for Developmental. The developmental milestones listed below are one version of the milestones first created by Stanley Greenspan, M.D., the creator of the DIR model, and later contributed to by many others, most prominently by his longtime collaborator Serena Wieder, Ph.D.

The Functional Emotional Developmental Milestones (FEDM)
1.   Staying calm and regulated, and shared attention
2.   Engagement and relatedness
3.   Basic intentional interaction and communication, five to ten circles of communication
4.   Problem solving, co-regulated interactions with a continuous flow
5.   Creative and meaningful use of ideas and words
6.   Building logical bridges between ideas
7.   Multi-causal, comparative thinking
8.   Grey area thinking
9.   Reflective thinking with a sense of self and internal standard

I drew a line after the first six milestones, because every kindergarten in this country assumes, and sadly most nursery schools now in our ill-conceived rush to "teach" kids, that you have reached FEDM 6 before you enter. If we can get our kids to the sixth level, they will do fine in school and life, and so we focus on these first six. In parenthesis at each level I will put when a neurotypical kid reaches the milestone, roughly.

Milestone I: Staying calm and regulated, and shared attention (zero to three months). This first level is where a newborn gets organized. No one sleeps in the house of a zero to three month old. But as their neurological systems begin to get organized they become calm and available. "Regulated" is a word we use a lot in DIR, and it means available to interact, neither too low nor too high. In working in the DIR model, you need kids be regulated so that you can work with them developmentally. If a kid is not regulated, you can't work on answering "why" questions, or work on shared social-problem solving, or anything else. It makes sense, you can't work on your taxes if you're furious at your partner for something, or if you are asleep. Kids can't work at higher developmental levels if they aren't regulated.

Milestone II: Engagement and relatedness (two to nine months). If a kid is calm and available, then we can work on engagement. To be engaged in the DIR sense means to be related to another, not engaged in some self-absorbed interest. We want kids to be engaged with us, we want to be the most fun and interesting thing in their world. Our goal at this level is to get kids hooked, and we will use that engagement and relatedness to build on the child's developmental milestones, within the relationship we are creating.

Milestone III: Basic intentional interaction and communication, five to ten circles of communication (four to nine months). When you offer some communication, and a child accepts your offer, that's a circle of communication. You open a circle verbally, gesturally, maybe with a glance, and you can close them up in just the same ways. It doesn't matter. This is the beginning of a real conversation, the opening and closing of circles, where I'm really thinking about you and you're really thinking about me. Since the core deficits of autism are all about social relationships, this is where the work on those core deficits begins to become apparent.

Milestone IV: Problem solving, co-regulated interactions with a continuous flow (nine to eighteen months). This, and the following, level is where the real action is in autism spectrum disorders and the DIR model. At this level, you need to be able to open and close sixty or more circles of communication, with you "crunching" what's in the kids head, the kid crunching what's in your head, in a continuous flow. You know when you are in a continuous flow; you will feel it. You know that feeling when you are talking with someone you met at a party, and you are on a topic you both like, and you feel heard, and time passes without you noticing; that's continuous flow. Conversely, if you are at the same party with a different person and the conversation lags, and you look for reasons to leave the interaction, "Oh, I have to go freshen my drink"; you are not in a continuous flow. This fluidity and connection is essential, as it lays the groundwork for the next level—the essential level where kids enter the world of abstraction.

Milestone V: Creative and meaningful use of ideas and words (eighteen to thirty months). In a word, abstraction! This is the level that you must get to if you are to enter a world where you don't have to use your memory to navigate the world. Kids on the spectrum have great memories, (a gross generalization, but follow me). They are using their memories to navigate the world, because they are not able to form symbols in their heads; they have not entered into the world of abstraction. Think about it. How many of you know kids on the spectrum who can tell you the arcane details of things that should not matter, such as what you wore the first time they met you, every word of a Disney movie, etc.? They are using their good memories to negotiate the world, because autism spectrum disorders are not disorders of memory! No intervention aimed at memory tasks is useful in attacking the core deficits: relating and communicating.

If you are operating out of your memory, you could do fairly well in school until second-and-a-half grade. At that point, the curriculum turns from memory tasks, to abstraction. In third grade you need to reflect on the reasons for things, and so kids with neurodevelopmental disorders of relating and communicating begin to fail. A developmental pediatrician who sees lots of kids on the spectrum came up to me after a talk and said, "I never realized before why so many of my referrals come at the beginning of third grade!" This is the level at which you can begin to answer emotionally meaningful "why" questions, and when you get there, you are off and running.

How you get to this level is the subject of many books, but Stanley Greenspan, M.D., and Serena Wieder, Ph.D. have written and published much about how to get to the abstract level. Dr. Wieder's work on fantasy play is particularly relevant, and is a lot of fun too.

Milestone VI: Building logical bridges between ideas (thirty to forty-eight months). At this level, you can take what the teacher is saying at the front of the class, think about it, add it to your thought, and put it back out as a new mix of your mutual ideas. You need to be able to do this to function in the typical classroom, and if you are not there, you will really struggle. This level is the result of strength developed at all the previous levels.

The "I" in DIR

"I" stands for Individual differences, and in DIR, individual differences in the way the kids process the world is key. That is why you will find so many occupational therapists who are conversant with the DIR model. The trans-disciplinary nature of the DIR model is one of its great strengths. Every one of us has differences in the way we process the world. I may like a loud rock concert; you may avoid loud places. Derek Jeter is able to quickly process visual stimuli, create a motor plan, and process feedback from his vestibular and proprioceptive system. This is how he is able make the play at first, even after a bad hop, whereas I would just get hit in the face by the ball. Differences in sensory systems are the norm, or else we would all be playing shortstop for the Yankees. If we allow that all of us have sensory processing differences, why wouldn't we allow that our kids do also? DIR pays particular attention to each child's sensory processing differ-ences. It is one of the most important features of the model, and it is one reason why this model succeeds where others fail. Imagine what it must be like for one student of mine who cannot process visual information with fluidity, so the world appears in flashes; cannot tell where her body is in relationship to gravity; cannot tell where her arms and legs are at any given time, or where the boundaries of her body are. Life for her must be like being thrown out of a plane, at night, in a thun-derstorm. How can you work on anything with this child if you don't address her sensory processing? The DIR model is particularly strong here, and it is a part of the model that the average person, and the average therapist, knows little about. I will leave descriptions of how to work on these systems to the volumes of writing that already exist about it, much of it in the occupational therapy literature.

The "R" in DIR

"R" stand for Relationship-based, and everything in the model is done in the context of a human relationship. This is how human beings evolved, how human beings have treated their children since they first stood up, and is currently backed with good neuroscience. Humans develop in the context of a relationship, first with mom, as they harness her executive functioning during the first three months of life (look back at FEDM I), and then in their surrounding human community. In this model, everyone needs to think about personal variables they bring to the relationship with the child. They need to think whether they like one emotional state over another one, whether they like boisterous play more than quiet, or vice versa, and whether what is going on in their lives is impacting their relationship in the moment. This model is difficult on practitioners and families alike, as there is no technology, no beeping machine, no screen, no clipboard or data sheet, between you and the child. You are the toy, you are the most important thing in the intervention, and it pulls a lot out of you. However, it is the Relation-ship in the DIR model that makes it the most effective, most rewarding, and most evidence-based of all the interventions. It is based upon the evidence of at least ten thousand years of documented human history. Kids develop in relationships, this is a disorder of relating and communicating, and so there is really only one sensible, evidence-based way to go.

A Note on Floortime

Floortime is the play-based intervention in the DIR model, and people often use DIR, Floortime, and the Greenspan Model interchangeably to talk about the process. I have outlined my own understanding of the DIR model above, and as you can see, it is much more than Floortime. Floortime is play with a purpose. When you are playing with a child in this model, you need to keep the FEDM in mind. Is the child calm and available? If not, you work to get him regulated. If he is, you look to see if you can get him engaged. You work hard at it, around his interests, which you work hard to understand. If he is engaged solidly, you look to see if he is able to open and close circles with you, and if he can, you work toward continuous flow at level IV. This is simplistic I know, but I hope you get the idea that the Floortime, the play in DIR, is play with a purpose, and that you will need to keep in mind where the child is developmentally, where he is in terms of his sensory system and where he is in terms of joy.

This intervention needs to be fun and meaningful. If you find yourself generating all the ideas, you are on the wrong track. If it feels like you are dragging the kid, you are on the wrong track. Affect is your greatest friend, your greatest ally, and you need to harness it. Dr. Greenspan just gave a great lecture on exactly this subject, and you can access that through DIR's governing body, The Interdisciplinary Counsel on Developmental and Learning Disorders (ICDL). Their website provides all the appropriate links, and is the real authority on the intervention.

Have fun, be child-centered, be curious, and you will be on the right track.

DIETARY INTERVENTIONS FOR AUTISM

BY KARYN SEROUSSI AND LISA LEWIS, PH.D.

Adapted from the book, *The Encyclopedia of Dietary Interventions for the Treatment of Autism and Related Disorders* (2008)
by Karyn Seroussi & Lisa S. Lewis, Ph.D. (available at www.sarpsborgpress.com)

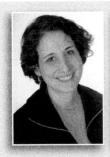
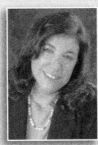

Karyn Seroussi and Lisa S. Lewis, Ph.D.

The Autism Network for
Dietary Interventions: www.autismndi.
com
The Encyclopedia of Dietary Interventions for the Treatment of Autism and Related Disorders: www.sarpsborgpress.com

Karyn Seroussi is the author of *Unraveling the Mystery of Autism and Pervasive Developmental Disorder*, the story of her son's autism recovery through dietary and other biomedical interventions. Lisa S. Lewis, Ph.D. is the author of *Special Diets For Special Kids, I & II*, the foremost books on gluten- and casein-free diets for children with disabilities. In 1995, Karyn Seroussi and Lisa Lewis created an international parent network that has educated thousands about dietary and biomedical interventions for autism spectrum disorders. Thirteen years, three books, countless conferences, and over fifty thousand emails later, they decided to put it all together. In 2008, they gathered the sum of that knowledge and co-authored *The Encyclopedia of Dietary Interventions for the Treatment of Autism and Related Disorders* (www.sarpsborgpress.com).

*P*lease *be advised that we are not giving medical advice. We have gathered this information so that you can make an informed decision in partnership with your medical practitioner. All changes to your child's diet should be done under the care of a qualified nutritionist or medical professional.*

Dietary intervention is quickly losing its status as an "alternative" therapy for autistic disorders. It is supported by several peer-reviewed studies, thousands of documented case studies, and a number of new, well-funded research projects.

But why would autistic patients need special diets?

Dr. Derrick MacFabe and his colleagues at the University of Western Ontario concluded that certain gut and dietary factors may worsen symptoms in autism spectrum disorders, epilepsy, and some inheritable metabolic disorders.[1]

Research by Dr. H. Jyonouchi of the Autism Center at the New Jersey Medical School found that, relative to a control group, children on the autism spectrum have an abnormal immune response to cow's milk protein, wheat protein and soy protein. The reaction in the autistic population was strongest to milk; in many cases, the reaction to soy was even more pronounced than the reaction to wheat.[2,3,4]

Dr. Kalle Reichelt at the University of Oslo/Rikshospitalet found opioid peptides derived from food proteins (exorphins) in urine of autistic patients.[5] These peptides, primarily casomorphin and gluteomorphin (gliadorphin), are close enough in structure to drugs in the morphine class that they have been long suspected of causing some of the more inexplicable symptoms of autism, such as self-absorption, self-stimulatory behaviors, sensory disturbances, bowel irregularities, and insensitivity to pain.

Dr. Timothy Buie, a pediatric gastroenterologist at Harvard/Mass. General Hospital, has performed over four hundred gastrointestinal endoscopies with biopsies on autistic children. In a preliminary study in 2002, he noted the frequent presence of chronic inflammation of the digestive tract, including esophagitis, gastritis, and enterocolitis. He found that 55 percent of the autistic children he examined showed disaccharide/glucoamylase, lactase, and sucrase enzyme levels below normal. These children were thus far more likely to suffer from impaired starch metabolism, carbohydrate malabsorption, and undiagnosed bowel disorders than their neurotypical peers. He concluded that more than 50 percent of autistic children appear to have symptoms of gastrointestinal illness, including abdominal pain, gas, bloating, and chronic diarrhea or loose stools, food allergies, and maldigestion or malabsorption issues.[1] This helps to explain why so many well-fed autistic children, upon medical examination, are sometimes found to be severely deficient in several essential vitamins and minerals.

Regardless of the complex cause, or causes, of these food intolerances, the outcome is simple. When you put these children on special diets, many of them will improve, sometimes dramatically. Dr. Ted Kniker of the Autistic Treatment Center in San Antonio, Texas, Dr. Ann-Mari Knivsberg at the University of Stavanger in Norway, Dr. Sandra Lucarelli at the University of Rome, Italy, and other researchers around the world have published studies demonstrating that some children and adults with autism show improvement after elimination of dairy products and wheat gluten from their diets.[2,3,4,5]

Unfortunately, autistic children are rarely tested for gastrointestinal illnesses, even when they present with symptoms that would raise alarm bells if seen in a typical child. Unusual test results may be disregarded, possibly because there already is a diagnosis: *autism*. Sometimes it is difficult, even for physicians, to remember that children with autism are also children. They may suffer silently from diseases or disorders that may, or may not, be related to their "primary complaint."

Some high-functioning people on the autism spectrum attest to the fact that dietary restriction relieves a great deal of pain or physical discomfort, as well as the "noise" that makes it hard for them to learn and to perform socially. It is impossible to judge the level of silent suffering that is going on in the autism population as a whole, because so many of these children cannot tell us how they feel. However, those of us who have experienced severe diarrhea, constipation, or intestinal disease will greatly sympathize with those in this group who are known or suspected to have these problems, and cannot express their pain to their caregivers.

Children with autism as a group have notoriously poor nutrition coupled with vitamin and mineral deficiencies. This may be due, in part, to extreme eating habits (they are notoriously picky). Deficiencies are also likely due to the above-mentioned tendency toward malabsorption. This is why physicians who specialize in the biomedical treatment of autism start out by addressing malabsorption issues, adding digestive enzymes to the diet, eliminating problematic foods (usually including gluten and casein), stabilizing the condition of the gastrointestinal tract by removing allergens and harmful organisms, and introducing nutrients not being properly absorbed and utilized by the body. This approach has resulted in significant improvement in cognitive function, and in some cases, a full recovery from many of the symptoms of autism, if not the underlying disorder.

Priorities

- There can be no "one size fits all" approach to treating autistic patients because there is no intervention that will make them all better. But here are some of the most common treatment priorities on the medical checklist:
- Improve the quality of the diet, reducing sugars, additives, and environmental pesticides and impurities
- Remove gluten, casein, and other proteins that likely cause physical and behavioral symptoms and/or distress

- Identify and address any food allergies and intolerances
- Identify and correct deficiencies or poor utilization of nutrients with vitamin/mineral supplements, such as vitamin B6 plus magnesium, glutathione, selenium, zinc, essential fatty acids, and amino acids
- Check for signs of gastrointestinal distress, and investigate and treat any illness
- Use antifungal and/or antibacterial medications, in conjunction with probiotics to correct gut dysbiosis
- Depending on test results, other recommendations might include digestive enzyme tablets, melatonin, thyroid medication, sulfation support, heavy metal detoxification, and immune system regulation.[6]
- This approach can be challenging for parents. Changes in diet and supplementation are not usually expensive, but can be hard to implement. There are no guarantees, but thousands of parents will tell you that it is worth the effort. Changes in behavior, improvements in bowel function, increased language, and decreased self-stimulation are common responses to biomedical interventions.

A Single Step

Dietary intervention often begins the moment that the first glass of potato, nut, or rice milk is poured. However, we all know that it actually begins earlier, when parents or caregivers make a commitment, sometimes against great odds, to give biomedical interventions a try. Changing diet may change your life, but then, so will autism and related illnesses. With any luck, you'll end up with a healthier lifestyle and a well-functioning child.

Most newcomers fear that dietary intervention will be an uphill battle. However, the ground does level off much sooner than you might expect. The diet will get much, much easier, and once improvement is evident, the support you receive from those around you—including spouses, doctors, and educators—will also increase.

One should never make an important decision without having as much information as possible, and an informed decision cannot be properly made without a good trial. Some children will respond quickly and noticeably within days, but many will take longer. Give dietary intervention a good chance before making up your mind that it will or won't help your child.

The "Three Stages" of Dietary Intervention

It is always less daunting to attempt a complicated task if it has been broken down into manageable stages. The following three stages will remove the mystery and difficulty of starting dietary intervention.

Stage 1: Getting Started

Identify the Pre-Diet Diet: Make a list of all the foods your child likes and eats. What do they have in common? Perhaps they are all starchy, sweet, salty, dairy-based, or wheat-based. Perhaps they are all the same types of foods. A child eating ice cream, bananas, grapes, chocolate pudding, sweetened yogurt, apple juice, and ketchup is not eating a varied diet—he is eating milk and sugar. A child who only eats bagels, crackers, cereal, pretzels, and waffles is not eating a varied diet; he is mostly eating one food: wheat. Foods that are craved are highly suspect, especially dairy- and wheat-based foods. Next, make a list of your child's physical symptoms. Does he get rashes? Does he get red cheeks or red ears after meals? Is his stomach bloated? Does he have diarrhea or constipation? Is he insensitive to pain? Note how these symptoms are associated with food, for example, does your child get red cheeks shortly after eating a particular food? Are bowel problems associated with any particular types of food? Are his behaviors worse at certain times of day, before or after meals?

> *"It's hard work, as you know better than we do. But when you see the results, it's truly incredible. And to think, our pediatrician scoffed at the idea, saying, 'that diet doesn't do a thing.'"—Garth Stein*

Since you are going to further limit the diet of a child who may already be on a limited diet, begin giving a multivitamin and mineral formula that is both low allergen and free of gluten and casein (common additives in vitamins). There are several available that are appropriate for children with autism made by specializing companies.

If possible, ask your pediatrician to do a blood test for celiac disease (CD) *before* removing gluten. To be thorough, they should check total IgA, gliadin IgA, and IgG, and tissue transglutaminase IgA. It is likely to come back negative, since the blood test for CD is targeting only one specific type of gluten allergy.

Commit to a three-month trial of dietary intervention. Join an online support group such as the one at www.gfcfdiet.com. Choose a date, planning a day or two's meals at a time.

Start a food diary—this will turn out to be an important tool and should not be overlooked. Get a spiral pad or notebook, and list each food your child eats on the left side of the page. On the right side of the page, list any changes you observe. Make a note of things like aggression, crying, whining, red ears, itchiness, bowel changes, or sleep problems.

Your food diary will help you see patterns, e.g. if your child has a delayed reaction to a food. This can help you determine why your child is experiencing a rollercoaster of good and bad days. You can also use your diary to note the impact of soy, corn, eggs, nuts, starches, citrus, fruits, sugars, and brightly colored foods; these foods are often poorly tolerated.

Remove all dairy products from the diet, and within a week or two, all gluten. Using sugars, rice, potatoes, and other starchy foods to achieve this transition may be necessary, but keep in mind that they will probably need to be reduced or even removed later on. A sugar and starch-based diet has shown to be problematic for many of our children, such as those with abnormal gut pathologies and/or immune abnormalities. Consider removing soy and corn at the same time gluten is removed. Many parents have given up on the gluten-free diet because they saw no change or a regression in their children, after having substituted soy for milk or corn for gluten. These two foods are almost universally problematic when starting the diet. They can always be added back later on a trial basis.

It is common to see crankiness, regression, or withdrawal symptoms during these first few days. Stay the course, and let your child know that you mean business.

Keep it Simple: Instead of providing homemade or commercially available chicken nuggets, teach your children to eat plain chicken that has been baked or broiled. Cut the chicken into child-friendly strips and serve with a simple dipping sauce that you can make from scratch quickly and cheaply. Teach your children to eat fruits and vegetables that are raw or gently steamed, again, using a simple sauce at first if they won't even try them plain, or blending them into pasta sauce or soup.

Find the recipes that work for you, create shortcuts so that they can be made in a snap, make large batches, and freeze portions for later use.

Time and Money: Some parents worry that dietary intervention will be very expensive, and worry that it won't be worth the trouble and expense. It is true that if you rely on convenience foods like frozen waffles, dietary changes will cost more than buying "regular" food. Although many parents are short on time and energy, making these from scratch is easy and inexpensive. For those who are accustomed to using lots of prepackaged snack foods and baked goods, and who try to replace these with store-bought alternatives, dietary changes will be relatively costly and will probably contain more starches than is generally optimal. For those who are willing to learn to follow some simple recipes at home, dietary intervention shouldn't increase your family's food bill by very much. In fact, it may save you quite a bit of money, since you are far more likely to pack healthy, safe foods before leaving the house, and far less likely to grab a meal at a fast-food restaurant.

Get support: Compile a few articles on diet that you can give family members, teachers, and other caregivers. Tell them what you are doing, and why. Ask for their support.

Stage 2: Testing and Record Keeping

After the diet is underway, some simple testing could yield some good results. An IgG multiple food allergy ELISA (enzyme-linked immunosorbent assay) panel could provide a guideline for other foods that may be causing inflammation, and a blood or skin test could identify "regular" IgE-mediated food and environmental allergies. An organic acids test can check for yeast and bacteria, and metabolic abnormalities. Ask your doctor to do a stool test to check for parasites, since this has proven to be a surprisingly common problem. If indicated, treat the child with antifungal or antibacterial medication, and remove any offending foods. *Remember: Just because the child does not test positive for wheat and dairy allergy does not mean that these foods are tolerated.* Only re-introduction of the foods can give you that answer, but try not to do a deliberate challenge at this stage. It is important to give the diet a fair trial first.

When your child appears to be stabilized after the initial withdrawal, introduce bottled probiotics and/or probiotic foods.

Stage 3: Evaluating the Response

After your child has been on the diet for a few weeks, you should have a good idea of whether or not it will be an important tool in your fight. If there has been improvement, you will want to continue. Although it may seem paradoxical, you will also want to continue if your child's behavioral or physical symptoms have worsened. A regression is very common when offending foods are removed from the diet, and generally indicates that the child will benefit from dietary intervention. If you see no change at all after several weeks or months, it is possible that diet will not be a significant intervention for your child. After your child has stabilized, you may want to tweak the diet he is on, or go further, exploring some of the "advanced" dietary interventions. Detailed information about all of these approaches can be found in *The Encyclopedia of Dietary Interventions for the Treatment of Autism and Related Disorders* by Karyn Seroussi and Lisa S. Lewis, Ph.D.

What To Expect, When to Move On

Most of the overall gains seen in children using these diets are in improved health and GI (gastrointestinal) function, and in cognitive and learning abilities. Some will begin to experience normal feelings of hunger or fullness. Some will begin to react normally to pain, or respond to the feeling of having to use the bathroom.

Sometimes changing the diet can lead to striking results within a short period of time. Younger children who are drinking large quantities of milk or eating primarily dairy or wheat-based foods may exhibit changes within a week. But for most, the change won't be apparent until a few weeks later—often after accidental ingestion, when there is a noticeable regression. You may notice changes within a few days, but if not, be patient.

Keep in mind that if a regression lasts more than three weeks, it may be the result of an increased quantity of an unknown allergen (for example, when corn is heavily substituted for wheat, or dairy is replaced by soy). If you need to rely heavily on starchy foods just to get your child off gluten and casein, a yeast overgrowth may have occurred or been made worse (another reason to keep it simple). For some children, it may be necessary to simultaneously remove other foods, especially soy, corn, and even rice. Some children will require the elimination of all complex carbohydrates and others will need to reduce oxalates (see *Encyclopedia*).

For children who do not show immediate or rapid improvement, it is tempting to slip or go back to the old diet entirely. In most cases, this is a mistake, especially for the children who self-limited their diets or had bowel problems. Although this subgroup is not the only one to benefit from dietary intervention, it describes children who ultimately respond well. Frequently, children with bowel problems are sicker than they appear, and dietary changes, while necessary, are just the tip of the iceberg.

Often parents who report no improvement have not really eliminated all the sources of gluten or casein from the diet. There are many hidden sources; for example, most cheese substitutes contain some form of casein. It can even be found in tuna fish and other canned foods. Many wheat-free cereals contain malt (from barley) and thus are not gluten free. Chewing gum, stickers, play clay—all of these can be sources of gluten and casein. In short, you need to be a detective and investigate everything that goes into your child's mouth. Remember that, especially with small children, nonfood items often end up there too. Just a trace can make a world of difference in your results.

Parents who have given dietary intervention a trial of at least three months, and who are certain that no hidden ingredients have been missed, may reasonably consider that food is not affecting their children. For those whose children's autism is not coming from these foods, do not give up your search for answers. Test immune function, look at issues like yeast and bacteria in the gut, and look into some of the other treatments that have proved useful to Defeat Autism Now! and other experienced and qualified professionals. There are some safe, inexpensive treatments that seem to be helping many autistic children for reasons that are only beginning to be understood. Remember, autistic behaviors are not a disease; they are a symptom, and there is no such thing as a symptom without a cause.

Different Approaches: "The Diets"

As stated above, some of the children who improve on a basic gluten- and casein-free diet still have a long way to go. The underlying problems in autism spectrum disorders usually have many layers. Opioid peptides from dairy and gluten may be just part of what is affecting your child. You may not see much improvement until all of the offenders have been addressed.

The Two-Tack Rule:
If you are sitting on a tack, it will take a lot of aspirin to make you feel better. If you are sitting on two tacks, removal of one tack will not result in a 50% improvement.
>—Dr. Sidney M. Baker, Defeat Autism Now! Co-founder; Author,
>Detoxification & Healing

What to Remove?

Dietary intervention in autism is usually referred to as "the GF/CF diet," but most children seem to need modifications that go well beyond gluten and casein free regimens. It is not unusual to hear a parent in the online support groups say that their child is on a "GF/CF/soy-free/corn-free/egg-free low-oxalate diet, with probiotic foods and limited sugars."

Therefore, it's no wonder that people have begun to refer to most of these dietary interventions simply as "GF/CF diets" or "gluten-free and restricted diets." As public awareness of celiac disease and gluten intolerance increases, this is probably the easiest explanation one can give.

There is much conflicting information on the Internet and on various support lists about which diets are "best." When one child does extremely well on a specific regimen, caregivers may become convinced that his diet will work just as well for other children, sometimes to the point of fanaticism. This can serve to inspire others, but it can also result in pressing for inappropriate adherence to one regimen when another might actually be more suitable.

Experience has shown that most people on the autism spectrum will benefit from a diet that is strictly free of gluten and dairy; therefore, the removal of these should be considered the foundation for dietary interventions. Additional changes are almost always needed for optimum improvement, but one size does not fit all. Every parent's goal is to find the ideal removal or rotation of foods for their child that will provide maximum benefit without being unnecessarily restrictive.

The most commonly restricted foods include gluten, dairy, corn, soy, yeast, oxalates, sugars, and starches. Other principles may apply, such as the use of probiotic foods, healthy fats, organic foods, and the restriction of food additives and artificial colors.

The most common dietary principles currently in use come from the Specific Carbohydrate Diet, developed by Elaine Gottschall, the low-oxalate diet introduced to the autism community by Susan Owens, and the Body Ecology Diet, developed by Donna Gates. None of these diets were originally developed to address autism spectrum disorders, so they usually must be modified to suit a child's individual needs. Detailed descriptions can be found in the *Encyclopedia of Dietary Interventions* by Karyn Seroussi and Lisa S. Lewis, Ph.D.

Gluten

Gluten is a protein found in members of the grass family including wheat, spelt, barley, rye and triticale. Gluten can also be found in products derived from these grains, such as malt, grain starches, hydrolyzed vegetable/plant proteins, textured vegetable proteins, soy sauce, grain alcohol, some natural flavorings, and some of the binders and fillers commonly found in vitamins and medications (see below). In their pure form oats do not contain gluten, but commercial oats are almost always contaminated with wheat.

Avoiding Gluten: This can be a challenge for two reasons. One is that it takes some time to become familiar with the rules of the diet and the lifestyle changes that are involved. The other problem has to do with getting your child on board; many children with autism will eat only wheat-based foods, such as bread, muffins, pretzels, crackers, noodles, and breaded chicken or fish (nuggets and fish sticks). At first, it may be hard to persuade a child to try anything new.

However, most people get the hang of the diet in a week or two, and many good substitutes are now available for traditional wheat products. There are commercially available gluten-free breads at many supermarkets and at all health food stores. Crackers without wheat or gluten are also widely available, made from grains, rice, and even nuts. If your child likes pasta, there are many excellent gluten-free alternatives; they come in different shapes and sizes and can be used in any recipe. Gluten-free baking, once you get the hang of it, is an economical way to prepare your family's favorite baked goods at home.

It is a good idea to accustom your child to meat, fish, and chicken prepared simply, either baked, broiled, or grilled. However, many children start the diet eating only breaded, fried "nuggets." You can prepare these by making your own breading out of acceptable cereals, flours, or ground nuts. Most commercially prepared and fast-food versions are unacceptable.

Be aware that ingredients change in prepared foods, and that what was acceptable six months ago may not be so anymore. It is a good idea to learn to read labels, and to call companies for information whenever you are unsure about an ingredient or food.

When you are avoiding gluten, it is important to know about "hidden" sources. For example, most of these diets allow coconut and dried fruits, but some brands contain traces of gluten. Look for fruits that have no sulfites (added to preserve color and retard spoilage), especially if phenols are a problem. Be aware that raisins sold in canisters may have traveled down a conveyor belt that was dusted with flour to prevent the fruit from sticking together. Because the flour is not an "ingredient" it does not have to be listed on the package.

Many foods are labeled "wheat free," but that does not mean they are gluten free. When in doubt, call the manufacturer. Almost all packaged foods have a toll-free number or website on the label. Find out whether they can guarantee that the product is free from gluten. If it's not, make sure to let them know that this will affect your decision to use the product.

"Hidden" gluten can also be found in some unexpected places, such as the glue on envelopes, Dixie cups, ground spices (some use flour to prevent clumping), appliances, fast-food fryers, and tropical fish food.

Foods and Ingredients That Always Contain Gluten:

Barley	Bleached Flour	Brown Flour
Barley Grass	Bran	Bulgur (Bulgar
(can contain seeds)	Bran Extract	Wheat/Nuts)
Barley Malt	Bread Flour	Bulgur Wheat
Beer	Brewers Yeast	Cereal Binding

Chilton	Hydrolyzed Wheat	Spirits (Specific Types)
Club Wheat	Starch	Sprouted Wheat or
Common Wheat	Kamut	Barley
Couscous	Malt	Hydrolyzed Wheat
Dextrimaltose	Malt Extract	Protein
Durum wheat	Malt Flavoring	Strong Flour
Edible Starch	Malt Syrup	Suet in Packets
Einkorn	Malt Vinegar	Tabbouleh
Emmer	Matzo Semolina	Teriyaki Sauce
Farina	Mir	Textured Vegetable
Farina Graham	Pasta	Protein - TVP
Filler	Pearl Barley	Triticale
Flour	Rice Malt (if barley or	Udon
Fu	Koji are used)	Unbleached Flour
Germ	Rye	Vegetable Starch
Graham Flour	Seitan	Wheat Flour Lipids
Granary Flour	Semolina	Wheat Germ
Groats	Semolina Triticum	Wheat Grass (can
Hydrolyzed Wheat	Shot Wheat (*Triticum*	contain seeds)
Gluten	*aestivum*)	Wheat Nuts
Hydrolyzed Wheat	Small Spelt	Wheat Protein
Protein	Spelt (*Triticum spelta*)	Whole-Meal Flour

Milk and Dairy

Milk consists of 87.4 percent water, 3.5 percent protein, and between zero and 3.7 percent fat. We all grew up with the idea that milk is a healthy food, and are naturally reluctant to take it out of our children's diets. But is it really good for everybody?

All mammal mothers feed their infants milk, but humans are the only mammal that ingests the milk of an unrelated species, and continues to do so long after weaning. This may be why dairy is one of the eight foods to which those with food allergies most frequently react.[1]

Although most American children get their required calcium and vitamin D from milk, there are many other sources for these vital nutrients. Therefore, pediatricians who insist that milk is necessary for good health are misinformed. Many perfectly healthy children do very well without it. In fact, many cultures consider cow's milk unfit for human consumption. Cows have evolved to produce milk that is most beneficial to its intended recipients: calves. The milk of every type of mammal has striking differences in composition, with variation in the contents of fats, protein, sugar, and minerals. Each evolves to provide optimum nutrition to the young of its own species.

Although milk is rich in calcium, it may not be the best way to obtain this mineral. Cow's milk contains 1200 mg of calcium per quart, compared to 300 mg per quart of human milk. Despite this difference, studies have shown that nursing infants absorb more calcium than those fed cow's milk-based formulas.[2] This seems to be due to the fact that cow's milk is much richer in phosphorus, a mineral that can combine with calcium in the intestines and prevent its absorption. (This is another reason to avoid drinking soda pop, which is extremely high in phosphorus.) Finally, research has shown that cow's milk protein intolerance (CMPI) is associated with a very high frequency of multiple food intolerance and allergic diseases.[3]

We all know that growing bones and teeth need calcium, but most of us have no idea where else to get these important minerals. Green vegetables such as kale, collards, and bok choy are excellent sources of calcium, with the added benefit of being low in oxalates (spinach, though high in calcium, should be avoided if oxalates are a problem). Certain fish, like salmon and perch, are also good sources of calcium, but take care to buy fish that is not high in mercury or other environmental toxins. A mere tablespoon of molasses contains 172 mg of calcium (as well as iron), so if yeast is not a big problem it is a good choice for sweetening baked goods. Some nuts, beans, and seeds (like sesame seeds) are rich in calcium, but they should be ground for best absorption. Calcium-fortified orange juice is equivalent to a glass of milk, although it is very high in fructose (fruit sugar). Finally, if a child will not eat enough nondairy sources of calcium, there are many good supplements available. Because vitamin D is required to properly absorb calcium, a good supplement will contain both.

With all these problems, why would anyone want to feed their children dairy products? First, it is hard to fight back years of thinking that milk is "the perfect food." The necessity of milk is perpetuated by every advertising medium currently in use, so it is certainly understandable that most parents believe that it is their duty to feed their children as much cow's milk as possible. Despite all the celebrities who sport "milk mustaches," dairy is not necessary for good nutrition, and can actually be harmful for some children.

How to Avoid Dairy: Removing dairy from the diet is not as difficult as it sounds, but you need to understand a few basic principles. First of all, you must remove *all* sources of dairy. This includes obvious sources such as butter, cheese, cream cheese, and sour cream, but it also includes some "hidden" sources. There are several packaged foods that surprisingly contain some form of milk protein, such as canned fish and bread. Even soy and rice cheeses generally contain some form of casein or sodium caseinate. It is imperative that you learn to read and understand labels, and that you continue to check them each time you buy a food. Food manufacturers often switch out ingredients due to price or availability, so a once-trusted item must be considered suspect until you have double-checked the ingredients. In many cases, food manufacturers are allowed to use up old food labels even if minor changes have been made in the ingredients. If you think you see a reaction to a food that formerly produced no problem, call the company to verify that the ingredients listed are indeed correct. If not, you can inform them that you will no longer be able to use the product, and that you will be sharing this information with others who have the same dietary requirements. Customer feedback will sometimes persuade them to revert to an older recipe.

Foods to Avoid (always contain dairy):

Butter	Casein/caseinates
Cheese (all types)	Lactose
Skim milk	Milk chocolate
Whole milk	Yogurt
Buttermilk	Kefin
Powered milk	Ice cream/ice milk
Evaporated milk	Cream
Condensed milk	Sour cream
Goat's milk	Cottage cheese
Sheep's milk	Whey

Foods to Be Wary Of (often contain dairy):

Baked goods (even if GF)	Chicken broth
Bologna	Creamed vegetables
Broth (canned)	Margarine/buttery spreads
Candy	Mashed potatoes
Canned foods	Nougat/caramel/toffee
Salad dressings	Pudding/custard mixes
Candies	Scrambled eggs
Cakes/cake mix	Soy cheese
Chewing gum	Tuna fish (canned)

Keep in mind that "non-dairy" does not mean milk-free. It is a term the dairy industry invented to indicate less than 0.5 percent milk by weight, which could mean fully as much casein as whole milk.

SUPPORT GROUPS

If you are new to dietary interventions, you will find it to be a valuable use of your time to join a support group. There may be one in your area, but if not, there are some wonderful groups online. Those who have never been on an online support group will be amazed at how quickly their questions can be answered, and at the quality of support they can get from others who are more experienced. Just remember, every child is different, and what worked for your child may not work for all.

Some of the most popular autism-diet groups include:

Gluten-Free/Casein-Free Diet (GF/CF):

www.yahoogroups.com/group/gfcfkids

The Specific Carbohydrate Diet (SCD):

www.yahoogroups.com/group/pecanbread

The Low Oxalate Diet (LOD):

www.yahoogroups.com/group/Trying_Low_Oxalates

The Feingold Diet: www.yahoogroups.com/group/Feingold-Program4us

The Body Ecology Diet: www.bedrokcommunity.org

DRAMA THERAPY

BY SALLY BAILEY

Sally Bailey, MFA, MSW, RDT/BCT

129 Nichols—CSTD Department
Kansas State University
Manhattan, KS 66506-2301
(785) 532-6780
sdbailey@ksu.edu
www.dramatherapycentral.com

Sally Bailey is an associate professor in the Theatre Department at Kansas State University where she directs the drama therapy program. She is the author of three books: *Wings to Fly: Bringing Theatre Arts to Students with Special Needs, Dreams to Sign: Bringing Together Deaf and Hearing Audiences and Actors,* and *Barrier-Free Drama.* She has worked with clients on the autism spectrum using drama therapy for the past twenty-five years. Her chapter on "Theoretical Reasons and Practical Applications of Drama Therapy with Clients of the Autism Spectrum" was recently published in *The Use of the Creative Therapies with Autism Spectrum Disorders.* She is a past president of the National Association for Drama Therapy and recipient of NADT's Gertrud Schattner Award for distinguished contributions in the field of drama therapy.

Drama therapy applies techniques from theatre to the process of psychotherapy. The focus is on helping individuals grow and heal by taking on and practicing new roles, creating new stories through action, and rehearsing new behaviors which can later be implemented in real life. Drama therapy involves participants in informal drama processes (games, improvisation, storytelling, role play) and/or formal products (puppets, masks, plays/performances) to help clients understand their thoughts and emotions better, improve behavior, and learn social interaction skills.

Drama therapy is effective because it involves action methods which can be rehearsed or repeated until a skill is learned. An embodied, concrete experience makes skills easier for clients on the autism spectrum to grasp, remember, and implement (Bailey, 2007, 2009b). While literature on autism suggests that people with ASD are not creative and have little interest in connecting with others, drama therapists find that the ASD clients they work with are imaginative, highly motivated to participate in dramatic activities, and crave social connection, but are not sure how to make those connections. Drama therapy helps in this connection process as drama is all about human relating and relationships.

Neuroscientists looking at the arts, learning, and the brain have discovered that the arts are motivating for children because they create conditions in which attention can be sustained over longer periods of time (Posner, Rothbart, Sheese, & Kieras in Ashbury & Rich, 2008). An additional benefit of the arts, particularly drama, is that participants receive feedback in the process of enacting a scene from the other actors, and from the audience, as well as afterwards when the group discusses the scene and/or when they replay the scene with corrections (Bailey, 2009a; Jensen & Dabney, 2000; Posner et al., 2008).

Temple Grandin (2002), a professor of animal science who has autism, says when she was growing up, she viewed many cultural customs and behaviors of neurotypical people as ISPs—Interesting Sociological Phenomenons. Role play can be the perfect way for people with ASD to come to a better understanding of the neurotypical world's ISPs. Practicing putting themselves in another person's or character's shoes can become the first steps toward understanding how the rest of the world feels, thinks, and relates; a way to begin developing and testing out a theory of mind.

Drama strongly engages the mirror neuron system in actors and audiences alike (Blair, 2008; McConachie, 2008). There are neuroscientists who suspect that autism may relate to deficiencies in the mirror neuron system (Ramachandran & Oberman, 2006) and others who believe that our empathic abilities and our abilities to learn cognitively and emotionally through observation relate directly to our mirror neurons (Iacoboni & Daprette, 2006; Iacoboni, et al., 2005; Oberman & Ramachandran, 2007). If this is true, then drama therapy could be extremely effective in promoting repair of weaknesses and disconnections in the mirror neuron system.

Drama therapy has been developed by a wide variety of practitioners. Most trained originally in theatre, then after recognizing the healing powers of drama, trained in psychology and psychotherapy. Early 20th century: Jacob L. Moreno in Austria and the U.S.; Peter Slade in the U.K.; Vladimir Iljine and Nikolai Evreinov in Russia. Late 20th century: Gertrud Schattner, Eleanor Irwin, David Read Johnson, Renee Emunah, and Robert Landy in the U.S.; Sue Jennings and Marian Lindkvist in the U.K. (Bailey, 2006).

Beginning in the early 20th century, drama was used by occupational thera-pists in hospitals and by social workers in community programs to teach clients social and emotional skills through performing in plays. The field began to inte-grate improvisation and process drama methods, emerging as a separate pro-fession in the 1970s. In relation to treatment of clients on the autism spectrum, drama was one of the very first techniques used. Hans Asperger, the German doctor who first described Asperger's syndrome in 1944, created an educational program for the boys he was treating which involved speech therapy, drama, and physical education (Attwood, 1998). Sister Viktorine, director of the program, was killed when the ward on which she was working was destroyed in an allied bombing attack in World War II, so no record of exactly how she used drama survives (Attwood, 1998). At the very least, this early use of drama indicates an appreciation for the strengths it offers as an intervention. Currently, many drama therapists across the U.S. and internationally are involved in the use of drama therapy with children, teens, and adults on the autism spectrum.

Success rate

Grady Bolding (2007), a drama major at Kansas State University who is on the autism spectrum, says about his experience in theatre, "The world of theater helped bring me out of my shell, since I got free crash courses in interpersonal communications with every script. Today, I speak like anybody else" (Bolding, 2007, p. 3). He reports that his theater training has helped him learn how to make eye contact, show emotional expression during conversations, and read the emo-tional messages in others' voices and body language. He credits the characters that he has played on stage and the script analysis work he has done in classes with teaching him how to carry on a conversation off-stage. He has been able to take that understanding and apply it to the real people he encounters in everyday life. He says, "I can interpret the way someone else is feeling somewhat—just a little bit now. Back then [before drama training], people were just objects" (Personal communication, 2009).

A participant in The Spotlight Program, one of many dramatic arts pro-grams springing up around the country for students with ASD, attests to this when he says, "I've gained friendships and learned new games, how to be more mature and how to interact with others" (North Shore ARC, 2008, p. 1). Another says, "I've learned to recognize myself in others" (North Shore ARC, 2008, p. 2).

When the drama activities are led by a trained drama therapist who knows how to target specific therapeutic goals, even more success can be achieved. The mother of an adolescent with ASD who I worked with told me:

I have seen the child we knew was inside, but which we rarely saw at home, come out on stage. . . . On stage she is at her most confident, most assertive, her most centered self. Being in the plays gives her something *entirely* her own. She decides for herself—she chose to participate, she helps write the play, she decides what role she's going to play. . . . In class you model appropriate and respectful behavior for the children and they pick it up and model your behavior back. You treat the children as young adults and you listen to their ideas. They learn by your actions how to treat others with respect. . . . Most adults tell our children to be quiet—they don't want to hear what they have to say. But [in drama therapy] what they have to say matters. . . . It's very hard for kids with special needs to have a large group of friends. They tend to be very isolated. I see her involvement [in drama therapy] as a great social experience. . . . At the end of the year she has created and maintained many social relationships and she has a sweet taste in her mouth, looking forward to *next* year (Personal communication, 1993).

Depending on the age, functioning level, and abilities of the client, drama therapists also use puppets, sandtrays, role play, masks, and many other dramatic activities to help clients safely and meaningfully practice new communication, social, and expressive skills.

Risk and/or side-effects

Drama is not for everyone, just as basketball is not for everyone. Not every person who is on the autism spectrum will want to participate in drama, but more may want to than might at first be suspected. See the documentary *Autism: The Musical* if you have doubts. If a client is open and willing to participating in drama therapy, there are no risks or negative side effects.

The National Association for Drama Therapy (NADT) is the professional organization for drama therapists in the U.S. and Canada. To find a drama therapist in your area, you can contact the NADT office at nadt.office@nadt.org or 571-333-2991 or you can send out a request on the Dramatherapy Listserve by e-mailing dramatherapylst@listserv.ksu.edu.

EARLY START DENVER MODEL

BY DR. SALLY ROGERS

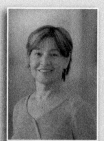

Sally J. Rogers, Ph.D.

The M.I.N.D. Institute
2825 50th Street
Sacramento CA 95817
(916) 703-0264
sally.rogers@ucdmc.ucdavis.edu

Dr. Sally Rogers is a developmental psychologist and a professor of psychiatry at the M.I.N.D. Institute, University of California Davis. She has spent her career studying cognitive and social development in young children with disabilities. She has published over 150 papers, chapters, and books. Her current research focuses in three areas: developing effective interventions for infants and toddlers with autism that families and professionals can deliver, earliest identification of autism in infancy, and imitation abilities in ASD. The intervention model that she developed with Geri Dawson, the Early Start Denver Model, is internationally known, and the book, *Early Start Denver Model For Young Children With Autism: Promoting Language, Learning, And Engagement* (The Guilford Press, 2009) and accompanying instrumentation for this approach have been recently published.

The ESDM was developed to target the core autism deficits seen in toddlers and preschoolers with autism: social orientation and attention, affect sharing and attunement, imitation, joint attention, language development, and functional and symbolic play. It uses an interactive, communication, and relationship-based framework that fosters active experiential learning by supporting child spontaneity and initiative. It works from a developmental curriculum, recognizing the current view of autism as a developmental disorder, and it incorporates teaching existing techniques that have received empirical support for improving skill acquisition in very young children with autism.

The ESDM[1] is based on a fusion of two well known approaches. First is the Denver Model, a comprehensive affective and developmentally based early intervention approach for preschool age children with autism originally developed by Rogers and colleagues.[2-3] The nature of the teaching interactions and the curricular priorities are heavily influenced by Stern's[4] model of infant interpersonal development and its successive developmental phases of the emerging social relationship between the infant and the caregiver.

The second is Pivotal Response Training (PRT). It involves a naturalistic application of applied behavior analysis to develop language and social skills, and has extensive empirical support developed by Laura Schreibman and Robert Koegel in the 1970s and '80s. [5-6]

An emphasis on eliciting strong positive emotion throughout interactions reflects Dawson and colleagues'[7] hypothesis that autism involves a fundamental deficiency in social motivation related to a lack of sensitivity to social reward. The resulting lack of social engagement, if not changed, can not only alter the course of behavioral development in autism, but also affect the way neural systems underlying the perception and representation of social and linguistic information are developed and organized.

History of development

The Denver Model began with a grant from the U.S. Department of Education to Dr. Rogers in 1981, and its effects as a group preschool intervention were first examined in a series of papers examining pre-post test data.[8, 3, 2] Significant accelerations in developmental rates of young children with ASD were found in several developmental areas, including cognition, language, reduction in autism symptoms, symbolic play, and social engagement. As a group, the children with autism doubled their developmental rates while in active treatment. Four independent replications of the model carried out in rural Colorado school districts[9] demonstrated significant accelerations of developmental rates within six months of implementation of the Denver Model. These studies suggested that the Denver Model has the capacity to affect development in many areas.

The first study of the Denver Model as an individually delivered intervention used a single subject design and randomized minimally verbal children to either the Denver Model or the PROMPT treatment.[10] The delivery involved one hour of individual treatment and parent training weekly, and daily one-hour home parent practice sessions for twelve weeks. Eighty percent of children acquired functional speech at a frequency of from ten to two hundred words per hour demonstrated in generalized probe sessions involving only natural communication interactions. A recent study of parent-delivered ESDM has also documented the efficacy of parent delivery in rapid acquisition of words, imitation, and social engagement. [11]

Success rate

The most recent study[12] involved 48 toddlers with ASD between eighteen and twenty-four months of age, randomly assigned to one of two groups: (1) The intervention group received, on average, twenty-five hours of the Early Start Denver model weekly, for two years; and (2) a community group who received community-based treatments. Groups did not differ at baseline in severity of autism symptoms based on ADOS scores, gender, IQ, or SES. Analyses documented that the intervention is effective for increasing children's IQ and receptive and expressive language ability, with results evident after only one year in intervention. After two years, children in ESDM showed a statistically significant average increase in overall learning composite scores (similar to IQ) of 17.6 points, whereas the control group showed an average increase of 7.0 points. Similar outcomes were also evident on receptive and expressive language, and on parent reports of communication, daily living skills, and motor skills. Longer-term follow-up studies are ongoing. In the last three published studies, acquisition of useful, communicative multiword speech has occurred with 80–90 percent of children enrolled in ESDM, in both parent-delivered intervention and twenty-five-hour per week home visitor intervention.

Content of intervention: developmental objectives

Each child's plan is defined by (1) **a set of short-term objectives** that represent what is to be taught over a twelve-week period and (2) **a set of activities** carried out daily to teach the objectives. The objectives are derived from a curriculum assessment carried out each twelve weeks using The Early Start Denver Model Curriculum Checklist. [1] The Curriculum Checklist covers the following ten domains: receptive communication, expressive communication, social interaction, imitation skills, cognitive skills, play skills, fine motor skills, gross motor skill, independence/behavior, and joint attention.

Process of intervention: teaching procedures

There are both general and specific aspects to the teaching process. General aspects of the teaching process, quantified in the ESDM Fidelity Tool, 1 involve the use of varied, naturalistic, child-initiated activities in which to embed instruction because of the empirically demonstrated gains in spontaneity, motivation, maintenance, and generalization that this kind of teaching supports for skills in which there are intrinsic reinforcers. [13-14] These are specified in the fifteen teaching behaviors assessed on the fidelity tool. Adults freely choose materials and activities in which to teach the targeted objectives to maximize attention and motivation, while considering the child's preferences and learning style.

Joint activity routines [15] are the vehicle for teaching. A joint activity routine involves a series of interactions between child and adult that allows for a shared activity to be begun, developed, elaborated, and completed. Inside a joint activity, objectives from at least two different developmental domains are taught. A joint activity routine typically lasts from two to five minutes, and involves multiple acts by both therapist and child. The materials and activities are generally chosen by the child, though the adult may offer choices and suggestions. Learning opportunities occur approximately every ten to fifteen seconds during treatment interactions. Transitions between activities are responsive to children's needs for a change and are carried out in a fashion that fosters child independence, motivation, and choice.

Tailoring the treatment: Response to Intervention (RTI)

A systematic decision process is used to "tailor the treatment," by systematically altering teaching procedures to improve progress if children are not progressing rapidly. This decision tree allows for the entire "toolbox" of teaching practices demonstrated to be effective for children with autism to be used if needed, but it prescribes **how** and **when** to alter teaching processes. While the teaching process favors naturalistic teaching, varied activities, intrinsic reinforcers, and shared control, no empirically supported teaching approach is "off limits."

Role of the family

Parents are an integral part of the intervention, influencing objectives, curriculum, and teaching practices. Parents are coached to fidelity in the ESDM intervention teaching approach to build their skills in incorporating the Early Start Denver Model approach in their natural caretaking and family routines as well as play activities throughout the day with their child. The goal of parent coaching is to empower parents via skill acquisition to promote a satisfying parent-child relationship and sense of parent competency and to generalize the skills across all daily family activities.

Risks or side-effects

The use of child choice, curriculum assessment, and decision tree minimize risks or side effects involving poor progress, child stress, and unwanted behavior because the approach can be tailored to each individual child's preferences, needs, and learning styles. The flexible delivery style (group education, parent delivery, 1:1 intensive, and 1:1 weekly therapy models) allows for the approach to fit into many different delivery systems. One risk involves cultural specificity. ESDM has not been tested outside of the US and outside of highly skilled directed settings.

ENHANSA: ENHANCED CURCUMIN SUPPLEMENT

BY ALAN ISRAEL

Alan Israel, R.Ph.

Lee Silsby Compounding Pharmacy
OurKidsASD.com (Supplements for Autism)
3216 Silsby Road
Cleveland Heights, OH 44118
(800) 981-8831 (Lee Silsby)
(877) 533-7457 (OurKidsASD)

Alan Israel is a board-certified pharmacist and has been in practice for more than thirty years. He obtained his pharmacy degree from Ohio Northern University and has been the owner of Lee Silsby Compounding Pharmacy since the early 1980s. Although Lee Silsby also compounds medications for several other specialties, Alan Israel has chosen to make autism the primary focus of the pharmacy. Since then, he has been to countless autism conferences around the country and has worked with several DAN! practitioners to compound medications according to their specifications. Besides compounding prescription medications, Lee Silsby also researches and develops its own nutritional supplements, such as ASD Vitamin & Mineral and Enhansa.

Enhansa is a proprietary blend of curcuminoids derived from the rhizomes of *Curcuma longa*, a plant from the ginger family. Curcumin is the principal curcuminoid in Enhansa. A wealth of promising research on the anti-inflammatory, antioxidant, and immune-enhancing properties of curcumin exists. However, most research has not been conducted through human trials, but instead has been conducted on cell cultures. Several studies have been done to assess the potential for curcumin to be absorbed by the gastrointestinal tract, into the body. The conclusions from these studies are that curcumin is poorly absorbed into the body.

If not for the poor absorption, curcumin would be an ideal candidate for use by patients with autism because it has the potential to restore levels of intracellular glutathione, reduce the inflammatory mediators that have been shown to be abnormally elevated in autism, and normalize the immune system so that it can begin to combat the fungal and viral infections that are so prevalent in autism.

Recognizing this, Lee Silsby Compounding Pharmacy developed a highly absorbable form of curcumin called Enhansa. Enhansa was first used in conjunction with a small group of Defeat Autism Now! practitioners and their patients. In this setting, it was easy for the practitioners to closely monitor their patients and learn what effects Enhansa had on their patients.

It was quickly observed that the use of Enhansa in autistic patients led to beneficial improvements in behavior, cognition, speech, and social skills, as well as improvements in the reduction of yeast- and viral-related issues. These findings have been found to be true in thousands of children with autism.

When using Enhansa, there are a few issues to be aware of. Because Enhansa can have such a strong effect on eradicating fungal and viral infections, die-off reactions often occur when first beginning the supplement. These reactions can range from mild irritability to regression and skin rashes. It is important to remember that these reactions are not to be viewed as negatives, but rather as a sign that the immune system is "waking up," allowing the body to better fight off fungal and viral reactions. Negative reactions usually subside in a matter of a few days to a few weeks. As the dosage of Enhansa is increased, these reactions can temporarily resurface. However, these reactions always subside after a little while. It can often be beneficial to use an activated charcoal supplement during the die-off phase. Activated charcoal has been reported to absorb and eliminate some of the products of yeast die-off that are responsible for the negative reactions.

The following is a typical example of what one may expect when using Enhansa with a child with autism:

"Just wanted to post how we are doing on Enhansa. We started out per the instructions at 150 mg and my kids had a huge reaction. We backed off and restarted at 75 mg and they did much better. [One of my children had some rashes, some blisters and low-grade fevers] and then an explosion in speech!! He is even talking to peers in class and making small talk! He even told off his teacher the other day for telling him no! (She gave him a time out but said she was secretly so thrilled!) He is caught up to age level in speech and is at a five-year-old level in motor skills!! His teachers report that he has friends and they said the kids love him and he is very popular. Enhansa has been awesome for his viral issues and yeast too."

ENZYMES FOR DIGESTIVE SUPPORT IN AUTISM

BY DR. DEVIN HOUSTON

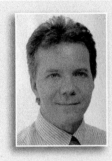

Devin B. Houston, Ph.D.

www.houston-enzymes.com
(866) 757-8627

Dr. Devin Houston founded Houston Enzymes in 2001 after many years of enzyme research in academia and industry. He invented the first enzyme product targeted to the autism community in 1999, and has since improved on that first effort. Dr. Houston continues to educate the public on enzymes and speaks on a regular basis at many autism conferences and parent groups.

The term "enzyme" refers to a broad class of specialized proteins that catalyze chemical reactions. Without enzymes these reactions would not occur or proceed at a rate not conducive to sustaining life. As catalysts, enzymes are not destroyed during the reaction. This allows a very small amount of enzyme to perform a large amount of work.

Digestive enzymes are a subset of enzymes specialized to break down foods after ingesting. These enzymes are necessary to derive nutrition from food. Specialized enzymes exist for different food proteins, carbohydrates, and triglycerides. The end result of their action is the provision of amino acids, glucose, and short-chain fatty acids to the body for production of compounds required for human metabolism.

The human body provides a fair amount of different enzymes for digestion, mostly from the pancreas and cells lining the gut wall. The bulk of the enzyme work occurs within the first part of the small intestine, or duodenum. It is here that protease enzymes begin the process of breaking proteins into smaller fragments called peptides, and carbohydrase enzymes start cleaving large carbohydrates into simple sugars. The duodenum and rest of the small intestine are also the site of absorption of nutrients into the systemic circulation.

Enzymes are present in raw foods but only in amounts sufficient to degrade the food over a period of several days. Many feel that enzymes in raw foods can supplement the digestion of food. Since digestion occurs within hours, not days, the actual contribution of food enzymes towards digestion is minimal. Enzymes can be supplemented in much more concentrated form. Fermentation of certain nonpathogenic fungi produces prodigious amounts of enzymes. Specific enzymes can be selected for production by altering the conditions under which the fungi are grown. The enzyme is then purified from the fungi, through many biochemical procedures resulting in a homogenous enzyme protein containing no fungal residue. The concentration of these enzyme blends is increased some billionfold over what is found in raw foods.

Many doctors have noted that children with autism often have gut problems. Inflammation can be a major problem. Tissues that are inflamed are damaged. Damaged cells don't produce enzymes, therefore, many children with autism may present with deficiencies in some enzymes until the gut is healed and operating normally. Malabsorption may present as well. Food intolerance and outright food allergies may also manifest in these children.

The most common food intolerance plaguing those with autism appears to be related to food proteins producing opioid-like peptides during digestion. Wheat and dairy products containing gluten and casein, respectively, are especially noted for producing exorphin peptides after contact with pepsin and elastase enzymes during the digestive process. This is a normal occurrence during digestion, however, some with autism exhibit stereotypical behaviors after ingesting wheat or dairy foods. One school of thought is that there may be an inappropriate interaction between opiate ligands and their receptors, however, this has not been substantiated. However, many parents found that diets that restrict wheat and dairy seemed to diminish the behavioral problems. The gluten-free/casein-free diet (GF/CF diet) is strongly recommended by many health care givers to their patients struggling with autism. The diet is not easy and requires a major lifestyle change for the patient and often the entire family.

Attempts were made in the 1990s to find an enzyme that would address the "peptide problem." Only when several protease enzymes were combined with a specific peptidase enzyme called dipeptidyl peptidase IV, or DPP-IV, was a degree of success obtained. DPP-IV was a known enzyme but not documented in commercially available enzyme blends until 1999. DPP-IV specifically degrades exorphin peptides and is produced by human gut cells. The fungal form is acid-resistant, as are most fungal enzymes. The actions of DPP-IV provide a possible mechanism of action and rationale for using protease enzyme supplements as a possible alternative to the GF/CF diet.

With the exception of alcohol, water, B vitamins, and some drugs, very little is absorbed from the stomach. Proteins and peptides are not absorbed until the food mass enters the small intestine. The stomach does not empty its contents into the duodenum until approximately two to three hours after ingestion. This provides a window of opportunity for addressing the problem proteins before their break down and absorption can occur in the small intestine. Plant-based enzymes are quite acid-resistant, unlike their pancreatic counterparts, and so may start working on foods within the stomach once in solution. A potent formulation of appropriate protease and peptidase enzymes can alter the pattern of protein breakdown such that exorphin peptides are not produced. If such peptides are produced, DPP IV peptidase can specifically degrade the exorphin peptides prior to food moving into the gut. However, the proper approach is to combine the DPP IV with other potent proteases to present a two-pronged attack: 1) change the manner in which the parent protein is broken down and, 2) use DPP IV to degrade any peptides that happen to form. It is interesting to note that this same approach is being used to develop an enzyme-based therapy for celiac disease.[1]

Enzymes may be helpful in other ways for those with autism. Keeping the gut free of undigested material prevents putrefaction that may lead to pathogenic bacterial blooms and yeast problems. Gas and bloating may be minimized by using carbohydrase enzymes such as lactase and alpha-galactosidase. Some vegetables contain carbohydrates such as stachyose and raffinose that are difficult for humans to digest. The human gut lacks the enzymes to degrade carbohydrates that become a food source for gas-producing bacteria. Alpha-galactosidase enzyme supplements can make up for the deficiency and ease the bloating. Chronic diarrhea may also be helped through the addition of enzymes such as amylase and glucoamylase that degrade starchy foods.

Other enzymes, such as xylanase, may modify some plant polyphenolic compounds by removing certain sugar groups that are attached to these compounds within the plant cells. These "phenolic compounds" are sources of antioxidants and other nutritional substances, and may play a role in modifying oxidative stress.[2] Removal of the sugar groups allows absorption of many polyphenolics and their subsequent metabolism by human cells.[3]

Enzymes are very likely one of the safest dietary supplements available. No upper limit has been established for dosing of any food-grade enzyme. No amount of plant-based digestive enzyme has been found to cause toxicity or side effects. Dosing of enzymes is not based on body weight or age as most of the ingested enzyme stays in the gut and is eliminated or broken down in the colon by microbial proteases. Enzymes are optimally given at the beginning of each meal to allow more contact time with the food in the stomach. Enzymes will not interfere with most medications, unless the medication is made of protein, carbohydrate, or triglyceride.

Well-controlled studies of enzyme use for the digestive problems associated with autism will eventually happen. The long history of safe use of enzymes in the food industry, however, should provide optimism and encouragement to try enzyme supplements without worry of significant side effects.

EQUINE THERAPY

BY FRANKLIN LEVINSON AND DR. NICOLA START

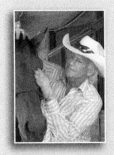

Franklin Levinson and Nicola Start, Ph.D.

www.WayoftheHorse.org
franklin@WayoftheHorse.org
(808) 572-6211

Franklin is a member of the North American Riding for the Handicapped Association (NARHA) as well as the Equine Facilitated Mental Health Association (EFMHA). Turning 64 this year, Franklin has been an equine professional for over 40 years. Some of what sets Franklin apart from other trainers/teachers is that, first and foremost, Franklin's goal and agenda with any horse is the development of "trust." No relationship can develop and flourish without mutual trust and respect at its very core. Franklin teaches the skills, attitudes, and paradigms essential to developing this sort of successful relationship with horses, and between humans as well. He recently created "Beyond Natural Horsemanship: Successful Training through Trust, Compassion, Wisdom, and Skill." He is published as an equine expert in horse publications in many countries.

The power of the human-animal bond has been described in sources as diverse as ancient literature, modern fiction, and recent research reports in the professional literature. The benefits, identified through research into social support and attachment, suggest that human-animal companionship may promote health and positive well-being in ways similar to human-human companionship. Specifically, researchers have discovered that companion animals are shown to lower blood pressure, decrease heart rate, moderate stressful situations, reduce feelings of loneliness and depression, and improve self-esteem. Studies have also shown positive results in the treatment of psychological and physical symptoms associated with autism spectrum disorders and other conditions when pets are employed as part of the therapeutic framework.

Hippotherapy (from the Greek *Hippos* for horse) is defined as a physical occupational or speech/language therapy treatment strategy incorporating the movement of the horse. The three-dimensional movement of the horse is used during a treatment session to challenge the patient, as the patient is not learning how to ride or control the horse. Rather, the movement of the horse is used as a dynamic surface, imparting forces to which the patient must accommodate and therefore train/retrain neuromuscular responses. A review of quantitative studies suggests that recreational horseback riding therapy and licensed-therapist-directed hippotherapy are individually efficacious, and are both medically indicated as therapy for gross motor rehabilitation.

In 1997, McCormick & McCormick explored in depth the therapeutic impact of key aspects of equine therapy such as touch, accurate nonverbal communication, fear, aggression, moral relationship, mirroring, empathy, compassion, and mutual trust.

Another study conducted by Ewing et al. (2007) allowed at-risk youths with severe emotional disorders to participate in a nine-week equine-facilitated learning program where the horses acted as therapeutic co-facilitators and education enhancers. The study stated the rationale behind the use of the horse as a more effective therapy animal involves the physical attributes of the horse. For the emotionally and cognitively disabled child, "the challenge of working with a 1,000-lb. snorting creature which both concentrates the mind and, when successfully met, stokes the dampened fires of pride" (Melson, 2001:115). McCulloch (2001) described a case study in which therapeutic horseback riding was beneficial in the rehabilitation of a boy with traumatic brain injury.

Horse riding can be an enhancing and empowering experience for many children who often come to psychotherapy feeling insecure and insignificant, as they are all too familiar (either consciously or unconsciously) with their own vulnerabilities. They hypothesize that much of a child's experience is looking up to the taller adult and so always being peered down onto. When a child is on top of a horse, he or she is looking down onto an adult for the first time. Furthermore, the child can experience the power of the body of the horse as it moves and is given an enhanced sense of his or her own body and thus, his or her sense of "self."

Therapy with a horse is viewed as a short-term, collaborative effort between a therapist and a horse professional. One of the purported goals of human-horse learning/therapy is to encourage client insight through horse examples. Horses have a variety of characteristics that are similar to humans, and they respond to nonverbal behavior of the human interacting with them. Individuals are often unaware of their behavior until they can understand it through the way in which the horse reflects it back to them. Interventions or activities are planned around the concept of the horse's reflective behavior, and are tailored to each individual and their needs as assessed by the psychotherapist, and the child and/or parent.

However, Ewing et al. (2007) consider first and foremost that equine facilitated learning or therapy is not a riding class. It is a therapeutic approach aimed at teaching life skills to children considered difficult to reach. In this approach, the horse is a vehicle that enables young adults to open up and to verbalize their problems and their fears. It is easier for children to learn empathy with animals because children view them as peers.

Researchers have suggested that these and other quintessential constituents of the horse—power, grace, vulnerability, and a willingness to bear another "combine to form a fertile stage for psychotherapeutic exploration" (Karol, 2007:77). The stature of a horse alongside a child solicits respect, a frequent problem area with at-risk children. Paying special attention to awareness of one's own body is essential for safety, which is used as a demonstration of how it is in the rest of the world. A therapist might instruct them how to approach the horse—remaining in their line of vision until the horse can see who is coming—the child experiences their place in relation to others within their environment.

Brown (2004) also identified that the horse is used successfully as a self-object, that is, a provider of self-cohesion, self-esteem, calmness, soothing, and acceptance through idealizing or twinship (which sustains the self by providing an essential likeness of another's self, Wolf, 1988). The child making connections with the horse can also facilitate vulnerability. They may be in a large enclosure with the horse, and be instructed to encourage the horse to move using their tone of voice and body language. This allows the child to move from powerlessness to seeking support to feelings of success.

Equine Facilitated Learning

The horse attracts people of all ages through its beauty, grace, power, and majestic stature. It has been clinically documented that just being around horses changes human's brain wave patterns. When we are with horses, we tend to calm down and become more focused. It is, therefore, no wonder that interaction with horses should prove therapeutic to grownups and children alike.

I first discovered Equine Facilitated Learning many years ago when I began researching, via the Internet, various ways people were interacting with horses. NARHA, a nonprofit, national organization here in the United States, had a new offshoot called the EFMHA. These particular programs centered on the emotional and mental health development of children and adults around guided interaction with horses. Startling improvement was observed in children with various mental and emotional challenges, from attention deficit disorder (ADD) and autism to antisocial violent behavior. This interested me a lot as I have always believed that horses can produce positive mental and emotional effects in humans when the interaction with the animal was appropriate. So I visited several places that offered training in this field and took the courses on offer.

Upon returning to my ranch on Maui, I began The Maui Horse Whisperer Experience, an interactive, hands-on experience of horses for non-horse people (experienced horse people and horse owners were invited as well). The positive effects of this type of successful interspecies communication were immediate, life-altering in certain cases. The confidence and self-esteem of individuals who were able to bond and communicate with the horses immediately and dramatically improved. People would drop their projections, misconceptions, and judgments about the horse and themselves once the communication became conscious and mutual.

For children with mental and emotional disorders in particular, interaction with the horses frequently yielded positive results. Children with ADD would magically focus on the horse for long periods of time when either grooming or leading the animals. They soon understood how to ask for and receive cooperation from the horse, which did wonders for their self-esteem. What a wonderful sight it is to see a shy, withdrawn, fearful child standing tall and confident as s/he leads a 1,200-lb. animal through an obstacle course of a series of twists, turns, and stops. Autistic children who had come to me, withdrawn and very much in their own world, began to say new words and attempt to express themselves in a manner that had not been previously seen by their parents and therapists. Given the lead rope of a horse, they would proudly lead the horse around the ranch for extended periods of time. Observing parents stood there, mouths agape and tears streaming down their faces, amazed at such a profound and wonderful response in their children and wards.

The principles of Equine Facilitated Learning are easy to understand. A horse will mirror the human in its company. The horse always seeks safety and peace. This is because the horse is a prey animal, always having to watch out for potential predators. A human trying to control a horse can make it fearful. If the human is disrespectful of the horse (inappropriate touching, movements, sounds, thoughts, or feelings), this can scare the horse, too. However, when the human makes conscientious and appropriate requests, rather than demands, the horse will cooperate. In order for the interaction to be successful, a human should be attentive to the horse's reactions. It is the human's responsibility to approach the horse as a parent approaches a child: with love, patience, and consistency.

In the wild, the horse gets its sense of peace and safety from the herd leader. Unfortunately, for the domesticated horse, there usually is no great human leader filling that role of the herd leader. Relationships between domesticated horses are often abnormal, as stables and barns are an unnatural environment. If there are no humans making appropriate requests that the horse can follow and comply with, horses miss the good leadership. It is often substituted with bad leadership, including obtaining compliance through food bribes or fear induction. A child, even one with mental or emotional disorders, when given a little insight into positive interaction with a horse, becomes the natural leader the horse is looking for. When the communication from the human is kind and appropriate, the horse is happy to cooperate and comply. Children often get good results more rapidly with horses as younger humans can be more comfortable with non-verbal forms of communication than adults, who are more likely to seek control.

Horses respond well to simple commands: go, stop, back up, turn this way, etc. When the horse complies with a request, thanking it: "Good boy/girl!" is sufficient; horses understand acknowledgment. Humans must be careful as there is a balance to be struck between excessive praise and not expressing sufficient appreciation: the communication with the horse must be balanced and human responses appropriate. The relationship will strike a natural balance when consideration, thoughtfulness, awareness, and kindness direct the interaction.

When I teach these gentle horse training techniques through the "Way of the Horse/Training Through Trust" seminars of Equine Facilitated Learning, children who come for emotional or mental health development experience Equine Facilitated Learning. The benefits of simple, successful interaction with horses are immediate and profound. I hope to bring Equine Facilitated Learning to other parts of the world, to enrich the lives of many more individuals—and horses!

FMRI-GUIDED TRANSCRANIAL DIRECT CURRENT STIMULATION TO RESTORE LANGUAGE

BY DR. HARRY SCHNEIDER

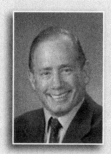

Harry D. Schneider, MD

146A Manetto Hill Road, Suite 207
Plainview, NY 11803
(516) 470-1930
491 North Indiana Avenue
Sellersburg, IN 47172
(516) 477-7682
hds7@columbia.edu or debra@harrydschneidermd.com

• Advanced degrees in language and linguistics • An upcoming doctorate in Speech-Language Pathology, 12/2010 • An excellent conventional and integrative medical specialist and diagnostician, having attended Columbia University's College of Physicians and Surgeons for his medical degree and Northwestern University for postgraduate studies • World Health Organization, Pan American Studies and Research • A neuroscientist at Columbia University Medical Center, where he has specialized in understanding the language circuits of the brain, having sent his research on these topics for publication to eminent peer-reviewed journals (www.fmri.org) • A research fellowship in Neuroimaging at the Program for Imaging and Cognitive Sciences, Columbia University Medical Center, New York, New York • Specialized training in diagnosing and managing autism at the Neurologic and Psychiatric Institute in New York, New York • Investigational studies and clinical trials using novel forms of language therapy combined with investigational use of music, cerebellar-based physical activities, and neuromodulation (transcranial electromagnetic stimulation) to restore language function in minimally verbal ASD children

I often hear statements like: "Autism is on the rise and a treatment needs to be found"; I agree! I can now state, after years of hard work, that we have developed a treatment therapy for autism that works *toward* restoring functional language to nonverbal children. We have learned how to stimulate dysfunctional language areas and their neural interconnections within the brain in order to reactivate them. This treatment research will be formalized for publication within a year or two, in an effort to make it available for *everyone's use.*

I think it is important to try to *understand* rather than to recite what a definition of autism is. I could quote a textbook definition of autism, "a disorder of neural development that is characterized by impaired social interaction and communication and by restricted and repetitive behavior." Our therapy volunteers tell me, however, that what they have read is not what they see when they actually meet the children at our office: "You really have to see a child with autism to understand what it's all about and how it affects their parents who take care of them day and night." On a recent radio show I did in Louisville, Kentucky, I was asked to define autism in simple, straightforward language, but I felt "simple" just wouldn't get the message across; I just spoke extemporaneously. I referred to autism as a horrific epidemic, a scourge of 21st century humanity, which has finally caused us all to open our eyes about the welfare of our children; autism didn't kill children, but would cause many to be lost to residential placement. I emphasized that we are not aware enough of what autism does, and that we need to learn much more about this dilemma.

I used an allegory to explain autism. I asked listeners to imagine the mothers of two boys standing in the snack section of a market. One boy I called "Robbie" and the other "Dylan." Robbie's mother told her son to go over and say hello to Dylan, who seemed like any other normal kid. Robbie said hello to Dylan, but received no answer. Robbie tried again and again, but Dylan did not even look at him. It was as if Dylan did not know that Robbie was there. Robbie asked some questions, and Dylan did not respond to them in any way. Then Dylan suddenly started to flap his hands as if something were stuck to them and began to shriek in an unusual way; Dylan even threw boxes of cookies on the floor. Robbie's mom asked Dylan's mom what was wrong with Dylan. Was he mentally retarded, did he have something wrong with his brain? His mom, accustomed to this type of question, simply said: "My son Dylan has autism."

Dylan's mom was referring to the nonverbal end of the autism spectrum. There are several types of autism spectrum disorders (ASDs): higher-functioning patients with Asperger's syndrome and savants (like "Rain Man," for those who saw the movie). We even have one patient who is thirty-one years old, who was in a special needs home for ten years after unsuccessful treatments. He came to my office for therapy and began to speak and improve socially within months. We wonder now how many others like him are put into a home somewhere. This is the heart of the ASD story: The financial drain of treating and placing these children is enormous, especially when they are deemed hopeless; the price for this thinking is staggering! We have decided to write a case study about this older patient, not for the purpose of showing our success (other than to reinforce the idea that this treatment can work at *any* age), but rather to say that there must be thousands of others put in some facility who may not have to be there.

My personal involvement with autism began about five to six years ago. I had met several patients at an alternative medicine conference in New York, who subsequently came to my office as patients; some of their children were on the spectrum. They complimented me by saying that I was very good at conventional and alternative medicine, but that I should also become a DAN! doctor. I looked perplexed and actually asked them who "DAN" was. They gently explained that Dan was not a *who* but a *what*—an acronym for a protocol called Defeat Autism Now! I went to California and became a certified DAN! doctor. After completing the DAN! training, however, I felt compelled to tell audiences that to effectively treat children on the spectrum, we had go beyond the current thinking of DAN!, which addresses biochemical irregularities in a child with autism, and promotes dietary interventions, such as a gluten-free/casein-free diet, vitamin supplementation, digestive enzymes, probiotics, and intravenous chelation to detoxify the body, just to name a few. I think some of the foundations of the DAN! protocol have a decent scientific base, but it is my opinion that the DAN! protocol is still a bit too structured and regimented and needs to be expanded and individualized for each child. I soon had a thought about what had to be done.

I brought my idea to my neuroscience lab at Columbia University Medical Center's Program for Imaging and Cognitive Sciences (PICS) We maintain a multi-investigator neuroimaging environment that investigates the neurocircuitry of the brain that underlies cognition, perception, and action; we look at how the brain functions for many of the things we do in life. We have an alphabet soup of technologies—fMRI, EEG, VEP, TMS, and tDCS—to draw from. We conceded it was now time to use our time-tested, cutting-edge technology to see what we could bring to the table to better understand this epidemic, which now affected more than 1 in 150 children. We decided to use functional magnetic resonance imaging (MRI) to "map out" the language areas in the brains of these children in an effort to see what was wrong. Regular MRI looks only at the anatomy of the brain: malformations, tumors, blockages. To see what parts of the brain are actually working, the child in the scanner needs to hear language, perhaps from a recording made by his parents. Active, working nerve cells in language areas of the brain increase their consumption of oxygen when processing the language; they extract oxygen from the hemoglobin in the red blood cells that carry it to them. In 1990, Dr. Seiji Ogawa made an important discovery: The MRI signal from hemoglobin without oxygen (deoxyhemoglobin) was different from hemoglobin that still had its oxygen. This small difference in MR signals formed the basis of the blood oxygen level-dependent (BOLD) signal used in fMRI that allows the computer to see what areas of the brain are using more oxygen than other areas when the brain is processing a task. It shows us the brain areas that are active. Then we look at how these active areas are interconnected using a sophisticated technology called diffusion tensor imaging (DTI). If brain areas are not properly connected to each other, then the entire network might not work. (For example, if there is a short circuit in your TV or PC, the whole unit might not work!)

The findings of these brain images are soon to be published, and will demonstrate "the autistic brain" (sounds like a bestseller). We demonstrated that normal

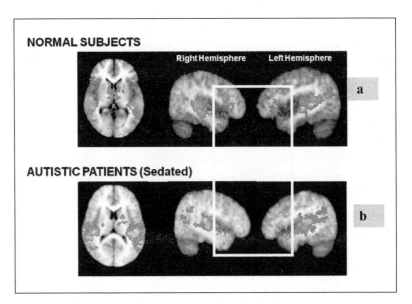

Figure 1. Brain areas for language, Broca's and the supplementary motor area (motor planning) are activated in normal subjects (top row), but those same areas do not activate in children with ASD (bottom row).

language production areas, such as Broca's "speech production" area, did not always activate for language, but did sometimes respond to music. The connections from Wernicke's "language reception" area in the back of the brain did not often connect all the way to Broca's area in the front of the brain. This investigational research used cutting-edge technology to demonstrate *partial causal explanations* regarding the problems with language in children with ASD. When published, it will not only be informative and heuristic in nature, but will also be an excellent early diagnostic tool for young children. That was the original purpose of the paper. Look at Figure 1 below to see what we saw.

The parents looked at the images of their children and said: "These are informative pictures. Thank you. I understand the nature of the problem. Now, what are you going to do for my child?" *My treatment idea, born of desperation, became a reality!*

My preliminary response to the parents was actually an introduction to linguistics. Their children couldn't speak, and I thought the parents needed to know more about how the brain controls language. I asked them how they themselves learned to speak; they looked confused. I reminded them that no one really taught language to them. There was no *explicit* teaching, no behavioral interventions, and no speech therapy. I suggested they all probably just looked and listened to all the language around them and one day they all began speaking. I proposed that all of us went from *"ga ga goo goo"* to "I refuse to do my homework, because I want to watch TV": our own way of speaking, after about two years. I explained that the reason a neurotypical child has such rapid language development was best described by Stephen Pinker: "Because languages can be *infinite* (70,000–500,000 + words) and a childhood is only *finite,* children cannot *just memorize language,* they must leap into the linguistic unknown and *generalize* to an infinite world of as-yet unspoken sentences." (Pinker, 1994) They do this because these neurotypical children *unconsciously* acquire grammar learning that all sentences (in English, at least) begin with a subject, then a verb, and finally an object (subject-verb-object, or SVO), such as "Mommy pours the juice." It takes them about two to three years to form a kind of "grammar template."

The child is a "naturalist," passively observing the speech of others, and the child "osmoses" this new grammar, not explicitly as I pointed out, but "implicitly" (unconsciously). Infants do not "learn" it, they *unconsciously* "acquire" the grammar part of language from birth to about age two, with an unconscious process that does not involve teaching. About age three, they then begin to consciously memorize things such as nouns, using the explicit system, and add them onto their grammar template. *All humans have two different learning/memory systems: an explicit and implicit one,* each using different parts of the brain. Until age three or four, this unconscious implicit system is still stronger than the conscious learning system. To better understand these two memory systems, I offered an example using retrograde amnesia: People cannot consciously remember what happened in the past, i.e., things they explicitly or consciously learned, but they can remember how to *unconsciously* drive a car, eat, use a keyboard, or play piano by ear.

What about an autistic child's language acquisition? Their grammar machine (implicit memory system) was partially damaged by autism. Kids with low-functioning autism (LFA) *have to consciously memorize almost all the language they can produce,* whether it's five or five hundred words. (If any of us tried to memorize a second language and then went to a foreign country, we would have a hard time.) These children never fully acquired their grammar, and if a language is only memorized, it may not lead to full language recovery. Moms usually tell me they know their child's entire verbal repertoire. With respect to language production, there is *in general* an inability to initiate and maintain language conversationally using colloquial conversation, and an inability to recount an event or tell a coherent story. With respect to language comprehension, we need to ask, "How much do they really understand?" Have they acquired the procedural grammar "template" to help them? If they can understand "The boy hugs the girl," can they understand "The girl is hugged by the boy"? The answer to the last question is usually an emphatic No! A child with ASD will also have difficulty with *prepositions, adjectives, adverbs, and pronouns.* I suspect most parents already know this.

After my linguistics lecture, the parents were still waiting for an answer to their original question: "How are you going to help my child?" I told them that the fMRI neuroimaging study was the first part of my journey. The Columbia research work I had co-investigated led me to develop a treatment plan for autism, which I currently employ in my private practice on Long Island. I explained that this treatment protocol applies cutting-edge technology called transcranial direct current stimulation (tDCS). It is the application of weak electrical currents (1–2 mA) to modulate the activity of neurons in the brain. When the electrode sponges are placed on the scalp, the amount of electricity produced in the brain is exceedingly small, changing the activity of the nerve cells minimally. In 1998, it was demonstrated that even a weak direct current delivered over the scalp can influence the excitability of the underlying cerebral cortex. These effects were reported to last for an appreciable amount of time after exposure.

TDCS is not "stimulation" in the same sense as conventional electric shock treatment for depression (it is 1/1,000—one millionth of that dose). It does not appear to cause nerve cell firing on its own and does not produce discrete effects such as the muscle twitches associated with classical stimulation. If a part of an existing speech network is not functional, we try to make it become functional, or create a different neural network to do the job; neurons are plastic and can take over the functions of other neurons, and it is possible to stimulate a brain's white matter and cause it to rewire. Currently tDCS is being studied for the treatment of a number of conditions, including major depression, brain injury affecting muscle movement, and memory. tDCS has been used to enhance *associative verbal learning,* a process by which a word is learned through association with a separate, preoccurring word (e.g., king-queen). This is an implicit skill, crucial for both acquiring new languages in healthy individuals and for language reacquisition after neurological damage. Therapeutic cortical stimulation in general has become applicable to many conditions, from motor disorders (e.g., Parkinson's disease) to depression. In this study, we are attempting to restore function to those areas of the brain that deal with the acquisition of grammar. These sites of action can be distant from the site of stimulation with tDCS, because axons with remote projections are more prone to be activated than local cell bodies. We have also noted that functional and clinical effects occur both during and beyond the time of stimulation, which relates to processes of synaptic plasticity induced by the stimulation. The cortical stimulation we use may activate, various cortico-subcortical networks (the grammar machine), depending on what part of the brain we attempt to stimulate.

We met with the parents the following week, and discussed using the images of their children's brains to guide the tDCS therapy. On the one hand, we were learning how to restore speech in patients who suffered stroke and some with traumatic brain injuries, but these patients had been born with neurotypical brains. On the other hand, we now had a "road map" of sorts of their children's "autistic" brains: all the areas and connections that were not working. I asked them if they wanted me to try this cutting-edge technology we had used on other types of patients on their children, in an effort to get them to speak. I told them that it would be a "work-in-progress," and we would all put our heads together. The good news I promised them was that, based on twenty years of research, there would most likely be minimal side effects (some itching and some skin redness); it would work, or it would not. They all agreed to try. We began our treatments within the next several weeks.

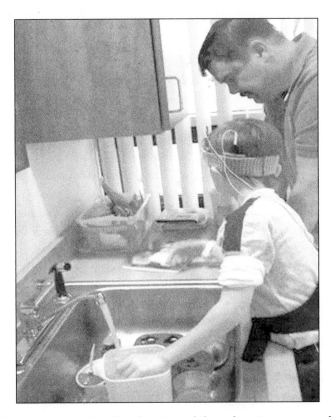

Figure 2. An example of implicit learning while undergoing neuromodulation therapy: Bryce plays in the sink while his dad reads *Goldilocks and the Three Bears*. **Bryce inadvertently hears what dad is reading and will join in if dad's book is more fun than his water toys.**

What kind of results have we had since that first meeting? We have found that children who came in with minimal language began to recover their grammar in a manner similar to how neurotypical infants might have acquired theirs. We noticed increased spontaneous vocalizations, often followed by increased spontaneous "consonant-vowel (CV) babbling" and then usually utterances containing multiple repetitions of CV syllables (e.g. *dadada*).

Grammar acquisition progressed with implicit learning training. We used a linguistic measurement, the mean length of utterances (MLU), as a measure of linguistic productivity in children. We calculated the number of utterances spoken by a child, and divided them by the number of morphemes (the smallest linguistic unit that has semantic meaning). Increasing MLU indicates a higher level of language proficiency. The MLU increased by >50 percent within four months. For example, ball (MLU = 1); balls (MLU = 2); *two* balls (MLU = 3); I want ball (MLU = 3); Daddy's speaking (MLU = 4). We documented the beginnings of a functional grammar template: the correct use of subject, verb, and object. For example, we saw the Subject and Verb: "Daddy hit" and the verb and object: "hit ball" progress to a more complete sentence "Daddy hit the ball." We noted improvement in other core deficits of autism, such as improvement in nonverbal communication skills, including eye-to-eye gazing, appropriate facial expressions, and the use of pragmatics: "*You* do it for me, mommy"; "Do I have to say something now, mommy?" We documented children's increases in interest in sharing enjoyment and achievements with other people: "Mommy, the cat ate the bird." (A child came into mother's room to tell her about a video.) We also noted some increase in interests in activities or play with others; improvement in obsessive-compulsive disorder (OCD) behaviors as language improved; a decrease in stereotyped behaviors (e.g., hand flapping); a need to use sign language less; and a wider range of things to enjoy, such as increased desire to play outside.

A thorough knowledge of neuroscience and brain pathways is of utmost importance when attempting to treat autism successfully, as well as lots of hard work, a dedicated team of scientists, totally involved parents, and infinite prayer. The initial challenge of what brain areas and connections to stimulate has been fruitful and rewarding. We are getting it right—nerve cells are plastic, and white matter pathways can rewire. As we have discovered at Columbia, and as Dr. Marcel Just, Director of Carnegie Mellon's Center for Cognitive Brain Imaging (CCBI) says: "We can begin to treat children's disabilities, such as autism."

I believe we have found the first of many successful treatments: the ability to begin to restore functional language for children on the spectrum. I hope all researchers eventually work together to share their ideas and thoughts, so that we may conquer this horrible affliction affecting our children.

FOOD SELECTIVITY AND OTHER FEEDING DISORDERS IN AUTISM

BY DR. PETULA VAZ AND DR. CATHLEEN PIAZZA

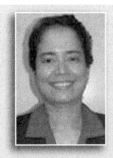

Petula C. M. Vaz, Ph.D.

985450 Nebraska Medical Center
Omaha, NE 68198-5450
(402) 559-8863
Fax: (402) 559-5004
pvaz@unmc.edu

Dr. Petula Vaz is an Assistant Professor at the Center for Autism Spectrum Disorders, Munroe-Meyer Institute at the University of Nebraska Medical Center. Her primary research interests are in the area of pediatric feeding disorders. Dr. Vaz is a licensed and certified speech-language pathologist. She is also a certified provider of VitalStim therapy for swallowing disorders. Dr. Vaz received her Ph.D. from Ohio University specializing in dysphagia and voice disorders. She has extensive predoctoral, doctoral, and postdoctoral research and clinical training in swallowing and feeding disorders. Dr. Vaz has several years of graduate and undergraduate level teaching and clinical mentoring experience.

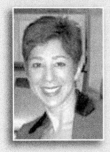

Cathleen C. Piazza, Ph.D.

Cathleen C. Piazza received her Ph.D. from Tulane University. She is Professor of Pediatrics and Director of the Pediatric Feeding Disorders Program at the University of Nebraska Medical Center in Omaha, and she previously directed similar programs at the Marcus Institute in Atlanta and at the Johns Hopkins University School of Medicine in Baltimore. Dr. Piazza and her colleagues have examined various aspects of feeding behavior and have developed a series of interventions to address one of the most common health problems in children with disabilities. Her research in this area has been among the most systematic in the field and has firmly established behavioral approaches as preferred methods for assessment and treatment. In her roles as clinical, research, and training director, Dr. Piazza has mentored a large number of interns and fellows who have gone on to make significant contributions to the field. Highly regarded for her general expertise in research methodology, Dr. Piazza is currently editor of the *Journal of Applied Behavior Analysis*.

Introduction

Feeding disorders in children involve the inability or refusal to consume sufficient amounts of liquid and solids to meet hydration and nutritional needs. Feeding problems occur in up to 90 percent of children with autism (Kodak & Piazza, 2008), and over 60 percent of these children exhibit selective eating behavior (Twachtman-Reilly, Amaral, & Zebrowski, 2008). The high incidence of pediatric feeding problems in children with autism have led some researchers to suggest that feeding difficulties in infancy may be an early sign of autism (Keen, 2008; Laud, Girolami, Boscoe, & Gulotta, 2009; Twachtman-Reilly et al.). The triad characteristic of autism—impairments in social interaction, communication deficits, and repetitive or stereotyped behavior—usually remain undetected during the first year of a child's life and are frequently missed until the child's second birthday. The presence of feeding disorders with selective eating behavior in children could potentially be a diagnostic precursor of autism. Therefore, early identification and management of feeding disorders in children is crucial. In addition, failure to address feeding disorders in a timely manner may lead to malnutrition and dehydration that may hinder physical growth and brain development, and it may also lead to other serious medical conditions such as failure to thrive, and even death.

Pediatric Feeding Disorders Program

The Pediatric Feeding Disorders Program (PFDP) at the University of Nebraska Medical Center's Munroe-Meyer Institute is one of the leading pediatric feeding disorders clinical, research, and training centers in the country. The assessment and treatment strategies used in the program focus on an interdisciplinary, empirical approach to feeding problems. A major component of the assessment and treatment strategies are based on the principles of applied behavior analysis, but the integration of the expertise of other disciplines such as medicine, speech, and occupational therapy, and nutrition are critical as the majority of feeding problems in children have a multifactorial etiology (Rommel, De Meyer, Feenstra, & Veereman-Wauters, 2003). The PFDP is well recognized for its commitment to high quality, interdisciplinary clinical care, to the teaching of health professionals, and to research related to pediatric feeding disorders. Dr. Piazza, the director of the PFDP, and her team have presented and published numerous research papers in this area.

Philosophy

The PFDP's interdisciplinary team consists of physicians, psychologists, nurse practitioners, nutritionists, speech-language pathologists, occupational therapists, physical therapists, social workers, feeding behavior technicians, and aides. Parents and caregivers are active participants in the child's feeding program. Research suggests that interdisciplinary treatment such as the type provided by the PFDP is the most effective and appropriate method of treating children with severe feeding problems (Cohen, Piazza, & Navathe, 2006; Kerwin, 1999; Volkert & Piazza, in press) including children with autism.

Program Structure

Children with autism between the ages of zero and twelve years with feeding problems of varying severity that compromise growth and/or nutrition are seen at the PFDP. Children over the age of twelve years are considered for admission to the program on a case by case basis. The PFDP has three different levels of service where the intensity of services provided vary along a continuum: a day treatment program, an intensive outpatient program, and an outpatient program. Children whose feeding problems are life-threatening or who have not progressed sufficiently with less frequent therapy are good candidates for the day treatment program. Children attending the day treatment program receive daily intensive therapy from Monday through Friday from 8:30 AM to 5:00 PM for approximately eight weeks. The program involves intensive feeding therapy sessions five to six hours per day, nutritional monitoring, and caregiver training. Once children have met their goals in the day treatment program, they are transitioned to the intensive outpatient program. The intensive outpatient program is for children who continue to require services after the day treatment program or whose feeding problems would respond to less intensive therapy. The intensive outpatient component of the program involves therapy sessions three to five days per week for approximately one to four hours per day. Once a child's treatment is stabilized in the intensive outpatient program, he or she is then transitioned to the outpatient program to maintain treatment gains, and progress the child to age-typical eating patterns. In the outpatient program, children are typically seen once or twice a week for approximately one to three hours of therapy. Depending upon the severity of the child's feeding problem, the entire course of treatment (i.e., to progress the child to age-typical feeding) may take up to two years.

Program Development and Monitoring

During the admission, the interdisciplinary team and the parents/caregivers develop specific goals for the child, which are the focus of assessment and treatment. Thus, all assessments and treatments are goal oriented and data driven. Common goals include increasing caloric intake, increasing acceptance and consumption of solid food and liquids, decreasing supplemental feedings (e.g., gastrostomy [G-] tube feedings), increasing texture and variety of consumed foods, decreasing inappropriate mealtime behavior, and caregiver training. The long-term goal of the program is for the child to become an age-typical eater. The team meets at least once a day to discuss the data and to revise the assessment and/or treatment plan as necessary. The program differs from the traditional interdisciplinary team model in that individual, discipline-specific (pull-out) therapy is not provided. Instead, the team develops a protocol that is individualized for the child. This protocol is followed by everyone who feeds the child. Therefore, the feeding therapy occurs during meals, in the presence of solids and/or liquids, under very specific conditions that have been developed beforehand by the entire team.

Assessment

The initial evaluation begins with the caregiver feeding the child as he or she would at home. Data are collected on child and caregiver behavior, which include how the caregiver prompts the child to eat and how the caregiver responds to child-appropriate and -inappropriate behavior. The child's responses to various textures and type of food and liquids and use and need for types of utensils are assessed. These data are used to develop hypotheses about current environmental events that may maintain child-appropriate and -inappropriate behavior and the child's current level of oral motor skills. Children with high levels of inappropriate behavior during caregiver-fed meals participate in a functional analysis (FA) to determine how specific environmental events affect child behavior (Piazza, Fisher, Brown, et al., 2003). The results of the FA result in a specific, prescribed treatment for the child.

Children with high levels of inappropriate behavior in the presence of specific foods or textures often participate in a food-preference (Munk & Repp, 1994) or texture-preference assessment (Patel, Piazza, Layer, Coleman, & Swartzwelder, 2005; Patel, Piazza, Santana, & Volkert, 2002), respectively. A hierarchy of food or textures the child refuses to eat is developed. The results of the assessment are used to develop individualized treatment protocols to facilitate the acceptance of target foods or textures as indicated.

Treatment

Individualized treatment protocols consistent with current research literature are developed that meet specific needs of these children. For example, a treatment based on negative reinforcement is used with children whose inappropriate behavior is maintained by escape from presentations of liquids or solids. Typical negative reinforcement-based treatments include providing a break following appropriate behavior (e.g., acceptance, swallowing) and elimination of escape for inappropriate behavior (escape extinction; Gulotta, Piazza, Patel, Layer, 2005; Kelley, Piazza, Fisher, Oberdorff, 2003). A treatment based on positive reinforcement is used with children whose inappropriate behavior is maintained by attention. Typical positive reinforcement-based treatments include providing attention or tangible items following appropriate behavior (e.g., acceptance, swallowing) and the elimination of attention for inappropriate behavior (attention extinction; Bachmeyer et al., 2009; Piazza, Patel, Gulotta, Sevin, Layer, 2003; Reed, Piazza, Patel, et al., 2004).

These types of treatments typically focus on increasing acceptance of food and decreasing inappropriate behavior. However, there may be other variations of these treatments that are implemented for children who show resistance to escape and/or attention extinction, such as blending preferred and nonpreferred foods together to increase acceptance of nonpreferred foods (Mueller, Piazza, Patel, Kelley, & Pruett, 2004; Piazza, Patel, Santana, et al., 2002); fading or altering some component of the mealtime environment gradually (Freeman & Piazza, 2002; Patel, Piazza, Kelly, Ochsner, & Santana, 2001) for a child who is cooperative with some aspect of the feeding situation, but not others; preceding presentation of a food or liquid with a low probability of acceptance, by a food or liquid with a higher probability of acceptance (Patel, Reed, Piazza, et al., 2006) for a child who demonstrates acceptance of some foods or some aspect of the feeding situation (e.g., acceptance of an empty spoon) but not others.

Increases in acceptance for some children might be accompanied by increases in expulsion (spitting out food). Such a response would necessitate the addition of treatment components designed to reduce expulsion. For example, the therapist might re-present expelled food (Sevin, Gulotta, Sierp, Rosica, & Miller, 2002). The therapist also might evaluate how texture of food affects expulsion (Patel, Piazza, Santana, et al., 2002). Some children hold or pocket accepted food, a behavior known as "packing." There are a variety of treatments used to reduce packing and increase swallowing. One treatment involves "redistribution" of packed food with a spoon or a Nuk brush to place packed food back on the child's tongue (Gulotta, Piazza, Patel, et al., 2005). In other instances, it may be necessary to reduce the texture of one or more food items (Patel, Piazza, Layer et al., 2005).

Caregiver Training

Research studies have shown that caregivers can be trained successfully to implement treatment protocols (Mueller, Piazza, Moore, et al., 2003; Najdowski, Wallace, Doney, & Ghezzi, 2003; Werle, Murphy, & Budd, 1993). The long-term success of a feeding program depends on the accuracy with which caregivers follow through with treatment procedures. Therefore, once an effective treatment is identified, caregiver training to monitor treatment integrity is a crucial final component of treatment.

Outcomes

Our empirically based, interdisciplinary treatment program is highly effective. The program has an 86 percent success rate with severe feeding problems (based on outcome data collected in the PFDP at the Kennedy Krieger and Marcus Institutes, where Dr. Piazza was the director). The costs associated with behavioral treatment are significantly less than those associated with alternative means of nutrition such as G-tube feeding. Data from studies on treatment of feeding disorders suggest that treatment of feeding problems results in improved quality of life for the child and family, reduced overall health care usage and costs, and reduced family stress.

GASTROINTESTINAL DISEASE: EMERGING CONCENSUS

BY DR. ARTHUR KRIGSMAN

This chapter is reprinted with permission from *The Autism File* magazine (Issue 35, 2010).

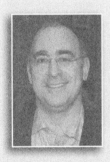

Arthur Krigsman MD

148 Beach 9th Street
Far Rockaway, New York 11691
(516) 239-4123

Dr. Krigsman is a pediatrician and board-certified pediatric gastroenterologist, and an assistant professor of pediatrics at New York University School of Medicine in New York. He has extensive experience in the evaluation and treatment of gastrointestinal disease in children with autistic spectrum disorder and participates in the growing field of research designed to better understand GI disease in this group of children. He has presented his findings in peer-reviewed journals and has shared his experience at scientific and lay meetings, and at a congressional hearing dealing with autism and its possible causes.

The presence of chronic gastrointestinal (GI) symptoms in children with autism spectrum disorder (ASD) has been well established. Prospective reviews of the frequency of these chronic and often intense GI symptoms, based upon careful questioning of the parents, reveal that they occur in as many as 70-80% of ASD children. The GI symptoms in these children are of a wide variety and include abdominal pain, diarrhea, constipation, abdominal distention, and growth failure ("failure to thrive"). In my experience with over 1400 such patients, I have often heard the parent state, "I can live with the autism, but I can't stand to see my child suffer with pain and severe constipation." Because the communicative and behavioral aspects of the disease are the most obvious, and because the GI symptoms frequently begin during infancy (prior to the onset of the behavioral and cognitive problems), parents are often unaware of the impact of the GI problems on their child's health until years later.

Historically, when parents do finally bring these GI complaints to the attention of their general practitioner or pediatric gastroenterologist, their significance is often minimized or dismissed. There are many reasons for this, including lack of familiarity with the GI diseases frequently seen in ASD, uncertainty on the part of the physician about how to properly proceed in the evaluation of these diseases, and long-standing beliefs in the medical world that GI symptoms in the "mentally handicapped" are due to a mysterious, poorly defined, and difficult to treat problem similar to those seen, for example, with mental retardation. Lastly, the political controversy and unending media misinformation swirling around the three scientists who were the first to describe bowel disease in ASD patients has given rise to doubts in some academic circles as to whether anything is really wrong at all with the bowels of these children.

Fortunately, the GI problems of children with ASD are now getting attention. First was a full-day conference jointly sponsored by NASPGHAN (North American Society for Pediatric Gastroenterology, Hepatology, and Nutrition), the American Academy of Pediatrics, and Autism Speaks. It was dedicated solely to the GI disease in these children. In addition there are two consensus statements published in a January 4, 2010 supplement to the journal Pediatrics, offering guidance to clinicians as to how best evaluate gastrointestinal symptoms within the setting of ASD.

The two most important points to keep in mind are that (a) GI symptoms should be evaluated no differently in children with ASD than they would in neurotypical children, and (b) problem behaviors may be the sole manifestation of a gastrointestinal problem. Let us explore these two statements.

The presence of chronic (i.e., long-standing) GI symptoms demands medical evaluation. The fact that the child has autism is merely an interesting sidebar item. The clinical story typically begins with the parents' concern over the chronicity and intensity of their child's GI symptoms. It is this that brings them to the pediatrician or gastroenterologist. The symptoms typically consist of any (or all) of the following:

- abdominal pain
- diarrhea (defined as unformed stool that does not hold its own shape but rather conforms to the shape of the container/nappy/diaper that it is in)
- constipation (defined as infrequent passage of stool of any consistency or passage of overly hard stools regardless of frequency)
- soft-stool constipation
- painful passage of unformed stool
- rectal prolapse
- failure to maintain normal growth
- regurgitation
- rumination
- abdominal distention
- food avoidance

An additional layer of complexity appears when there is an observed correlation between the intensity of the GI symptoms and the level of cognitive-behavioral dysfunction. In the non-ASD world of pediatric gastroenterology, the GI pathology responsible for these varying symptoms is often difficult to determine from the symptoms alone. The same holds true in the ASD patient group. In both cases, numerous underlying GI problems can cause these symptoms. In my experience with ASD children, the following diagnoses have been endoscopically confirmed and determined to be causing some or all of these symptoms:

- eosinophilic esophagitis (EoE)
- esophageal hypereosinophilia (EH)
- reflux esophagitis
- Candida esophagitis
- esophagitis of unknown origin
- Barrett's esophagus
- peptic gastritis
- eosinophilic gastritis
- lymphocytic gastritis
- autoimmune gastritis

- gastric ulcer
- gastropathy of unknown origin
- Helicobacter pylori gastritis
- peptic duodenitis
- duodenal ulcer
- white-spot (micro-erosive) duodenitis
- H. pylori duodenitis
- non-specific enteritis
- celiac disease
- non-specific colitis
- Crohn's disease

Of course, ASD children may suffer from the same common GI ailments as neurotypical children (e.g., constipation, reflux, transient stomach virus infections, etc.), so a GI complaint in an ASD child does not automatically suggest the presence of the above-mentioned diagnoses. It is certainly appropriate to undertake a trial of empiric (that is, treatment of a suspected disorder without prior confirmation of the true diagnosis) therapy for any of the common childhood GI problems (e.g., reflux, constipation, etc.). However, if the symptoms prove resistant to conventional empiric therapies or if the suspected diagnosis is that of a chronic disorder that will require long-term treatment (i.e., inflammatory bowel disease), empiric therapy is inappropriate and contraindicated. The fact that most ASD children experience chronic GI symptoms, and that most ASD-GI-symptomatic children have demonstrable causal pathology of the types listed above, has led many to conclude that GI pathology occurs with increased frequency in ASD children when compared to neurotypical children. This is certainly the conclusion I have drawn in working with these children.

The approach to evaluating these chronic symptoms should be the same as those employed to diagnose and treat neurotypical children. Established diagnostic algorithms exist for all of the above-mentioned symptoms and include a careful taking of the history, physical examination, blood tests, stool tests, urine tests, abdominal imaging studies, nutritional assessment, and assessment of growth patterns. These tests should be designed to cover as broad a spectrum of potential diagnoses as possible, including metabolic diseases such as mitochondrial disorders. Needless to say, these tests are most useful when they provide strong evidence of a specific diagnosis. However, more often than not, even the most comprehensive non-invasive evaluation does not shed light on the cause of the symptoms in the ASD-GI patient. These are the cases that usually require direct visualization of the GI tract via endoscopy. Endoscopy not only provides direct visualization of the lining of the GI tract but also the ability to obtain a small sample of tissue (biopsy) for microscopic examination by a pathologist. The recent introduction of wireless capsule endoscopy (commonly referred to as the "pillcam") allows direct visualization of the small intestinal lining not accessible to more conventional endoscopy and has contributed greatly to our understanding of bowel disease in ASD children. ASD-GI patients who have undergone diagnostic endoscopy and biopsy frequently have more than one of the diagnoses listed above, and the precise order in which they need to be treated, as well as the nature of their relationship to each other, has to be further studied.

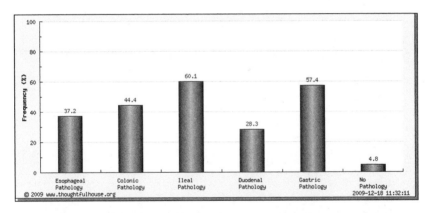

Figure 1. Frequency by Anatomic Location of Various GI Pathologies in ASD-GI Symptomatic Children Undergoing Endoscopy and Colonoscopy. Performed by Arthur Krigsman, MD. 2003–2009. Reported by Independent Pathologists (Mount Sinai Hospital NY, Lennox Hill Hospital, NY, and CPL Labs, TX.)

For the most part and for the sake of simplicity, the various diagnoses of the esophagus and stomach listed above are also seen in the neurotypical population but the ASD-associated enterocolitis (ASD-EC) present in the majority of ASD-GI patients, and well described in the medical literature, appears to be unique to ASD patients. (The exception to this appears to be a focal enhanced gastritis described only within the population of ASD-GI patients.) Because of this, established treatments for the esophageal and gastric (stomach) diagnoses exist, but the best treatment for the ASD-associated enterocolitis is unknown.

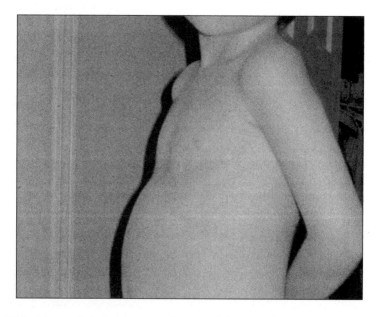

A child without a bowel movement for several days will develop a distended belly.

It is uncertain whether treatment of non-specific enterocolitis may also treat some of the esophageal and gastric pathology. Much work needs to be done in this area. It does seem clear, though, that ASD-associated enterocolitis is, in many cases, a chronic disease. Because academic interest in the area of autism-associated bowel disease is increasing, it will be interesting to see the results of clinical trials aimed at determining the treatment outcomes of a variety of pharmaceutical and dietary interventions for autism-associated enterocolitis. Many researchers believe that these clinical trials should include established therapies for other inflammatory bowel diseases (IBDs) such as Crohn's disease and ulcerative colitis. The rationale for this is that preliminary data demonstrate an interesting overlap between the clinical presentation, laboratory findings, and endoscopic/histologic findings of autism-associated enterocolitis and IBDs. As in Crohn's disease, the symptom presentation of ASD-associated enterocolitis may consist of abdominal pain, diarrhea, abdominal distention, and growth retardation. Interestingly, constipation and difficulty in passing soft or unformed stools is a frequent presenting symptom in ASD-associated enterocolitis though this is not thought to be typical of the symptoms of Crohn's disease (though there are reports of just such presentation in Crohn's disease as well). Abdominal x-rays of ASD children presenting with chronic GI symptoms characteristically show fecal loading, meaning a colon loaded with stool. The colon in these patients does not typically appear distended on x-ray, thus providing reassurance that there is no obstruction. Obstruction would represent a medical emergency and requires urgent medical attention. In such cases, the patient is quite ill and toxic looking. The constipation most typical in ASD-GI children is best referred to as "soft stool constipation." This means that the child will go many days (often up to a week or more) without a bowel movement. During this period, the abdomen becomes progressively more distended. Parents often report that the progressive retention of stool correlates with progressive worsening in the child's behavior (e.g., "stimming," aggression, self-injurious behaviors, hyperactivity) and cognition (i.e., focus, processing, thought, and language, etc.). The stool that is finally produced after many days is semi-formed or unformed and is often produced only with great straining.

Other interesting overlaps in the clinical presentation of ASD-associated enterocolitis and Crohn's disease exist as well. Disturbance in growth patterns is often noted at presentation. Interestingly, the deviation from normal growth affects linear growth (height) more often than weight. It is tempting to hypothesize that if a caloric insufficiency exists in these children, it is not to the extent that linear growth is stunted. There are reports of decreased bone mineralization in ASD children, independent of their being on any specific restrictive diet. This too suggests the presence of malabsorption or maldigestion. Reports of duodenal brush border enzyme deficiencies (not associated with known genetic defects) in ASD-GI patients further suggests a possible underlying mucosal inflammatory process and may contribute to growth retardation.

Overlap in laboratory testing between ASD-associated enterocolitis and IBD includes the finding of an elevated erythrocyte sedimentation rate, C-reactive protein, and platelet counts as well as the presence in the stool of lactoferrin, calprotectin, and lysozyme. The latter three stool markers are considered specific for the presence of intestinal inflammation. The relative frequency with which these markers of inflammation are present in ASD-associated enterocolitis as compared to IBD has not yet been determined. Perhaps most interesting in terms of laboratory overlap is the frequent presence of elevated IBD-specific serologic markers. These markers are serum antibodies to both bacterial and fungal gut flora that are statistically associated with the presence of IBD and are rarely found in the non-IBD population. It is important to point out that these markers are not considered to be a diagnostic test for IBD. They are most appropriately used when a clinician is trying to distinguish Crohn's disease from ulcerative colitis. However, their frequent presence in ASD-GI children suggests that a similar mechanism of disease might be present there as well and provides potential avenues of further research.

In patients undergoing clinically indicated diagnostic endoscopy for the above symptoms, there is the frequent occurrence of a non-specific mucosal inflammation. The term "non-specific" indicates that the features seen under the microscope, though not normal, do not indicate the presence of a specific disease. It implies that the finding is not normal, but that many causes are possible. Though there are specific microscopic features of Crohn's disease that allow one to make a definitive diagnosis, it is not unusual for Crohn's disease patients to produce biopsies that are non-specific in nature. Such is the case with ASD-associated enterocolitis where the majority of the patients demonstrate non-specific findings upon biopsy. However, there are a number of ASD-GI children whose intestinal biopsies demonstrate the changes strongly suggestive of Crohn's disease.

These clinical, laboratory, and endoscopic/histologic overlaps provide strong preliminary support for clinical trials that investigate the efficacy of pharmaceuticals commonly used to treat IBDs. It is our hope that such clinical trials will be undertaken soon.

Moving on to the second of our statements made at the outset of this article, parents, physicians, and therapists must realize that difficult-to-treat ASD behaviors or behaviors that have not been responsive to standard behavioral interventions may be the sole manifestation of a GI diagnosis. This means that unprovoked aggression, violent behavior, and irritability may have an underlying GI cause, and this must be taken into consideration prior to the reflexive desire to begin a psychotropic drug such as risperidone (despite its FDA approval for the treatment of autism). Gastroesophageal reflux disease, gastritis/gastric ulcer, and constipation are just three examples of GI diagnoses that are known to cause such behavioral symptoms. In addition, poor focus and an inability to make significant academic or communicative progress despite intensive interventions may indicate the presence of treatable bowel disease that, once treated, can significantly improve the child's degree of disability. The concept of behavioral problems as a symptom of GI disease was strongly supported in the consensus article published in the January 4, 2010 supplement of the journal Pediatrics.

The take-home messages are as follows:

1) Treatable GI disease is exceedingly common in ASD.

2) The signs and symptoms that alert one to the possible presence of GI disease are both conventional (e.g., diarrhea, abdominal pain, etc.) and ASD-specific (e.g., behaviors, aggression, poor response to therapies, etc.).

3) The approach to the GI evaluation of these signs and symptoms should be no different from a child without autism.

4) Parents and therapists who note such signs and symptoms must strongly advocate for the child regarding the need for a comprehensive GI evaluation.

5) Treatment of GI disease should follow established treatment protocols for the particular diagnosis.

6) GI diagnoses unique to ASD require further study to determine best treatment practices.

7)   Empiric treatment for common, transient childhood conditions is appropriate but should be halted if the patient demonstrates non-responsiveness.

8)   Empiric treatment for suspected chronic disease in inappropriate and contraindicated.

HELMINTHIC THERAPY

BY JUDITH CHINITZ

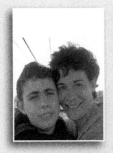

Judith Hope Chinitz, MS, MS, CNC

New Star Nutritional Consulting
(914) 244-3646
www.newstarnutrition.com
judy@newstarnutrition.com

After her son's diagnosis with autism in 1996, Judith Chinitz has spent the last fourteen years searching for answers. After saving her son's life through diet, and seeing firsthand the healing power of food, Judy earned a second master's degree in nutrition after having previously worked as a special education teacher. Judy is the author of *We Band of Mothers: Autism, My Son, and the Specific Carbohydrate Diet,* which also contains commentary by Dr. Sidney Baker. She also assisted Dr. Baker in founding Medigenesis, an Internet-based, interactive medical database.

Autism, Immune Abnormalities, and Parasite Therapy

In 1964, Dr. Bernard Rimland published his book, *Infantile Autism: The Syndrome and Its Implication for a Neural Theory of Behavior,* proving that autism was a physiological—as opposed to a psychological—condition. By the 1970s, researchers began to note immune system abnormalities in autistic children. In the 1980s, researchers such as Dr. Reed Warren, for example, demonstrated that those with autism had abnormal lymphocyte responsiveness (that is, their white blood cells don't respond normally to germs) and abnormal levels of various types of immune cells, including low levels of natural killer cells. (This means that children on the autism spectrum have a hard time fighting pathogens, like yeast, viruses, and bacteria.)

In 1998, Dr. Sudhir Gupta of the University of California, Irvine, published a paper in the *Journal of Neuroimmunology* entitled, "Th1- and Th2-like cytokines in CD4+ and CD8+ cells in autism." This paper states that the "... data suggest that an imbalance of Th1- and Th2-like cytokines in autism may play a role in the pathogenesis of autism."

To date, a few of the specific abnormalities found in individuals with autism include:

a.   In an unstimulated state, individuals with autism have higher levels of proinflammatory cytokines (chemical messengers of the immune system) than control groups.

b.   With stimulation of the immune system (i.e., with the introduction of pathogens), individuals with autism spectrum disorders (ASDs) have markedly higher levels of proinflammatory cytokines than controls.

c.   Specific proinflammatory cytokines that have been found to be high in people on the spectrum include tumor necrosis factor-alpha (TNF-α) in both the blood and the gut; interferon gamma (IFN-γ) in both the blood and the gut; and higher levels of interleukin-12 (IL-12) in the blood.

d.   Individuals with ASD have lower levels of regulatory cytokines (those chemicals that turn off inflammation) like interleukin-10 (IL-10) than control groups.

These proinflammatory chemicals appear to affect not just how these individuals respond (or don't respond) to disease-causing microbes; they also affect the health of the digestive system and the function of the brain itself.

Dr. Martha Herbert, an Assistant Professor of Neurology at Harvard Medical School, and a pediatric neurologist at the Massachusetts General Hospital in Boston, a foremost authority on autism, has stated repeatedly that the brain is downstream from the digestive system, meaning that if the latter is compromised, the former suffers. The lining of our digestive system comprises about 60 percent of the immune system. Our bodily systems are not separate entities, but all parts of a whole. If one part is compromised, the rest are affected.

Also evident from the medical literature is the finding that many individuals with ASD have abnormal gut microbiota. What does this mean? The human body contains trillions of microbes, far more than there are cells in our bodies. No one really knows exactly what the composition of these microbes should be. However, we do know that there should be something like 400–500 different types of bacteria living in our intestines. Multiple researchers have now demonstrated that individuals with ASDs have not only abnormal amounts of bacteria living in their digestive systems, but also seemingly abnormal kinds as well. It's a chicken-and-egg scenario: abnormal gut microbiota leads to abnormal gut conditions compromising the immune system, but the reverse is also true. Abnormal immune functioning within the gastrointestinal tract will lead to abnormal microbiota.

The hygiene hypothesis, which was first proposed about twenty years ago, conjectures that we have become "too sterile." With the advent of germ theory a century ago (the recognition that many diseases arise from specific germs), we have concentrated our efforts on eradicating bacteria, yeasts, and parasites from our environment and ourselves. However, the fact is that many species of these organisms were normal parts of human flora for all of evolution, and without our "old friends," as they are called, we may have tipped our immune systems into a chronic state of imbalance.

So, where does this leave us? Many individuals with autism have abnormal gut microbiotia and abnormal immune functioning. How best to handle this is not yet known. Many doctors focus on killing off the bad stuff—antibiotics for bad bacteria, antifungals for *Candida*, etc. And this helps . . . sometimes. Another line of thought though is to shift the immune system and gut back into normalcy by *adding* good flora and fauna, rather than, or as well as, subtracting bad . . . especially when the lines between good and bad may be more blurred than originally thought.

Enter Parasites

The presence of parasites was natural for the evolving humanoid species up until seventy-five or so years ago. We lived on and with the soil, and thus our intestines were filled not only with bacteria and yeasts, but protozoa and other parasites too—including helminths. Helminths are a family of parasitic worms that include roundworm, hookworm, tapeworm and whipworm, among others.

With our current anti-germ way of thinking, many are immediately horrified when they first think about "infecting" themselves with parasites. "Aren't parasites bad?" is the typical first question from those first learning about this form of therapy. Well, yes, they certainly can be. A 20-foot tapeworm living in your intestines might be considered undesirable. Then again, we are all very well aware of the health benefits of yogurt, with its live bacteria. Do you equate this with eating salmonella on purpose? Like bacteria, some parasites are good and some are bad. And like bacteria, some are perhaps meant to be in us. An absence of good bacteria in the gut will seriously compromise the health of the individual. More and more research suggests that an absence of good parasites is a major factor in the development of certain disorders.

In 2007, Dr. Kevin Becker of the National Institutes of Health, published an article in *Medical Hypotheses* entitled, "Autism, asthma, inflammation, and the hygiene hypothesis." Dr. Becker concludes, "Altered patterns of infant immune stimulation may hypersensitize the early immune system not toward allergic sensitivity and bronchial hypersensitivity but to inflammatory or cytokine responses affecting brain structure and function leading to autism. It is well documented that immune cytokines play an important role in normal brain development as well as pathological injury in early brain development. It is hypothesized that immune pathways altered by hygiene practices in western society may effect brain structure or function contributing to the development of autism."

What do we know about beneficial helminths? Research thus far has shown that certain helminths raise levels of regulatory cytokines (those chemicals that turn off inflammation) and they lower levels of inflammatory cytokines, including TNF-α. That is, helminths may do exactly what is needed to improve the immunological functioning of individuals on the spectrum. There have now been several clinical studies done on individuals with asthma, allergy, multiple sclerosis (MS), and inflammatory bowel disease. Results have varied depending on the disease and the type of parasite tested and of course may have been affected by the length of the trial and the dosages used. Some trials have demonstrated a significant positive effect on pathological processes caused by the presence of helminths, while other studies have suggested the presence of helminths has little or no effect on underlying pathology. We are in the earliest stages of this science. At the time of this writing, several more trials are planned including testing human hookworm's effectiveness for multiple sclerosis and celiac disease. In fact, Mount Sinai Hospital in New York City is recruiting to do a clinical trial of *Trichuris suis* ova (TSO) in children with autism. Anecdotally, many people have now benefitted enormously from therapeutic doses of parasites for diseases such as MS, inflammatory bowel disease, asthma and allergy, Sjögren's syndrome, and of course autism.

Over the last two years or so, more and more parents have put their children on courses of TSO, which are porcine (pig) whipworm ova (eggs). As these are not native to humans, they live for only two to three weeks in the human gut. Anecdotal reports have been astounding, to say the least. The children are showing global improvements, which are sometimes dramatic. The incidence of negative side effects is extremely low, and consists of nothing more than reports of increased hyperactivity, some agitation, and sleep disturbances.

My son Alex is fifteen years old, and profoundly autistic. In 2002, an endoscopy/colonoscopy showed that he had horrific bowel disease (colitis) and his immune system was so compromised that to live he required intravenous immunoglobulin (IVIG human antibodies) IVs for seven years. I first read of parasite therapy and the hygiene hypothesis (the idea that we are too sterile, too devoid of normal microbiota) in 1999, in an article in *The New York Times*, which described the work being done with TSO by Dr. Joel Weinstock, who was then at the University of Iowa. Dr. Weinstock had tested these worms in seven individuals with inflammatory bowel disease, and had six of them enter remission. The seventh also dramatically improved. I tried to get the University of Iowa to treat Alex, but as he fit none of their criteria, they would not. It took me eight years of waiting to be able to get TSO for him, but when I finally did (in October, 2007) Alex's response was as dramatic as I always knew it would be.

Within ten weeks his perpetual stomach bloating began to disappear. His evening screaming attacks stopped as the pain from the gas subsided. His mood become more and more stable—he was happy almost all the time. The changes were remarkable, and this in a child who has rarely responded to any treatment.

Now, many children with autism have responded extraordinarily well to TSO: improved digestive functioning, increased language and cognition, improved social skills, better mood and mood regulation, and more. The average amount of time it takes to begin to observe the changes is about twelve weeks. Some children, however, have certainly taken longer, even up to eighteen weeks. TSO is taken orally: small vials of saline solution containing the invisible ova are drunk every two to three weeks. However, TSO is so expensive at the moment that it is beyond the reach of many families, especially considering that it must be done continuously.

Because of the expense, I looked for other parasites that would do the same and cost less. Alex (as do several other children on the spectrum), now hosts a small number of human whipworms (*Trichuris trichuria*) and hookworm, *Necator americanus*. It is too soon to comment on how the TTO (*Trichuris trichuria* ova) is working, but the hookworm caused similar benefits in the children: improved academic/cognitive functioning. In fact, within eight weeks of his first dose, Alex (who at the time was fourteen years old) demonstrated the ability to read for the first time.

Hookworm and whipworm cannot reproduce directly in their host. They live in the intestines and lay eggs, which are passed out in stool; under certain specific environmental circumstances, the eggs then mature to an infective stage, at which point they can enter the host. (When we lived without modern plumbing and hygiene practices, stool would end up on soil or in water.) Thus, there is no danger of being "infested." If any adverse symptoms do occur, the worms can be destroyed with a dose or two of an antiparasitic medication, such as albendazole.

That said, there have not yet been any formal studies done on children with autism, and not many on adults with different issues. Those contemplating trying this therapy should be aware that it is untested and that no one can guarantee safety 100 percent. (Then again, this is true for almost all therapies, both accepted and alternative.)

Parasites like TSO are not prescription medications. They are natural substances, purchased on one's own through companies like Ovamed (www.ovamed.org). However, it is a wise idea to proceed only with a doctor's approval and guidance, since albendazole is a prescription. (TSO will die in two to three weeks anyway, but it is always best to proceed with reasonable caution.)

There is far more we don't know than we do about the immunological causes of autism, the events that have triggered the abnormalities, and mostly the way to remediate the condition. We don't even know if these abnormalities I have described are the cause of autistic symptoms, and if they are, how they caused the developmental problems. Parasite therapy may seem radical to many, but after fourteen years of battling my son's tremendous immune and digestive disorders, and after many months of research on the topic, I made the decision (the right one, as it turns out) to proceed. My philosophy was beautifully expressed by Dr. Herbert at the Autism One conference in Chicago, in May, 2008: "When faced with prolonged scientific uncertainty, use your best judgment."

THE HOLISTIC APPROACH TO NEURODEVELOPMENT AND LEARNING EFFICIENCY (HANDLE)

BY CAROLYN NUYENS AND MARLENE SULITEANU

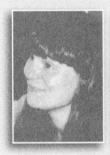 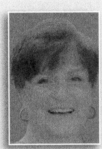

Carolyn Nuyens and Marlene Suliteanu,
OTR/L

The HANDLE Institute
7 Mt. Lassen Drive, Suite B110
San Rafael, CA 94903
(415) 479-1800
www.handle.org

Carolyn Nuyens, executive director of The HANDLE Institute, has extensive personal and professional experience in the autism community. She is a Certified HANDLE Practitioner and Instructor. She traveled to India in 2005 with the creator of HANDLE, Judith Bluestone, to introduce HANDLE to the autism community there.

Marlene Suliteanu, OTR/L, also a Certified HANDLE Practitioner and Instructor, with a therapy practice in Oceanside, California, is Judith Bluestone's sister. Judith authored *The Fabric of Autism: Weaving the Threads Into A Cogent Theory* as a semi-autobiographical, in-depth explanation of how HANDLE understands autism.

No two individuals diagnosed with autism present with exactly the same concerns or behaviors. Therefore nothing about HANDLE is arbitrary, standardized, or self-limiting. This article presents both what knowledge HANDLE practitioners share with others who would attempt to help folks on the spectrum, and how the unique HANDLE principles and practices differ from those others.

Characteristics, Commonalities

Although each person on the spectrum is unique, neurodevelopmental characteristics shared by many individuals with autism are:

1. Hypersensitivities, especially auditory, tactile, and vestibular—which means bothered by sounds and irritated by imposed touch sensations (think: seams in socks, tags in shirts, hugs and kisses), and "gravitational insecurity" because the vestibular system tells us how gravity is acting on our bodies.

2. Low muscle tone (throughout the body)—which is about the readiness to respond to task challenges, of which the first and uncontrollable one is gravity itself; and it's what we use to modulate movements (how fast, how hard, etc).

Another experience shared by many on the spectrum: digestive disorders. HANDLE practitioners consider it likely that hypersensitive ears contribute to that, because the jaw is next to the ears. When chewing anything sounds very loud (which it does if our ears are hypersensitive), we avoid chewing, and thus don't start the digestive process soon enough for the stomach to know what enzymes to create. This is only one simple example of how irregularities in one system can cause irregularities in others. There are typically multiple contributing factors to digestive problems that individuals on the spectrum experience.

A commonality considered vital is *language*, especially related to interpersonal relationships and as it affects how some professionals gauge intelligence. Producing intelligible and appropriate language is probably the most complex task anyone achieves: it requires oral-motor precision and learned patterns of movement, and all of that must happen synchronized with breathing. Remember that auditory issues and low muscle tone recur among many individuals on the spectrum; either or both can limit effective spoken communication. Adding in the need to partner right hemisphere (ideas) with left hemisphere (words and sentence structure) complicates the more "physical" elements significantly.

There is a crucial one not yet named: *stress*. When life is difficult—proportional to how challenged anyone feels at any given time—there is an internal experience of stress. For essentially everyone on the autism spectrum, the body/brain baseline level of stress is very high. Anything added to systems already struggling to create and maintain stability can be overwhelming. "Anything" can mean perfumes, crowds (especially of children), household cleaning products, even medications, and always includes performance and behavioral expectations beyond the person's ability.

Because HANDLE practitioners know that, they understand that a "tantrum" or "meltdown" is actually a call for help, a plea to notice that the stress level has overflowed its container. A word of caution to family members: Try to identify what pushed your loved one beyond endurance—and don't expect it to always be the same thing. It could be noise in high-ceilinged supermarkets; or maybe it was the crowds, or smells, or any combination of these things. Always trust that there *is* a precipitating cause.

Who provides HANDLE services? Where?

The HANDLE Institute (in San Rafael, CA) confers the credential of Certified HANDLE Practitioner on individuals who have completed (1) a sequence of post-graduate intensive and explicit training programs; (2) a supervised internship, the duration of which is not time-based but competence-based and therefore varies in length from nine months to several years; and (3) an exam for which there are no "right" answers, but rather engaging the intern in processing and reasoning from the HANDLE perspective, and to applying neuroscience creatively and always individually. There are also Certified HANDLE Screeners, but their clientele are usually not on the autism spectrum.

The practitioners represent diverse backgrounds: there are educators, counselors, occupational therapists, a chiropractic neurologist, and others from diverse fields of endeavor. There are practitioners on every continent. Two Canadian provinces have certified practitioners: Ontario and British Columbia. The environment in which HANDLE services occur varies too, but has in common the interpersonal relationship foundation of nonjudgmental respect, and a "physical" manifestation of the core HANDLE premise: stressed systems to do not get stronger. So each site in which you encounter a HANDLE practitioner will strive to minimize sensory disturbance. Practitioners even wear only all-natural clothing without dramatic patterns or harsh colors, and no scents. The site limits auditory or visual distractions. Work surfaces are wood. And you won't find reflective surfaces like mirrors.

What is a HANDLE program?

Although there are slight variations specific to the practitioner and the site, basically the program consists of a three-part start-up sequence, followed by six about-monthly Program Review visits.

The start-up sequence:

1. Evaluation

The HANDLE Practitioner provides a comprehensive and sensitive evaluation (usually employing the copyrighted Learning Foundations Inventory) involving interactive tasks; assessment of specific neurodevelopmental functions; and an extensive interview of client, plus in some cases parents and other caregivers, to gather information about particular concerns such as health problems, nutrition, sleep, and pertinent details of the developmental history. The initial evaluation is typically scheduled for two hours, but varies depending on the complexity of the situation and the client's participation.

The HANDLE practitioner observes the individual's response patterns during this unique series of tasks and rapport-building activities. The client's responses are never judged, and do not result in any scores or diagnostic labels. Instead, the responses provide information to help the practitioner see how the body/brain system is working. The practitioner analyzes how the client takes in, processes, and uses information. Seemingly perplexing behaviors come together like pieces of a puzzle, as the HANDLE practitioner analyzes both the individual systems and how the systems interact with each other.

Among the functions and systems considered are:
- Olfaction and gustation (smell and taste)
- Tactility and kinesthesia (touch and movement)
- Vestibular functions (balance, proprioception, muscle tone)
- Visual functions (including visual tracking, convergence, accommodation, and specific light sensitivity)
- Oral motor functions (dental factors, speech articulation)
- Hearing and auditory processing (sequence, syntax, meaning)
- Reflex inhibition and differentiation of movement/response
- Rhythm and timing
- Lateralization (right-versus-left)
- Midline crossing and interhemispheric integration
- Receptive and expressive language skills
- Visual discrimination and memory
- Visual-motor integration
- Visual-spatial processing
- Temporal-spatial organization
- Attentional priorities

2. Instruction: *Neurodevelopmental Profile and Recommended Program*

The practitioner assembles the findings of the evaluation into a chart of those interactive and interdependent sensory-motor systems: what's serving him/her well, and how it does; and what's getting in his/her way, interfering with efficient function. This image is the Neurodevelopmental Profile.

Based on that Profile, the practitioner recommends an initial program of seemingly simple activities, each of which is complex neurologically and addresses several aspects of what interferes with the client's ability to satisfy life's demands efficiently. Two examples: a Crazy Straw, used as instructed, supports focused vision, even bowel and bladder continence, as well as the more obvious oral motor skills; Face Tapping stimulates the trigeminal nerve to integrate all five senses, affecting speech and auditory sensitivity (especially important to folks on the spectrum). Nutritional recommendations may be made, as well as suggestions for environmental or lifestyle changes to improve functioning and reduce stress.

HANDLE routes each person toward his/her full potential with an individualized program of activities that require virtually no special equipment, to gently enhance functioning. The client is guided through each activity to help his/her brain/body system process and organize information more efficiently. Each HANDLE program is customized for effective implementation in the client's home or other supportive setting. The program usually requires less than a half hour daily to complete, doesn't have to be done all at once, or even in a certain order. Some activities may require support from a helper.

The HANDLE practitioner gives the client whatever materials are needed to do each activity, including written instructions. Both the assessment and the presentation are recorded and the client receives a copy as a DVD.

Among the key distinctions of a HANDLE program is the one principle guiding every kind of sensory-motor activity and other recommendation. It is called Gentle Enhancement. The objective of each recommended activity is to provide organized stimulation without producing stress. Weak, disorganized, damaged, or immature systems need to be "gently enhanced." The parent or caregiver is taught to recognize the signs of a stress state change and deal with it in an effective manner; and the client learns how to identify how the body conveys its needs, to respect them too. Gently enhanced systems get stronger; stressed systems shut down. It's a near-reflexive way that the brain fulfills its primal directive, namely to keep us safe. Honoring the body's signals of what input it can use and what exceeds its tolerance—at all times—earns from the body a comparable kind of respect: the client stabilizes, to enable him/her to function more efficiently.

3. Fine-tuning Follow-up

A week to ten days later the client returns to the practitioner to assure reliable familiarity with everything that was taught: *why* as well as how to implement the program independently. During this one- to two-hour appointment the practitioner watches the client perform all the activities in the program, making corrections or adjustments as needed. Just as importantly, the client is encouraged to give feedback about the program and what was experienced. Often it surprises clients and families that changes can have occurred within that first week, and the practitioner asks about those changes. Video recordings made of all clinical sessions provide the client and caregiver a tool for easy reference at home.

Program Review Visits

After approximately one month of the client-family's implementing the recommendations, they return to the practitioner to determine whether changes that have occurred due to the neurological reorganization, the creation of neural connections, and/or the kinesthetic learning warrant different activities. Often the initial program establishes prerequisites to higher level challenges. This sequencing logic applies thereafter. That is, as the client implements HANDLE recommendations, changes occur; those changes represent gains in systems that previously interfered with function; now those systems can accept additional challenges, toward full functional interaction with the other systems of the body.

Program reviews are usually scheduled every four to six weeks, depending upon client needs. Some clients choose to receive off-site program reviews, via Skype, or through e-mail discussion and videotapes/DVDs.

What Changes can you expect from a HANDLE program?

The most frequent report of post-HANDLE behavior changes are "more calm" and "sleeps better." Other gains: toilet training, eye contact, hair washing, balance, organization, focus—etc.!— including communication skills, both receptive and expressive language. Given the vast diversity among clients, there is no way to predict changes precisely. What always happens is gains in the interactive dynamism of all the sensory-motor systems, and that in turn, enables more efficient functioning, which means less stress. Combining the strengthened sensory-motor interaction with the client applying the principle of Gentle Enhancement, and it's easy to understand how a reduced stress level generalizes. Less stress clearly looks like a "more calm" life, and can allow the client to sleep better; it also often means better digestion, and a stronger immune system, thus less susceptible to illness.

A Book About HANDLE

You can find a more extensive explanation of how HANDLE understands autism, in *The Fabric of Autism: Weaving the Threads Into A Cogent Theory,* by Judith Bluestone.

HYPERBARIC OXYGEN THERAPY: LET'S PUT THE PRESSURE ON AUTISM FOR RECOVERY

BY Dr. James Neubrander

James A. Neubrander, M.D., FAAEM

Comprehensive Neuroscience Center
100 Menlo Park, Suites 410 and 200
Edison, NJ 08837
(732) 906-9000; (732) 906-7888
www.drneubrander.com
www.neuro-center.com
www.IBRFinc.org

Dr. Neubrander trained in pathology and laboratory medicine and is board certified in Environmental Medicine. He is the Medical Director of Autism Research for the International Brain Research Foundation and Medical Director of the Comprehensive Neuroscience Center in Edison, New Jersey. He serves on many scientific advisory boards dedicated to treating autism and neurodevelopmental disorders. He lectures many times each year at national and international conferences and physician training courses. His lectures are scientific, evidence-based, and emphasize newer treatments or modifications of established protocols that appear to enhance clinical outcomes beyond the results previously reported. He is the coauthor of several peer-reviewed articles, has been interviewed and filmed for many documentaries and television spots, has been referenced in many books written about autism, nutrition, and environmental medicine, and has been quoted innumerable times by scientists, researchers, clinicians, and lay persons, most notably for methylcobalamin, hyperbaric oxygen, and heavy metal detoxification.

Hyperbaric therapy, also known as hyperbaric oxygen (HBO) or hyperbaric oxygen therapy (HBOT), is a specialized therapy applying an increase in atmospheric pressure, with or without a concurrent increase in oxygen concentration, to incorporate more oxygen *onto* the red cells and to dissolve more oxygen *into* body water: plasma, lymph, cerebrospinal fluid, interstitial fluid, etc. This is accomplished by using specialized chambers, either *multiplace,* which treats many patients simultaneously, or *monoplace* in which only one person can be treated at a time.

Hyperbaric therapy is classically defined as the inhalation of 100 percent oxygen at greater than one atmosphere absolute (ATA) in a pressurized chamber. This definition is now popularly defined as the inhalation of varying degrees of oxygen at greater than one atmosphere absolute (ATA) in a pressurized chamber and referred to by the autism community as "HBOT."

Treatment pressures and oxygen concentrations are *always compared against values at sea level* where the pressure is one atmosphere and oxygen concentration is 21 percent. The basic principle of the gas laws states that the behavior of a gas is defined by the pressure, volume, temperature, solubility characteristics, and diffusion properties. In simple terms, the greater the pressure and/or the greater the oxygen concentration breathed, the more oxygen molecules that will be dissolved into the plasma. It is important to know that three factors are varied to achieve treatment protocols and clinical results for children with autism: a) how much pressure is applied, most commonly varying from 1.3 to 1.75 atmospheres; b) how strong the oxygen concentration is, most commonly varying from 24 percent to 100 percent; and c) how long the treatment session lasts, most commonly 1 hour to 1.5 hours per "dive" (the common term for a treatment). *Hyperbaric therapy is truly drug therapy* because too much is toxic, too little is ineffective, and the amount of time between dosing affects both its toxicity and effectiveness profiles.

Approved indications for HBO therapy do not include autism. They are intracranial abscess; anemia from severe blood loss; burns; carbon monoxide poisoning; compartment syndrome; decompression sickness (DCS); embolisms; gas gangrene; infections (refractory); injuries (crush, radiation); ischemias (acute and severe); wound healing, including skin flaps and grafts that are compromised. *Unapproved conditions* for HBO are many—autism being one. Each condition has shown HBO to be an effective adjunctive therapy as documented in published studies. Unfortunately, insurance companies rarely reimburse for these unapproved therapies.

The first known record for the use of hyperbaric therapy was in 320 BC, when Alexander the Great used a chamber that was submersed under water. In 1500, Leonardo da Vinci drew sketches of diving vessels but did not pursue the concept. In 1772, Karl W. Scheele discovered oxygen independently from Joseph Priestly, an amateur English chemist who in 1775 also discovered oxygen independently from Karl W. Scheele. Therefore, Scheele and Priestley are both given credit for its discovery. Priestly named it "dephlogisticated air." It was later renamed "oxygen" by Antoine Lavoisier.

In 1783, the French physician Caillens was the first doctor reported to use oxygen therapy as a remedy. In the mid- to late 1800s, the first severe problems with decompression sickness were seen in coal miners and caisson workers, many of whom died. In 1878, Paul Bert published *Barometric Pressure: Researches in Experimental Physiology*, describing caisson's disease and the bubble theory of decompression sickness (DCS) and oxygen toxicity. In 1889, Moir developed the first recompression chamber to treat DCS. In 1899, Lorraine-Smith described pulmonary oxygen toxicity. In 1921, Cunningham from Kansas City, Missouri built a 10-foot by 88-foot chamber that used compressed air to treat hypoxic states, hypertension, syphilis, cancer, and diabetes. This resulted in a successful challenge by the American Medical Association (AMA) in the 1930s. In 1928, Henry Timken from Cleveland, Ohio, built a six-story, seventy-two-room hyperbaric hotel, but the 1929 stock market crash caused the hotel to fail. Between the 1930s and 1940s, Behnke established oxygen tolerance limits for divers, which remain the basis for the oxygen recompression treatment tables still used today.

The recent history of hyperbaric medicine begins with Boerema, the father of modern hyperbaric medicine. In the late '50s, he filmed pigs, whose red cells had been removed, living with pure oxygen under hyperbaric conditions while only their plasma remained. This phenomenon was published in 1960 in *Life Without Blood*. In 1967, the Undersea Medical Society *(UMS)* was formed and considers itself to be the guardian of hyperbaric medicine. In 1977, Davis and Hunt published the first Hyperbaric Oxygen Therapy textbook.

The era of hyperbaric medicine for autism began in 2002 when Heuser published positive SPECT scan results from a four-year-old child with autism who had undergone HBO therapy. In 2005, though not directly related to autism, *Stoller* documented positive neurocognitive changes from hyperbaric oxygen therapy in a case of fetal alcohol syndrome sixteen years post injury.

The above two studies became the foundation upon which clinicians treating autism, at that time believed to be an untreatable "hard-wired" disorder, hypothesized that HBO may help their patients. In 2005, in an unpublished study, Buckley and Kartzinel described positive SPECT scan results and clinical findings after using low-pressure, low-oxygen concentrations in autistic children. From 2006–2009, Rossignol published several studies regarding HBO and autism. Included was the first double-blind placebo-controlled study from six centers (one of which was Neubrander's) that documented low-pressure, low-oxygen concentrations to be an effective treatment for autism. In 2007, at a think tank in California, Neubrander reported increased clinical responsiveness from a one-month diagnostic protocol he specifically designed for children with autism. In 2009, Thatcher and Neubrander published a paper which demonstrated, by quantitative EEG (qEEG) technique, the phase reset phenomenon that occurs in children with autism. Their study demonstrated that children with autism had a significantly *shortened* period of time for neuronal recruitment (phase shift) followed by a significantly *increased* amount of time necessary to process the information that was gathered (phase lock). Also in 2009, at a think tank in Chicago, Neubrander presented his and De Fina's preliminary findings demonstrating that his low pressure, low oxygen concentration "diagnostic protocol" and the standard high pressure, 100 percent oxygen protocols both began to correct the phase shift and phase lock abnormalities. The neuronal recruitment period was lengthened and the excessive processing time was decreased. However, at the same think tank, Granpeesheh and Bradstreet shared the findings of their double-blind, placebo-controlled study. Their study showed low-pressure, low-oxygen concentrations, similar to the ones used in the Rossignol study, to not be clinically significant. Those of us involved in the Rossignol study strongly disagree with their findings. In addition, their findings do not reflect my clinical experience after closely monitoring over 800 children and 75,000 treatment hours for children with autism using the specific protocols I have designed for this important subset of the population.

When it comes to the use of hyperbaric oxygen for children with autism, parents don't really care much about definitions, history, philosophy, or our scientific debates. What they want is enough preliminary science to support its use and demonstrate its safety. Though they prefer double-blind, placebo-controlled, crossover studies, what they require is strong anecdotal evidence by other parents who have children just like theirs and face the same challenges that they face everyday. Their main concern is not whether science has "dotted all its I's and crossed all its T's" beyond a shadow of a doubt, but rather there be a treatment that has the potential of helping their child now, not at some distant point in the future. Nor is their main concern whether or not their doctor will support them, but rather that have they attempted to do all they believe they could and should be doing before their child's window of opportunity permanently closes. Contrary to the popular wisdom of an old paradigm, parents who seek my colleagues' and my treatments are well-studied, well-read, and usually college-educated. They are definitely not a bunch of gullible, ill-informed lemmings, following charlatan Pied-Piper physicians who are just out to fleece them because they are desperate.

I could share *hundreds* of stories of children who responded positively to HBOT from my clinic. Should you be interested, you can see videos of parents talking about what HBOT did for their child at *www.drneubrander.com*. Though exceptions do occur, as a general rule, most children respond only mildly or mild-to-moderately within the first forty-hour treatment "set." However, HBO therapy, if continued intermittently for several cycles, is one of the most powerful treatments I have to induce language, increase awareness and cognition, and allow more normal socialization and emotional responses. As an example of "a best-case scenario," consider two boys from different families who came to my clinic August 2007. One boy was eight years old and the other boy was eleven years old. Both boys spoke with only two or three word utterances, had little socialization, and engaged in parallel play with minimal to no interaction with peers. Thirty days later, both boys were speaking in six- to nine-word sentences, with adjectives, adverbs, prepositions, pronouns, and conjunctions. In addition, not only would they now participate in interactive play, they would initiate it with other children. However, best-case examples do not paint the real picture that most parents will experience if they try HBOT for their child. The most common examples I see in my clinic are initially reported by parents to show mild or mild-to-moderate changes, not moderate to significant ones. The top twenty improvements most commonly seen include positive changes in language, eye contact, self-awareness, general awareness, independence, emotional responses, and gastrointestinal regulation.

Success does not occur in a vacuum. In my experience, in order to increase the benefit-to-cost ratio, pre-treatment with adjunctive therapies is required. Those I use to accomplish this goal, prior to initiating HBO, require six to twelve weeks of methyl-B$_{12}$ injections and key supplements.

You ask, *What are the risks?* The worst-case scenario occurred in Florida late in the spring of 2009 when an *old* monoplace chamber ignited and fatally burned a child and his grandmother. In general, HBOT therapy, as done in the United States using up-to-date chambers that are not homemade, boasts an incredible safety record, with only this one incident having occurred in the last forty years. This includes chambers used in clinics and at home. When parents follow strict safety guidelines and receive prerequisite medical and technical training courses, like the ones we require at our clinic, contrary to what some organizations tell their patients and post on the Internet using scare tactics, portable HBOT chambers can be safely used in the home setting. This allows a valuable treatment to be ongoing rather than intermittent, and a treatment that becomes less expensive rather than more expensive over time, for those who own their own chambers.

So, what are the real risks? Barotrauma, which occurs in 2 percent of individuals, is usually minor and analogous to "mildly spraining the eardrums." The risk of seizures, what parents worry about the most, increases by 0.01 percent to 0.03 percent. Perforated eardrums can occur when chamber operators pressurize too quickly prior to the ears being able to clear. The take-home message is that HBOT is as safe as flying in an airplane, when safety procedures are carefully followed.

There are many clinics in the country that will offer HBOT to children with autism. Hospitals will not offer this service because they are only allowed to use HBOT for the approved indications shown above. Private clinics do not have these restrictions, and are therefore more than willing to treat children with autism. Such clinics are not difficult to find by conducting a Google search. It is important to note that protocols from different clinics vary significantly. The variations include: 1) the pressures used, which vary all the way from 1.1 to 2.8 ATA; 2) whether oxygen is delivered by an oxygen concentrator or 100 percent pure oxygen; 3) the time used per session, commonly varying between sixty to ninety minutes; 4) the number of sessions used per day varying between one and two; 5) the time between sessions varying between two and twelve hours; 6) and the number of treatment hours per treatment "set," most commonly forty hours but as high as ninety hours. Parents rightfully ask, *What protocol or clinic is the best for my child?* The answer is, *No one knows*. Opinions abound. Clinicians do not agree. Unfortunately, the research needed to document that HBOT is a valuable treatment for children on the autism spectrum will require hundreds of thousands of dollars and no less then ten to fifteen years to complete and then to replicate prior to becoming an accepted practice that is reimbursable by insurance companies. Once that fact has been established, to determine which protocols are the most effective will require additional hundreds of thousands of dollars and an additional ten to fifteen years. Knowing that, the last question parents must ask themselves is, "How old will my child be by then and what do I want to do in the meantime?"

Therefore, parents wishing to investigate this treatment option for their children must be diligent in their research. They need to understand that the treatment is expensive and comes with no guarantees. If they want to do HBO, they need to look for a clinic that produces quality care, a clinic that has treated many children with autism, and a clinic that believes children with autism not only can be helped, but deserve to be helped today.

INTEGRATED PLAY GROUPS (IPG) MODEL

BY DR. PAMELA WOLFBERG

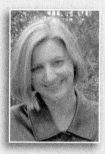

Pamela Wolfberg, Ph.D.

Autism Institute on Peer Relations and Play
Integrated Play Groups Training,
Research and Development Center
www.AutismInstitute.com or www.wolfberg.com
info@wolfberg.com

Associate Professor/Director, Autism Spectrum Program
Department of Special Education
San Francisco State University,
1600 Holloway Avenue
San Francisco,
CA 94132,
(415) 338-7651.
Wolfberg@sfsu.edu

Pamela Wolfberg, Ph.D. is Associate Professor and Director of the Autism Spectrum program at San Francisco State University and co-founder of the Autism Institute on Peer Relations and Play.. She received her doctorate from the University of California, Berkeley. As originator of the Integrated Play Groups (IPG) model, she leads research, training and development efforts to establish inclusive peer socialization programs worldwide. She is widely published and the author of *Play and Imagination in Children with Autism* and *Peer Play and the Autism Spectrum: The Art of Guiding Children's Socialization and Imagination*. She is the recipient of several distinguished awards for her scholarship, research and service to the community.

Integrated Play Groups (IPG) is an empirically validated model for promoting socialization, communication, play, and imagination in children on the autism spectrum, while building relationships with typical peers and siblings in natural settings. (Wolfberg, 2009, 2003) The model is grounded in current theory, research, and practice pertinent to addressing core challenges in autism that affect both social and representational aspects of play. Embedded in this model are methods for observing, interpreting, and building on children's play interests and social communicative abilities, and for designing environments conducive to social and imaginative play.

Conceptually, the IPG model is described as multidimensional, encompassing developmental and ecological features that are framed in sociocultural theory. (Vygotsky, 1966; 1978) In practical terms, an IPG brings together children with autism (novice players) in mutually engaging play experiences with more capable peer play partners (expert players) while guided by a qualified adult facilitator (play guide). Each IPG is individualized as a part of a child's comprehensive educational and therapy program. IPG programs take place in natural settings, including in the home, school and community. Group members range from three to five players with a higher ratio of expert to novice players. Each group meets twice weekly for thirty to sixty minutes sessions over a twelve-week period, or longer. Play sessions are tailored to the unique interests, developmental capacities, and sociocultural experiences of child participants.

Drawing on finely tuned assessments, the IPG intervention (guided participation) provides a system of support for maximizing each child's developmental potential and intrinsic motivation to play, socialize, and form meaningful relationships with other children. Equal emphasis is placed on guiding the typical peers to be more accepting, responsive, and inclusive of children who may present differing ways of playing communicating and relating to others. Moreover, novice and expert players are encouraged to mediate their own play activities with as little adult guidance as possible.

The IPG model was created by Pamela Wolfberg, Ph.D. (Associate Professor and Director of the Autism Spectrum Program, San Francisco State University, and cofounder of the Autism Institute on Peer Relations and Play). In its early conception, Dr. Wolfberg worked in close collaboration with Adriana Schuler, Ph.D. (Professor Emeritus, SFSU) and Therese O'Connor, MA (Co-founder of the Autism Institute on Peer Relations and Play). Over the years, the model has continued to evolve and expand, owing to the collective efforts of many other remarkable professionals, family members and the children themselves participating in local, national and international training, research, and development initiatives.

The IPG model was first initiated as a pilot research project in an urban elementary school, with a small grant from the San Francisco Education Fund. (Wolfberg, 1988) Based on the preliminary success of this project, the IPG model was expanded through a model demonstration and research project that was supported, in part, through a grant from the United States Department of Education. (Wolfberg & Schuler, 1992) In 2000, the Autism Institute on Peer Relations and

Play (www.autisminstitute.com) was established as a center for IPG training, research, and development. Opportunities for IPG training, research, and development are also offered as a part of the Autism Spectrum Graduate Program (Project Mosaic) at SFSU (www.sfsu.edu~autism), and in conjunction with our other major research projects with support from Autism Speaks (Wolfberg, Turiel & DeWitt, 2008) and the Alexander von Humboldt Foundation. (Julius & Wolfberg, 2009)

A wide range of professionals and family members have received initial preparation for applying the practices of the IPG model in inclusive settings. To become fully qualified to formally deliver the IPG model as a program or service with an official endorsement (i.e., certification) from the Autism Institute on Peer Relations and Play requires intensive training and supervision at the advanced level. Advanced training comprises a competency-based curriculum that draws on the foundational book: *Play and Imagination in Children with Autism* (Wolfberg, 2009) and the IPG Field Manual *Peer Play and the Autism Spectrum: The Art of Guiding Socialization and Imagination.* (Wolfberg, 2003)

Currently, the IPG model is being adopted by increasing numbers of schools and organizations at the local, national, and international level. The expansion of programs around the globe coincides with the IPG model having gained widespread recognition as among established research-based practices for children on the autism spectrum. (see for example: California Department of Education, 1997; Iovannone, 2003; National Autism Center, 2009) This is consistent with the recommendations of the National Research Council, (2001) which has ranked the teaching of play skills with peers among the six types of interventions that should have priority in the design and delivery of effective educational programs for children on the autism spectrum.

To address the growing need to support diverse learners on the autism spectrum and their families, extensions of the IPG model are also emerging through collaborative efforts. Incorporated into the model are such innovations as sensory integration, drama, art, video and other creative activities of high interest for children as well as teens. (see for example Bottema, 2008; Fuge & Berry, 2004; Neufeld & Wolfberg, 2009; Wolfberg & Julius, 2009; Wolfberg, McCracken & Tuchel, 2008) Another current initiative is focused on universal playground design and programming that supports the unique social, imaginative, and sensory needs of children on the autism spectrum in mutually engaging experiences with peers and siblings. (Wolfberg, 2010) These newer efforts are currently at various stages of development and investigation.

Success Rate

The IPG model has an established and growing research base documenting ample evidence of a high success rate. A series of small- and large-scale studies have been and are currently being conducted to evaluate and replicate the IPG model. (Gonsier-Gerdin, 1993; Lantz, Nelson & Loftin, 2004; Mikaelan, 2003; O'Connor, 1999; Richard & Goupil, 2005; Wolfberg, 1988; 1994; 2009; Wolfberg & Julius, 2009; Wolfberg & Schuler, 1992; 1993; Wolfberg, Turiel, & DeWitt, 2008; Yang, Wolfberg, Wu & Hwu , 2003; Zercher, Hunt, Schuler & Webster, 2001) Most investigations have been focusing on the effect of the intervention on the social, communication, and play development of children with autism, representing diverse abilities (mild to moderate to severe), ages (three to eleven years), settings (community, home, school) , geographic locations (Asia, Europe, North America) and languages (English, French, German, Chinese). Social validation measures assessing parent perceptions of the impact of the intervention on their children with autism have also been included.

Overall, outcomes for the children with autism consistently show relative gains in social, communication, and play development. Specifically, decreases in isolate and stereotypic play have been noted, along with collateral gains in increasingly socially coordinated play and representational play (functional and pretend). Language gains also have been noted in several cases. Further, the evidence suggests that skills may be maintained after adult support is withdrawn. The data also supports evidence of generalization beyond the specific IPG across peers/siblings, settings, and social activity contexts.

The attitudes, perceptions, and experiences of the expert players have been explored through observation and interviews with play guides and the children themselves. Findings to date suggest that the peers developed greater sensitivity, tolerance, and acceptance of the novice players' individual differences. They also articulated a sense of responsibility as well as an understanding of how to include the less skilled players by adapting to their different interests and styles of communication. Novice and expert players also reported having fun while forming mutual friendships extending beyond the IPG.

Risk and/or side-effects

There are no known risks or side effects associated with the IPG model when implemented with fidelity.

INTESTINE, LEAKY GUT, AUTISM, AND PROBIOTICS

BY DR. ALESSIO FASANO

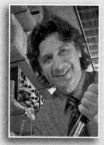

Alessio Fasano, MD

University of Maryland School of Medicine
Mucosal Biology Research Center and Center for Celiac Research
Health Science Facility II, Room S345
20 Penn Street
Baltimore, MD 21201
(410) 706-5501
Fax. (410) 706-5508
afasano@mbrc.umaryland.edu

Dr. Fasano is Professor of Pediatrics, Medicine, and Physiology at the University of Maryland School of Medicine and is the Director of the Mucosal Biology Research center at the same Institution. Dr. Fasano was born in Italy, where he completed is training as a pediatric gastroenterologist. In 1993, he was recruited at the University of Maryland and founded the Division of Pediatric Gastroenterology and Nutrition. In 1996, he established the Center for Celiac Research, a unique facility that offers state-of-the-art research, teaching, and clinical expertise for the diagnosis, treatment, and prevention of celiac disease. Dr. Fasano's research program encompasses both basic and clinical areas, including bacterial pathogenesis, intestinal pathophysiology, and prevention and treatment of both acute and chronic diarrheal diseases. In recent years, Dr. Fasano's research has focused on intercellular tight junctions (TJ) pathophysiology and its role in the pathogenesis of autoimmune diseases, with special emphasis on celiac disease. Dr. Fasano has published more than 170 peer-reviewed papers and his research quality and creativity is further reflected in the filing of more than 160 patent applications, many of which are approved. He is an elected member of the American Society for Clinical Investigation. Because of his translational science, he has been awarded several prizes, including the 2005 Innovator of the Year Award, the 2006 Best Academic/Industry Collaboration Award, the 2006 Entepreneur of the Year Award, the 2007 America's Top Doctor's Award, and the 2009 Researcher of the Year Award. His research has been funded by the National Institutes of Health since 1995. Dr. Fasano has been a permanent member of the NIH study section, and continues to serve as an ad hoc reviewer.

The Intestine and ASD

The human intestine is a deceptively complex organ. It is lined by a single layer of cells exquisitely responsive to stimuli of innumerable variety, and is populated by a complex climax community of microbial partners, far more numerous than the cells of the intestine itself. Under normal circumstances, these intestinal cells form a tight, but selective barrier to "friends and foes": microbes and most environmental substances are held at bay, but nutrients from the essential to the trivial are absorbed efficiently. (1,2) Moreover, the tightness of the epithelial barrier is itself dynamic, though the mechanisms governing and effecting dynamic permeability are poorly understood. What is becoming increasingly clear is that a leaky gut is associated with a large number of local and systemic disorders, including autism spectrum disorders (ASDs). (3)

ASD and Diet

ASDs are heterogeneous neurodevelopmental disorders that affect approximately 1 percent of the general population. (4) It is generally agreed that there are multiple causes for ASD, with both genetic and environmental components involved. Gastrointestinal (GI) symptoms are frequently experienced by subjects with ASD, but their prevalence, nature, and therefore best treatments, remain elusive. (5,6) The most frequent GI symptoms experienced by subjects with ASD include constipation, gastroesophageal reflux, gastritis, intestinal inflammation (autistic enterocolitis), maldigestion, malabsorption, flatulence, abdominal pain or discomfort, lactose intolerance, enteric infections, etc. Of the almost fifty treatments proposed for ASD, seven (antifungal therapy, chelation, enzymes, GI treatments, intestinal parasite therapy, nutritional supplements, and dietary options for autism) are specifically focused to the GI tract, and they will be addressed in detail in other parts of this book. It is worthwhile to note that in a recent survey conducted by the Autism Research Institute involving more than 27,000 parents of autistic kids, avoidance of gluten (~9,000 cases) and/or casein (~7,000 cases) were the most frequent treatments implemented in their children, with a better : worse ratio of 30:1 and 32:1, respectively.

Intestine, Microbiome, and Leaky Gut

A possible unifying theory to "connect the dots" of all the factors mentioned above would link changes in gut microorganisms ecosystem with leaky gut, passage of digestion products of natural food, such as bread and cow's milk that would activate immune inflammatory cells that cause inflammation both in the intestine (autistic enterocolitis) and the brain (ASD). Alternative to the inflammatory hypothesis, it has been proposed that the defect in the intestinal barrier in ASD patients allows passage of neuroactive peptides of food origin into the blood and then into the cerebrospinal fluid, to interfere directly with the function of the central nervous system (CNS). No matter which of the two theories turns out to be correct, changes in intestinal microbiome and the consequent leaky gut seem to be the common denominators. Therefore, it would be logical to consider manipulation of the gut microbiome as the most effective intervention to treat ASD. Among the different strategies currently available to change the gut microbiome, the use of probiotics seems to be the most promising and feasible long-term intervention.

Definition of Probiotics

Probiotics are nonpathogenic bacteria that are claimed to have several beneficial effects related to their capability to either reduce the risk or treat a series of diseases. (7) Most probiotics are bacteria, which are small, single-celled organisms. Bacteria are categorized by scientists with genus, species, and strain names. For example, for the probiotic bacterium *Lactobacillus rhamnosus* GG, the genus is *Lactobacillus*, the species is *rhamnosus,* and the strain is GG. Most probiotic products contain bacteria from the genera *Lactobacillus* or *Bifidobacterium,* although other genera, including *Escherichia, Enterococcus, Bacillus,* and *Saccharomyces* (a yeast) have been marketed as probiotics. The requirements for a microbe to be considered a probiotic are simple. The microbe must be alive when administered, must be documented to have a health benefit, and must be administered at levels shown to confer the benefit. Probiotic products should be safe, effective, and should maintain their effectiveness and potency through the end of product shelf life.

Formulation of Probiotics

Once destined for commercial use, these bacteria are purified, grown in large numbers, concentrated to high doses, and preserved. They are provided in products in one of three basic ways: (8)

- as a culture concentrate added to a food at medium levels, with little or no opportunity for culture growth
- inoculated into a milk-based food (or dietary supplement) and allowed to grow to achieve high levels in a fermented food
- as concentrated and dried cells packaged as dietary supplements such as powders, capsules, or tablets, and delivered at a range of doses

Probiotic bacteria have a long history of association with dairy products. This is because some of the same bacteria that are associated with fermented dairy products also make their homes in different sites of the human body. Some of these microbes, therefore, can play a dual role in transforming milk into a diverse array of fermented dairy products (yogurt, cheese, kefir, etc.), and contributing to the important role of colonizing bacteria. Dairy products may provide a desirable "probiotic delivery vehicle" for several reasons. To date, however, there is little research on the impact of delivery vehicle and probiotic efficacy for any of the possible formats. This is an important area for future research.

The table below lists some commercial strains currently sold as probiotics. (9) Species are listed as reported by manufacturer, which may not reflect the most current taxonomy. Note that to be legitimately called a "probiotic," a strain must have undergone controlled evaluation for efficacy. The strains listed in this table may or may not have been adequately evaluated. The purpose of this table is to give the reader a sense of what is commercially available, not to provide recommendations for probiotic strain use.

Strain	Commercial products	Source
L. acidophilus NCFM *B. lactis* HN019 (DR10) *L. rhamnosus* HN001 (DR20)	Sold as ingredient	Danisco (Madison, WI)
Saccharomyces cerevisiae (boulardii)	Florastor	Biocodex (Creswell, OR)
B. infantis 35264	Align	Procter & Gamble (Mason, OH)
L. fermentum VRI003 (PCC)	Sold as ingredient	Probiomics (Eveleigh, Australia)
L. rhamnosus R0011 *L. acidophilus* R0052	Sold as ingredient	Institut Rosell (Montreal, Canada)
L. acidophilus LA5 *L. paracasei* CRL 431	Sold as ingredient	Chr. Hansen (Milwaukee, WI)
B. lactis Bb-12	Good Start Natural Cultures infant formula	Nestle (Glendale, CA) Chr. Hansen (Milwaukee, WI)
L. casei Shirota *B. breve* strain Yakult	Yakult	Yakult (Tokyo, Japan)
L. casei DN-114 001 ("*L. casei* Immunitas")	DanActive fermented milk	Danone (Paris, France)
B. animalis DN173 010 ("Bifidis regularis")	Activia yogurt	The Dannon Company (Tarrytown, NY)

Strain	Commercial products	Source
L. reuteri RC-14 *L. rhamnosus* GR-1	Femdophilus	Chr. Hansens (Milwaukee, WI) Urex Biotech (London, Ontario, Canada) Jarrow Formulas (Los Angeles, CA)
L. johnsonii Lj-1 (same as NCC533 and formerly *L. acidophilus* La-1)	LC1	Nestlé (Lausanne, Switzerland)
L. plantarum 299V	Sold as ingredient; Good Belly juice product	Probi AB (Lund, Sweden); NextFoods (Boulder, Colorado)
L. rhamnosus 271	Sold as ingredient	Probi AB (Lund, Sweden)
L. reuteri ATCC 55730 ("Protectis")	BioGaia Probiotic chewable tablets or drops	Biogaia (Stockholm, Sweden)
L. rhamnosus GG ("LGG")	Culturelle; Dannon Danimals	Valio Dairy (Helsinki, Finland) The Dannon Company (Tarrytown, NY)
L. rhamnosus LB21 *Lactococcus lactis* L1A	Sold as ingredient	Essum AB (Umeå, Sweden)
L. salivarius UCC118		University College (Cork, Ireland)
B. longum BB536	Sold as ingredient	Morinaga Milk Industry Co., Ltd. (Zama-City, Japan)
L. acidophilus LB	Sold as ingredient	Lacteol Laboratory (Houdan, France)
L. paracasei F19	Sold as ingredient	Medipharm (Des Moines, IA)
Lactobacillus paracasei 33 *Lactobacillus rhamnosus* GM-020 *Lactobacillus paracasei* GMNL-33	Sold as Ingredient	GenMont Biotech (Taiwan)

Strain	Commercial products	Source
L. plantarum OM	Sold as Ingredient	Bio-Energy Systems, Inc. (Kalispell, MT)
Bacillus coagulans BC30	Sustenex, Digestive Advantage and sold as ingredient	Ganeden Biotech Inc. Cleveland, OH)
Streptococcus oralis KJ3 *Streptococcus uberis* KJ2 *Streptococcus rattus* JH145	ProBiora3 EvoraPlus	Oragenics Inc. (Alachua, FL)

Safety of Probiotics

Although the safety of traditional lactic starter bacteria has never been in question, the more recent use of intestinal isolates of bacteria delivered in high numbers to consumers with potentially compromised health has raised the question of safety. The safety of lactobacilli and bifidobacteria has been reviewed by qualified experts in the field. The general conclusion is that the pathogenic potential of lactobacilli and bifidobacteria is quite low. This is based on the prevalence of these microbes in fermented food, as normal colonizers of the human body, and the low level of infection attributed to them. However, reports of association of lactobacilli and bifidobacteria with human infection (commonly endocarditis) in patients with compromised health suggest that these microbes have rare opportunistic capability.

In many countries, the use of probiotics is not regulated by legislation comparable to that applied to drugs. Hence, the use of probiotics has become widespread despite the fact that their efficacy in clinical practice is not based on solid scientific evidence. For this reason, probiotics are often catalogued as "alternative" therapies.

Efficacy of Probiotics

While the initial use of probiotics was based on anecdotal reports of their beneficial effects, we have more recently witnessed a series of more rigorously designed clinical trials documenting the potential use of probiotics for the treatment of a variety of pediatric disorders, including enteric infectious diseases, allergic and atopic disorders, and intestinal inflammatory diseases. The two most studied probiotics are lactobacillus GG and bifidobacteria BB12, and there have been a large number of studies with these organisms in the pediatric population, with consistent good safety data (lack of side effects) but mixed efficacy.

The inconsistent positive therapeutic results may be related to the fact that each probiotic organism has different effects, and therefore they cannot be used indiscriminately for each disease. Indeed, different conditions may be triggered by different microbiota composition and therefore may require different probiotics to be effectively treated. By performing more detailed studies to link gut microbiota composition to certain conditions, such as ASD, we will be able to decipher the host-microbe cross talk and, therefore, we will be able to customize probiotic treatment for specific conditions (i.e., personalized medicine). Another strategy that may complement the use of probiotics is the treatment with prebiotics. Prebiotics are nondigestible oligosaccharides (i.e., sugars), which pass through the intestine into the colon, where they are fermented by the colonizing bacteria. (7). The fermentation products, short-chain fatty acids, produce an acid milieu, which facilitates the proliferation of health-promoting bacteria.

Despite the fact that in a recent survey involving 539 primary pediatricians, 19 percent of them suggested the use of probiotics for the treatment of their ASD patients, (9) no well-designed studies have been conducted to justify their routine use in autism. Ideally, all treatments should be based on principles of evidence-based medicine proving the efficacy of treatment judged on the basis of the strength of evidence, including randomized, controlled clinical trials, which are at the peak, followed by cohort studies, case control studies, and then case reports.

Probiotics are available in the United States in foods, dietary supplements, and medical foods. There are no drugs approved for human use in the United States. In the past few years, the diversity of food products containing probiotics has expanded considerably. Not all products, even those claiming to be "probiotic," deliver adequate levels of probiotic microbes that have been documented to have health benefits. Nevertheless, probiotics represent very promising strategies and, therefore, it would be desirable to perform well-designed, multi-center studies to establish the microbiota of ASD patients in order to choose the proper probiotics to reestablish a healthy gut ecosystem able to decrease or completely ameliorate the clinical presentations of ASD.

INTRAVENOUS IMMUNOGLOBULIN (IVIG)

BY DR. MICHAEL ELICE

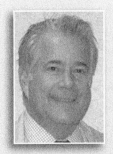

Michael Elice, MD

Autism Associates of New York
77 Froehlich Farm Boulevard
Woodbury, NY 11797
info@autismny.com
(516) 921-3456

Dr. Elice is a board-certified pediatrician and has been in practice for thirty years. Dr. Elice is a graduate of Syracuse University and the Chicago Medical School. He completed his pediatric residency at the North Shore University Hospital in Manhasset, New York. He has academic teaching positions and is on the staff of North Shore University Hospital and Schneider Children's Hospital. He is an associate professor of pediatrics at the New York University Medical School and the Albert Einstein School of Medicine. He is on the medical advisory board of the New York Families for Autistic Children (NYFAC) and is a member of the National Autism Association New York Metro Chapter. He has lectured at Defeat Autism Now! conferences around the country.

Autism spectrum disorders (ASDs) are currently defined as a syndrome of impaired social interaction, impaired communication skills, and restricted repertoire of activity and interests. The diagnoses contained within the spectrum range from attention deficit disorder (ADD), with hyperactivity (ADHD), obsessive compulsive disorder (OCD), tic disorders (such as Tourette's syndrome, aka TS), pervasive developmental disorder, not otherwise specified (PDD–NOS), and oppositional defiant disorder (ODD). These diagnoses are usually made prior to age three years, and have been on the rise over the past thirty years. The current statistics released by the Centers for Disease Control (CDC) and state health departments report the incidence of autism is 1:58 to 1:110 children, depending on geographic location, making autism spectrum disorders one of the greatest epidemics in pediatric medicine.

Intravenous immunoglobulin (IVIG) therapy has been used for common variable immunodeficiency syndrome (CVID), a disorder characterized by low levels of serum immunoglobulins and increased susceptibility to infections. The variability refers to the degree and type of immunoglobulin deficiency the patients had. Most individuals with CVID present first with recurrent bacterial infections. The underlying biomedical etiologies on children with autism have been under investigation. Genetic disorders possibly associated with epigenetic activity may lead to an increased incidence of multiple system disease in these children. Certain subsets of these children have a high incidence of immunological abnormalities and autoimmune disease. They also have markedly decreased serum immunoglobulin levels and impaired antibody responses. Based on the immunological abnormalities, a number of trials of IVIG have been utilized in autistic children. Gupta et al., in an open clinical trial, administered IVIG to ten children aged three to twelve years at four-week intervals for six months. Evaluations from the IV infusion nurse, physician, parents, and therapists showed clinical improvement in most of the patients. Younger patients showed greater improvement. Plioplys treated ten autistic children, ages four to seventeen years, with IVIG, four times every six weeks and found similar results. Delgiudice-Asch et al. administered IVIG monthly for six months to five autistic children. The sensory response Ritvo-Freeman scale showed a clinically meaningful response.

Based on this information, new research in autism spectrum disorders dictates the measurement of serum immunoglobulins, B and T cell lymphocyte levels, and anti-streptococcal antibodies. Patients who have received immunizations against polio, measles, diphtheria, tetanus, and strep pneumoniae may have low or absent antibody levels to one or more of these vaccines indicating a degree of immunodeficiency.

A subgroup of patients with OCD, ADD/ADHD, and tics or Tourette's syndrome has been identified who share a common clinical course characterized by dramatic symptom exacerbations following group A beta-hemolytic streptococcal (GABHS) infections. The term PANDAS has been applied to these patients, signifying Pediatric Autoimmune Neuropsychiatric Disorders Associated with Streptococcal Infections. The clinical symptoms are characterized by presence of the OCD and/or tic disorder, prepubertal onset of symptoms, intermittent exacerbations, neurological abnormalities such as motoric hyperactivity, adventitious movements, and the temporal association of the symptom exacerbations and GABHS infections.

In the 1980s, studies of childhood onset OCD and parallel investigations of rheumatic fever and its associated symptoms suggested a useful model of pathophysiology of these symptoms. It was thought that in certain children, susceptibility to genetic disorders possibly associated with epigenetic and transposon activity may lead to an increased incidence of multiple symptom disease in these children. Thus, certain strains of GABHS incite the production of antibodies that cross-react with central nervous system cellular components to cause inflammation of the basal ganglia in the brain resulting in these neuropsychiatric symptoms. Nearly 75 percent of these patients have symptoms of childhood onset OCD, worries about harm to self and others, violent images and behaviors, and ritualistic behaviors. These symptoms commence about four weeks prior to onset of the adventitious chorea-like movements, leading to the speculation that OCD might occur as a sequel of strep infections.

In a study by Swedo, et al. of fifty children meeting the PANDAS criteria, 40 percent met the DSM-IV (*Diagnostic and Statistical Manual of Mental Disorders, Fourth Edition*) criteria for ADHD, 18 percent ODD, 28 percent anxiety disorder. Exacerbations of OCD/tic symptoms were also accompanied by emotional lability and irritability, tactile/sensory defensiveness, motoric hyperactivity, messy handwriting, and symptoms of separation anxiety; a unique constellation of symptoms. The treatment for PANDAS is currently being studied including prophylactic antibiotics to prevent recurrent streptococcal infections and IVIG therapy. The children demonstrated dramatic improvements in OCD symptoms, anxiety, depression, emotional lability, and global functioning based on global change scores (41 percent). In contrast, placebo administration was associated with little or no change in overall symptoms severity. Side effects were limited to the duration of the procedure and included dizziness, nausea, and headache. In most cases, the discomfort occurred only during the first or second infusion and often persisted for twelve to twenty-four hours. Over 80 percent of patients who received IVIG remained much or very much improved at one-year follow-up, with their symptoms now in the subclinical range of severity. These results are particularly impressive in light of previous reports of the intractable nature of pediatric OCD and tic disorders. Long-term outcome studies in OCD have found less than one third of the patients with clinically meaningful symptom improvements.

In 2005 Boris, et al. published a study showing beneficial response of IVIG therapy in autistic children to whom 400 mg/kg IVIG was administered each month for six months. Baseline and monthly Aberrant Behavior Checklists were completed on each child in order to measure the child's response to IVIG. The participants' overall aberrant behaviors decreased substantially soon after receiving their first dose of IVIG. Total scores revealed decreases in hyperactivity, inappropriate speech, irritability, lethargy, and stereotypy (stimming, repetitive behaviors). This led to a reasonable rationale ratio to utilize IVIG therapy in children with autism.

The procedure of intravenous infusion of immunoglobulin is quite simple. The serum is sent to the doctor's office and remains frozen until the patient arrives, to ensure freshness. The volume to be infused is set up in a calibrated mechanical pump that begins the infusion at a slow rate to make sure the patient is tolerating the infusion. Depending on the volume to be infused, which is based on the weight of the patient, the procedure usually takes four to five hours.

Several days before the infusion, the patient receives information regarding premedication and hydration. Premedication might consist of oral ibuprofen and Benadryl at home or approximately one hour before arriving at the office. Sometimes it is necessary to administer IV Benadryl or Valium to relax the patient so that the IV catheter can be placed. This is a simple procedure, much like venipuncture to draw blood from a vein. The difference is that a catheter, a plastic extension of the needle, is threaded into the patient's vein and remains there for the duration of the procedure. The catheter allows a bit more flexibility of movement, so the patient may be more comfortable. In our office, the patient has the option of lying on an exam table with a comfortable backrest and pillow so they can sleep through the infusion or in a reclining chair so they can read or watch TV or a DVD of their choice. We encourage parents to bring these items for the comfort of the child.

A trained IV nurse is always present and will monitor vital signs; i.e., temperature, blood pressure, and pulse, as well as monitor the pump to be certain the infusion is proceeding efficiently. In the unlikely event that the patient demonstrates vital sign alterations or any other problem, the nurse will assess and report to the supervising physician. A crash cart for CPR/medications is always available. Thus far, we have never had any such incident.

Once the procedure is completed, the catheter is removed, instructions for at-home care are given, and the patient is discharged. There is a small possibility that the patient may develop fever, malaise, nausea, or headaches. These are rare and can be dealt with additional ibuprofen or Benadryl. The patient is instructed to make an appointment for the next monthly infusion. After the first infusion, seeing how simple it actually is, parents and children are very comfortable with the experience.

The treatment for common variable immunodeficiency characterized by low levels of serum immunoglobulins is similar to that of other disorders such as PANDAS. Intravenous immunoglobulin (IVIG) has led to improvement of symptoms. IVIG is a plasma product formed by taking antibodies from thousands of donors. The plasma undergoes processing for mixing, antibody removal, chemical treatment, and filtration to remove viruses, and then is freeze dried. This extensive processing dictates the high cost of the infusion, which is approximately $4,000 per child. This varies depending on the weight of the patient calculated based on 1 gram/kg of weight.

Intravenous immunoglobulin replacement combined with antibiotic therapy has greatly improved the outcomes of patients with PANDAS, CVID, and other autism spectrum disorders. The aim is to keep the patients free of infectious disease and to prevent the ensuing chronic inflammatory changes that may occur as a consequence of this immune system dysregulation. In our clinical practice, we have many children who have received IVIG. Based on anecdotal reports of parents, educators, and therapists, there have been improvements in focus and attention, and decreases in OCD/tic behaviors. In addition, these children—who are often sick with strep throats and other illnesses—have sustained longer intervals of health, compared to their previous history. Most recently, one of our patients visited Disney World, where he had been at least twenty times in his life. His older brother got strep throat and was treated with appropriate antibiotics. Forty-eight hours later, the patient became violent, started screaming, could not sleep, and was basically out of control. Within twenty-four hours of starting antibiotics, his behavior improved dramatically. Like "apples to oranges," said his father. This underscores the value to prophylactic antibiotics and IVIG which is the next step in treating this "autistic twelve-year-old male."

The results of these investigations, as well as clinical response noted in our practice, suggest that IVIG is highly beneficial to a subgroup of patients with tics and obsessive-compulsive symptoms. However, they do not provide support for routine use of immunomodulatory agents in OCD and tic disorders. IVIG is a potent immunological therapy. A NIH Consensus Statement asserted that the risks involved in the use of IVIG are minimal.

Other articles have confirmed their safety, after two decades of experience. Latov et al. reported that IVIG is used in the treatment of immunological diseases that affect the entire neuroaxis, including the brain, spinal cord, peripheral nerves, muscles, and neuromuscular junction. In prospective, controlled, double-blind clinical trials, IVIG was found to have proven efficacy in Guillain-Barré syndrome, chronic inflammatory demyelinating polyneuropathy, multifocal motor neuropathy, and dermatomyositis. It was found to probably be effective in myasthenia gravis and polymyositis, and possibly effective in several other neuroimmunological diseases. Further studies are needed to evaluate the use of IVIG for neuroimmunological diseases in which its efficacy is suspected but not proven and to elucidate its mechanisms of action.

33

LINWOOD METHOD

BY BILL MOSS

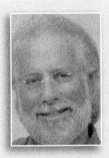

Bill Moss, M. Ed.

Executive Director
Linwood Center, Inc.
3421 Martha Bush Drive
Ellicott City, MD 21043
(410) 465-1352
www.linwoodcenter.org
admin@linwoodcenter.org
bmoss@linwoodcenter.org

Bill Moss is the executive director of the Linwood Center, a program that provides services and supports to children and adults living with autism. He has worked in special education and the developmental disabilities community for over thirty-five years. Moss received his undergraduate degree in psychology and sociology from the University of Maryland and his graduate degree in Special Education and Educational Management and Supervision from Loyola College. He is a licensed Residential Child Care Program Administrator in the State of Maryland and conducts lectures and trainings nationwide.

The Linwood Method has intrigued parents and professionals for many years. It has been studied, lauded and sometimes criticized. This discourse will take a brief look at what the Linwood Method is and how the staff at Linwood Center implements its procedures. We will then look at how Linwood came to be and what it has done for the children who have passed through its doors.

To understand the Linwood Method, one must accept a fundamental tenet which is at the heart of Linwood's approach: The only lasting change is that which occurs as an integral part of the child's overall development. Different than the often-used practice, of changing behavior as a mechanical response to repeated drill and training, the Linwood Method is more likely to produce lasting outcomes by implementing practices that motivate the child to learn. Applied Behavior Analysis (ABA) teaches us that, in order to bring about positive behavior change, one must be able to identify the pivotal elements in the child's environment that influence behavior. Like Koegel and Koegel's Pivotal Response Treatments, (Koegel & Koegel, 2006) Linwood relies on the fundamental aspects of observation, establishing relationships, and changing behaviors in the child's natural settings.

Learning occurs in the classroom, on the playground, in the lunchroom, in the child's own living room, and in the community. Rather than isolate the child in a therapy room to address a specific behavior, Linwood staff engages the child in learning events within activities identified as strong motivators for the child. Because each child has highly individualized needs, interests, and tolerance thresholds, he may not, for example, be required to sit at a desk in a classroom for prolonged periods of time. While one child can sit at a desk for twenty or thirty minutes, another child may only be able to sit for three or four minutes. Requiring that child to conform to "classroom rules" more often than not leads to a power struggle between the child and the adult. The more effective process is for the adult to devise a learning activity in which the child can successfully participate within the timeframe his threshold will permit. Once the child accomplishes the prescribed task(s), staff will reward him with his favorite item or activity. Basic principles of learning theory such as reinforcing successive approximations of the targeted response come into play here. The thoughtful staff member will ensure that the learning activity is laced with an abundance of positive social interplay, reinforcement, and needed breaks. The adult will adjust expectations accordingly by following the child's lead.

Determining the dynamics in the child's environment that influence behavior and motivate participation and cooperation are critical components of the Linwood Method. Determining these dynamics can only be accomplished through decisive and deliberate observation. In the above scenario, staff will have determined the child's threshold for sitting at his desk and actively engaging in a learning activity. The staff member, through observation, will have also determined those dynamics that motivate the child. The threshold may change from day to day, activity to activity and staff member to staff member. As the child demonstrates a readiness to accept increasing demands, this threshold will be carefully "stretched" and then stretched again, when it can be tolerated. At Linwood, the relationship (the social dynamics) between the child and the adult is essential and will dictate the effectiveness of any given learning activity.

Let's examine another scenario. The child's program plan calls for the child to learn to use a ruler. The child has few interests and many interfering behaviors. Observation reveals that one of his interests is to play with colorful yarn. As it becomes time to engage in the math lesson, rather than ask the child to put down his yarn, the teacher, through that very important positive relationship she has previously established with the child, will engage the child in a brief counting activity using his yarn. They will then compare the lengths of his yarn, identify the colors of his yarn, and then measure his yarn using a ruler. They will write the word, "yarn," they will incorporate the words and pictures into the child's picture exchange communication system, they will create silly stories with the yarn, and so forth. The point is that the adult will use whatever motivates the child in order to facilitate learning, develop communication skills, and build social relationships.

In 1955, long before "autism" was commonly known, and long before the advent of ABA, the Dutch therapist, Jeanne Simons, opened Linwood's doors to children who were destined at that time to be institutionalized. Simons created a school and residential haven for these children, the first and only program of its kind, to provide relief for the parents. Linwood's unique place in the short history of autism is defined by its very early connection to the first researchers in the field. Dr. Leo Kanner, who, in the 1940s, developed the nation's first child psychiatry program in a pediatric hospital, conducted his early autism research at Linwood. Kanner developed this program at Johns Hopkins School of Medicine in Baltimore, where he coined the term, "Early Infantile Autism." In 1965, Dr. Charles Ferster, an American University professor and researcher, obtained a federal grant to conduct research on behavior modification with autistic children. He developed the "Linwood Project," where he analyzed Simons's therapy, breaking the methods down to objective behavioral language, and defining "The Linwood Method."

Fundamental rights, courtesy, respect, dignity, individuality, and self determination are the concepts common to the language we use today in the developmental disabilities community. These words were not so commonly used in the early years when little was understood about the condition just being defined as "autism." However, Jeanne Simons understood these concepts; she practiced them and handed them down to her staff where they are now woven into the fabric of Linwood, and the approach as it is practiced today. Displayed on the walls at Linwood are the following words that Simons wrote, circa 1960:

> "And that's why we walk behind the child. He feels your protection when you walk behind. If you give him a chance to go any direction, he may be wrong when he goes this way or that. Just follow him. If it's

a dead end, pick him up gently and bring him to the main route. But never think that you know the answer, because you are dealing with an individual who may want to go very different routes, which for him may be better. That's why I feel more comfortable behind the children so I can see where they are going."

Linwood is a small program with roots emanating from its inception in historic Ellicott City, Maryland, halfway between Baltimore and Washington D.C. As the prevalence of autism increased and captured the attention of the public at large, a wide array of therapies and programs sprung up throughout the world. Linwood persisted in quietly, modestly and successfully providing programs and services to children and adults living with autism. Addressing the ever-increasing need for services throughout the lifespan for individuals on the autism spectrum, Linwood has developed what is widely considered some of the best and most innovative services in the region. In addition to basic educational and vocational education for students, Linwood provides community-based residential services for both children and adults on the spectrum, as well as vocational training and supported employment services for these individuals.

Jimmy's story perhaps best illustrates Linwood's impact on the autism community. At age seven, Jimmy could read, write, and do math. However, his days were characterized by screaming, flapping his hands, and spinning in panic. He was a danger to himself and destructive to his environment. Doctors were sympathetic, but could not help. At age eleven, after being turned down by twenty-three different programs, Jimmy's parents found Linwood. After ten years in Linwood's school and residential program, he gently transitioned into adulthood where he now receives both residential and employment support. Jim is a semi-independent adult. He lives in a beautiful home in a quiet suburban neighborhood and works full-time at Wal-Mart as the head "cart man"—nine years and counting. The negative and frightening "autistic behaviors" are gone. Jim has a delightful personality and is well-loved by family, staff, and co-workers.

34

LOW DOSE NALTREXONE (LDN)

BY DR. JAQUELYN McCANDLESS

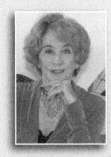

Jaquelyn McCandless, MD

www.lowdosenaltrexone.org

Jaquelyn McCandless MD is certified by the American Board of Psychiatry and Neurology and licensed in Hawaii and California, and has specialized in the bio-medical treatment of autism for the last twelve years. Dr. McCandless initiated the Defeat Autism Now! Physicians' Clinical Training in 2003, and is the author of the first clinical biomedical treatment book for autism, *Children with Starving Brains, a Medical Treatment Guide for Autism Spectrum Disorder,* first published in 2002, latest and 4th Edition published in February 2009, by Bramble Books.

In the last eleven years of working with children with autism spectrum disorder, I have learned—along with my colleagues in the Defeat Autism Now! organization focused on the biomedical aspect of autism—that children with this diagnosis are immunocompromised. This is shown by their inability to self-detoxify and low glutathione levels and abnormal immune parameters compared to neurotypical children. I conducted a private clinical study in 2005 on a medication to assess its help for immune status, a very low dose of an FDA-approved generic (1997) drug called naltrexone, an opioid antagonist used for adult opioid and alcohol addiction at usual doses of 50 mg or more per day. Studies over a decade earlier on full or higher dose naltrexone showed benefit in autistic self-injurious behavior (SIB) but at that time the connection between opioids and our immune systems was not widely known or understood. Autism researchers were hoping to counteract the opioid effects of casein and gluten with the opioid antagonism offered by naltrexone, rather than subjecting children to dietary restriction (GF/CF diets). Panksepp, Shattock and other early researchers noted variably better results with low doses; studies on higher doses were more equivocal in children, and noncompliance due to the bitterness of the drug posed a problem for autistic children, most of whom could not swallow capsules. After it was learned that most cases of SIB were due to pain from gut inflammation, which children were unable to describe, appropriate anti-inflammatory and other treatments for this gut condition decreased the use of naltrexone for SIB.

For private clinical studies in response to my request for a suitable transdermal form of low dose naltrexone (LDN), molecular pharmacologist Dr. Tyrus Smith then (2005) at Coastal Compounding Pharmacy in Savannah GA created a very effective transdermal cream compounded with emu oil. This allowed easy adjustment of dosing (some of the smaller kids did better with only 1.5 mg), the bitter taste was no problem, and the pleasant cream made in oil from the emu could be put on the children's bodies while they slept. The cream is put into syringes, with 0.5 ml providing 3 mg for children or 4.5 mg for adults; most adults prefer capsules; both are equally effective. Our use is of an ultra-low dose of pure naltrexone, less than 1/10 the recommended dose of 50 mg usually used for addiction, called low dose naltrexone, or LDN; it must be compounded (3 mg for children, 4.5 mg for adults) for "off-label" use to get these tiny doses. In private unpublished research studies I found that sixteen out of twenty children (80 percent) increased their CD4+ count in sixteen weeks of LDN usage and 70 percent of twenty-eight parents of children with autism raised their CD4+ count. LDN has shown itself to be a non-toxic, effective immune enhancer, nonaddicting, inexpensive (cost for month's supply of transdermal cream or oral capsule $25–$40, depending upon where you get it), and extremely easy to use (one capsule OR one transdermal application at bedtime, only once, daily). Many thousands of children with autism have been or are using LDN since I introduced it to the autism community in 2005; 75 percent of a 200-parent assay at that time rated LDN "overall beneficial." Though children are often prescribed this medication for immune benefit by their doctors, what parents appreciate most is increase in cognition, language, and socialization. I have dozens of letters and posts of grateful fathers telling me LDN has finally given them a relationship with their child and mothers who tell me that for the first time their child is playing with their siblings. Though many things about autism are heartbreaking, one of the saddest is the isolation and aloneness these children have. Very often they can be seen playing by themselves, seemingly preoccupied with an inner life or with repetitiously manipulating or lining up toys or objects, while totally oblivious of other children on a playground playing and relating.

History of LDN: Naltrexone is an extremely safe drug that was originally approved by the Food and Drug Administration in 1984 as a treatment for heroin, opium, and alcohol addiction due to its effectiveness in blocking the opioid receptors in the brain that drive the craving for these drugs. The dosage used is usually 50 mg/day for these disorders, and there is a current study using similar dosages to treat obesity. A New York physician, Bernard Bihari MD, in working with hospitalized AIDS patients in 1985, was giving some patients naltrexone to help addiction craving issues while they were being treated for AIDS. Cravings were helped, but their immune systems were responding negatively; he learned from a researcher at Penn State, Dr. Ian Zagon, that in his research work with canines, naltrexone actually helped the immune system more as the dose was lowered. Dr. Bihari did lower the dose, and determined that ideal dosing to help immunity was much lower than the dose needed for addiction therapy. Because naltrexone was able to block opioid receptors, it also was effective at blocking the reception of opioid hormones that are produced by brain and adrenal glands, including endorphins and enkephalins (specific types of endorphins that occur at the body's nerve endings and act as transmitters). Many of our body's tissues have receptor sites for endorphins, including nearly every cell in the immune system. This makes naltrexone an ideal treatment for managing pain, boosting immune function, and in many, boosting mood. Some parents call it the "happy cream," many noting that for the first time ever, after starting it, their children wake up happy. Dr. Bihari discovered naltrexone was able to accomplish these benefits in a low dose (between 1 to 4.5 mg, rather than 50 mg) taken once a day at bedtime, and the dose used most frequently for children under 100 pounds is 3 mg.

Since Dr. Bihari's discovery, LDN has been shown to have benefit for a wide variety of illnesses related to low immune function besides HIV/AIDS, including virtually every known cancer, as well as chronic fatigue syndrome, fibromyalgia, gastrointestinal disorders (celiac disease, colitis, Crohn's disease, irritable bowel syndrome), lupus, multiple sclerosis (MS), Parkinson's, rheumatoid arthritis, psoriasis, amyotrophic lateral sclerosis, and Alzheimer's disease. Many MS and other autoimmune patients have been on this medication for many years without progression of their disease, and the general consensus is that those with serious diseases such as MS and metastatic cancer should take LDN indefinitely. Some children with autism have been on LDN for two to four years, ever since I introduced it to the autism community in 2005 (including my beloved granddaughter

Chelsey, adorning the cover of my book, and inspiration for all my work in autism).

Although naltrexone is non-toxic and virtually free of side effects, occasionally it can cause sleep problems or hyperness during the first week or two of its use. If sleep problems persist, reducing the dose from 4.5 mg to 3 mg or in children from 3 mg to 1.5 to 2 mg is often helpful. The primary contraindication for LDN is the use of narcotic pain medications, and in children taking steroids, usually for gut inflammation, I request they not start LDN until they are down to 10 mg or less a day of prednisone on their way to going off steroids completely. It is not advised to administer LDN to someone who is taking immunosuppressants, as they will tend to counteract and neither be optimal.

As an effective, non-toxic, non-addicting, inexpensive behavioral and immuno-enhancing/modulating intervention, LDN is joining our biomedical arsenal to help more and more children recover from autism as well as helping many persons both adult and children with autoimmune diseases including HIV+ AIDS, MS, Crohn's, fibromyalgia, and cancer, or any disease that is caused by immune/autoimmune impairment or endorphin deficiency. Currently used in ultra small doses as an "off-label" FDA approved medication, LDN must be physician-prescribed and also compounded for the tiny dosing required. The filler medium carrying the medication is very important—it is required, in order to provide most benefit to be hypoallergenic and immediate-release to get the "jumpstart" for the brain to send the message out to the adrenal and pituitary glands to tell them to make endorphins. As to the carrier, I personally prefer emu oil for transdermal use and avicel for capsule preparations.

For more information on LDN, see www.lowdosenaltrexone.org, or you may join Autism_LDN@yahoogroups.com, and see www.LDNAfricaAIDS.org on my research on LDN for HIV/AIDS in Africa.

MEDICINAL MARIJUANA: A NOVEL APPROACH TO THE SYMPTOMATIC TREATMENT OF AUTISM

BY DR. LESTER GRINSPOON

Lester Grinspoon, MD

Harvard Medical School
35 Skyline Drive
Wellesley, MA 02482
www.marijuana-uses.com
www.rxmarijuana.com
lester_grinspoon@hms.harvard.edu

Dr. Lester Grinspoon is a professor of psychiatry emeritus at the Harvard Medical School and a well published author in the field of drugs and drug policy. He has authored more than 190 articles in scientific journals and ten books, including *Marihuana Reconsidered* (Harvard University press 1971, 1977, and American archives press classic edition, 1994) and *Marijuana, the Forbidden Medicine* (Yale University press, 1993, 1997), now translated into fourteen languages. Dr. Grinspoon is a frequent lecturer on drug policy issues and has appeared as an expert witness before legislative committees in many states and numerous committees of the U.S. Congress. In 1990 he received the Alfred R. Lindesmith Award for Achievement in the Field of Scholarship and Writing from the Drug Policy Foundation in Washington, DC.

Drugs have a place in treating autistic symptoms, but their uses are limited. Antipsychotic drugs and mood stabilizers may help autistic patients who repeatedly injure themselves. The older conventional antipsychotic drugs have serious side effects on body movements; the novel or atypical drug risperidone (Risperdal) has shown a glimmer of promise in recent research. Anticonvulsants may be useful in suppressing explosive rage and calming severe anxiety. About

20 percent of autistic people have epileptic seizures, and some researchers have suggested that unrecognized partial complex seizures, which cause changes in consciousness but not muscular convulsions, are one source of autistic behavior disturbances. In several control studies, selective serotonin reuptake inhibitors (SSRIs) have been found to relieve depression and anxiety and reduce compulsive ordering, collecting, and arranging. Unfortunately, little is known about the long-term effects of drugs in autistic children, and no known drug has any effect on the underlying lack of capacity for empathy and communication.

With the explosive growth of interest in exploring the medicinal capacities of marijuana, some courageous parents, dissatisfied with the usefulness and toxicity of the above mentioned drugs, and desperate to find pharmaceutical means of relieving their children of some of the harsh symptoms of autism, have been experimenting with oral doses of cannabis. The following anecdote was provided by Marie Myung-Ok Lee who teaches at Brown University. She is the author of the novel *Somebody's Daughter* and is a winner of the Richard J. Margolis Award for Social Justice Reporting.

My son J, who is nine years old, has autism. He's also had two serious surgeries for a spinal cord tumor and has an inflammatory bowel condition, all of which may be causing him pain, if he could tell us. He can say words, but many of them don't convey what he means.

J's school called my husband and me in for a meeting about J's tantrums, which were affecting his ability to learn. Their solution was to hand us a list of child psychiatrists. Since autistic children like J can't exactly do talk therapy, this meant sedating, antipsychotic drugs like Risperdal (risperidone).

As a health writer and blogger, I was intrigued when a homeopath suggested medical marijuana. Cannabis has long-documented effects as an analgesic and an anxiety modulator. Best of all, it is safe. A publication by the Autism Research Institute described cases of reduced aggression, with no permanent side effects.

After a week on Marinol, which contains a synthetic cannabinoid, J began garnering a few glowing school reports. But J tends to build tolerance to synthetics, and in a few months, we could see the aggressive behavior coming back. One night, at a medical marijuana patient advocacy group, I learned that the one cannabinoid in Marinol cannot compare to the sixty in marijuana, the plant.

Rhode Island, where we live, is one of fourteen states where the use of medical marijuana is legal. And yet, I hesitated. Now we were dealing with an illegal drug, one for which few evidence-based scientific studies existed precisely because it is an illegal drug. But when I sent J's doctor the physician's form that is mandatory for medical marijuana licensing, it came back signed. We underwent a background check, and J became the state's youngest licensee.

The coordinator of our medical marijuana patient advocacy group introduced us to a licensed grower, who had figured out how to cultivate marijuana using a custom organic soil mix. The grower left us with a month's worth of marijuana tea, glycerin, and olive oil—and a cookie recipe. We paid $80.

We made the cookies with the marijuana olive oil, starting J off with half a small cookie. J normally goes to bed around 7:30 PM.; by 6:30 he declared he was tired and conked out. As we anxiously peeked in on him, half-expecting some red-eyed ogre from Reefer Madness to come leaping out at us, we saw instead that he was sleeping peacefully. Usually, his sleep is shallow and restless.

When J decided he didn't like the cookie anymore, we switched to the tea. After two weeks, we noticed a slight but consistent lessening of aggression. Since we started him on his "special tea," J's face, which is sometimes a mask of pain, has softened. He smiles more. For the last year, his individual education plan at his special needs school was full of blanks because he spent his whole day in an irritated, frustrated mess. Now, April's report shows real progress, including "two community outings with the absence of aggressions."

The big test has been a visit from Grandma. The last time she came, J hit her. This time, she remarked that J seems calmer. As we were preparing for a trip to the park, J disappeared, and we wondered if he was going to throw one of his tantrums. Instead, he returned with Grandma's shoes, laying them in front of her, even carefully adjusting them so that they were parallel. He looked into her face, and smiled.

It's strange, I've come to think, that the virtues of such a useful and harmless botanical have been so clouded by stigma. Meanwhile, in treating J with pot, we are following the law—and the Hippocratic Oath: First, do no harm. The drugs that our insurance would pay for—and that the people around us would support without question—pose real risks to children. For now, we're sticking with the weed.

How is J doing now, four months into our cannabis experiment? Well, one day recently, he came home from school, and I noticed something really different: He had a whole shirt on.

Pre-pot, J ate things that weren't food. J chewed the collar of his T-shirts while stealthily deconstructing them from the bottom up, teasing apart and then swallowing the threads. His chewing become so uncontrollable we couldn't let him sleep with a pajama top (it would be gone by morning) or a pillow (ditto the case and the stuffing). The worst part was watching him scream in pain on the toilet, when what went in, had to come out.

Almost immediately after we started the cannabis, this stopped. Just stopped. J now sleeps with his organic wool-and-cotton, temptingly chewable comforter. He pulls it up to his chin at night and declares, "I'm cozy!"

Next, we started seeing changes in J's school reports. At one August parent meeting, his teacher excitedly presented his June-July "aggression" chart. For the past year, he'd consistently had thirty to fifty aggressions in a school day, with a one-time high of 300. The charts for June through July, by contrast, showed he was actually having days— sometimes one after another—with zero aggressions.

I don't consider marijuana a miracle cure for autism. But I do consider it a wonderful, safe botanical that allows J to participate more fully in life without the dangers and sometimes-permanent side effects of pharmaceutical drugs, now that we have a good dose and a good strain. Free from pain, J can go to school and learn. And his violent behavior won't put him in the local children's psychiatric hospital—a scenario all too common among his peers.

We have pictures of J from a year ago, when he would actually claw at his own face. That little child with the horrifically bleeding and scabbed face looks to us now like a visitor from another world. The J we know now just looks like a happy little boy.

We worried that "the munchies" would severely aggravate J's problems with overeating in response to his stomach pangs. Instead, the marijuana seems to have modulated these symptoms. J still can get overexcited if he likes a food too much, so the other day, we dared to experiment with doenjang, *a tofu soup that he used to love as a baby. The last time we tried it, a year ago, he frisbeed the bowl against a tile wall.*

We left J in the kitchen with his steamy bowl and went to the adjoining room. We heard the spoon ding. Satisfied slurpy noises. Then a strange noise that we couldn't identify. A chkkka bsssshhht doinnng! We returned to the kitchen, half expecting to see the walls painted with doenjang. *Everything was clean. The bowl and spoon, however, were gone.*

J had taken his dishes to the sink, rinsed them, and put them in the dishwasher— something we'd never shown him how to do. In four months, he'd gone from a boy we couldn't feed, to a boy who could feed himself and clean up after. The sight of the bowl, not quite rinsed, but almost, was one of the sweetest sights of my parental life. I expect more to come.

(Readers interested in a more detailed account of J's treatment with marijuana are referred to the section on Featured Patient Accounts on my Marijuana As Medicine website www.rxmarijuana.com).

Because autism is such a devastating and so far incurable disease and the available pharmaceutical products have such limited usefulness and serious side-effects, many parents—like Marie Myung-Ok Lee—seek out alternative therapies. I have had the opportunity to consult with and help a small number of these parents explore marijuana as a medicine, which can help to control some of the severe behavioral problems. (For the approximately one in five children with autism who suffer some sort of seizure disorder, it is important to note that marijuana is an excellent anticonvulsant, and was widely used as such in the last part of the 19th century and the early decades of the 20th.) Those who have persevered in the arduous process of both finding the correct oral vehicle and titrating the optimal dose, have been rewarded in more or less the same ways she has.

The first obstacle in the path of anyone who wishes to explore cannabis as a medicine is to overcome the widely held belief that it is a very dangerous substance. The misinformation campaigns of the United States government and such organizations as the Partnership for a Drug-Free America notwithstanding, marijuana is an unusually safe drug. In fact, after federal-court-ordered lengthy hearings before a Drug Enforcement Administration Law Judge, involving many witnesses, including both patients and doctors, and thousands of pages of documentation, Judge Francis L. Young in 1988 asserted that "marijuana, in its natural form, is one of the safest therapeutic active substances known to man . . . " Cannabis was much used in Western medicine from the mid-19th century until shortly after the passage of the Marijuana Tax Act of 1937, the first of the Draconian legislation aimed at marijuana. There has never been a recorded death attributable to marijuana. When it regains its rightful place in the U.S. pharmacopeia, it will soon be recognized as one of the least toxic medicines in that compendium. While there are no studies of the toxicity of cannabis in children, neither are there pediatric studies of the toxicity of risperidone and other conventional drugs used in the treatment of autism. However, to the extent that one can extrapolate the adult toxicity profiles of the antipsychotic drug risperidone and cannabis, the latter is the much safer drug.

It is often objected, especially by federal authorities, that the medical usefulness of marijuana has not been demonstrated by controlled studies, the rigorous, expensive, and time-consuming tests necessary to win approval by the Food and Drug Administration (FDA) for marketing as medicines. The purpose of the testing is to protect the consumer, by establishing both safety and efficacy. Because no drug is completely safe (nontoxic) or always efficacious, a drug approved by the FDA has presumably satisfied a risk-benefit analysis. The cost of doing the controlled studies necessary for FDA approval may run to about $800 million per drug, a cost borne by the drug company seeking it as a necessary prerequisite for the distribution of its patented product. Because it is impossible to patent a plant, pharmaceutical companies are not interested in developing this herbal medicine, and so far the cannabinoid products they have developed are not nearly as useful as whole herbal marijuana.

But it is doubtful whether FDA rules should apply to marijuana. First, there is no question about its safety. It has been used for thousands of years by millions of people, with very little evidence of significant toxicity. Similarly, given the mountain of anecdotal evidence which has accumulated over the years, no double-blind studies are needed to prove marijuana's efficacy. Any astute clinician who has experience with patients who have used cannabis as a medicine knows that it is efficacious for many people with various symptoms and syndromes. What we do not know is what proportion of patients with a given symptom will get relief from cannabis, and how many will be better off with cannabis than with the best presently available medicine. Here, large control studies will be helpful.

Physicians also have available evidence of a different kind, whose value is often underestimated. Anecdotal evidence commands much less attention than it once did, yet it is the source of much of our knowledge of synthetic medicines as well as plant derivatives. Controlled experiments were not needed to recognize the therapeutic potential of chloral hydrate, barbiturates, aspirin, curare, insulin, or penicillin. Furthermore, it was through anecdotal evidence that we learned of the usefulness of propranolol for angina and hypertension, of diazepam for status epilepticus (a state of continuous seizure activity), and of imipramine for childhood enuresis (bed-wetting) although these drugs were originally approved by the FDA for other purposes. Anecdotes or case histories of the kind presented here by Marie Myung-Ok Lee are, in a sense, the smallest research studies of all.

Anecdotes present a problem that has always haunted medicine: the anecdotal fallacy or the fallacy of the enumeration of favorable circumstances (counting the hits, and ignoring the misses). If many people suffering from, say, muscle spasms caused by multiple sclerosis take cannabis and only a few get much better relief than they could get from conventional drugs, these few patients would stand out and come to our attention. They and their physicians would understandably be enthusiastic about cannabis and might proselytize for it. These people are not dishonest, but they are not dispassionate observers. Therefore, some may regard it as irresponsible to suggest, on the basis of anecdotes, that cannabis may help some people with a variety of symptoms and disorders. That might be a problem if marijuana were a dangerous drug, but it is becoming increasingly clear that it is a remarkably safe pharmaceutical. Even in the unlikely event that only a few autistic children get the kind of relief that "J" gets, it could be argued that cannabis should be available for them because it costs so little to produce, the risks are so small, and the results so impressive.

While federal law is absolute in prohibiting the use of marijuana for any purpose, beginning with California in 1996, there are now fourteen states where it is possible to use it as a medicine, within specified limits. California, in addition to being the first state to make an accommodation to patients in need of cannabis, is also one of the states in which the legal interpretation of those needs and the means by which they can be filled is broad enough to satisfy the demands of patients with the wide variety of symptoms and syndromes for which this herb is useful. New Jersey, the latest state to adopt medical marijuana legislation, is unfortunately among the most restrictive. It is so restrictive, both with respect to the symptoms and syndromes for which a patient is allowed to use the drug and the means by which patients are allowed access to it, that only a relatively small percentage of the patients who would find marijuana more useful, less toxic, and less expensive than the conventional drugs they presently use will have access to it. Fortunately for her and her family, Marie Myung-Ok Lee lives in Rhode Island, where after presenting the appropriate credentials from "J's" physician, she was licensed to legally obtain marijuana. However, in most states patients or the people responsible for their care have to make, what for many of them, is a very difficult decision—whether to buy or grow cannabis outside of the law.

Beyond gaining access to marijuana, there are the problems involved in the preparation of this medicine in a form suitable for children. The most common way in which marijuana is used as a medicine is through inhalation of the smoke from a pipe, a joint, or a vaporizer. This is the preferred method for adults, because it makes it possible for the patients to precisely titrate the dose, because with this method of delivery they will perceive the therapeutic effects within minutes. However, inhalation is not an option for children who suffer from autism; for these patients, the best route for administration is oral, in the form of cookies, brownies, tea, etc. There are now available marijuana cookbooks from which a variety of edibles which appeal to children can be found. With ingestion, the therapeutic effects will not appear before one and a half to two hours, but the advantage is that they last for many hours. Beyond preparing the edible, are the challenges of determining the right dose (such as beginning with a fraction of a cookie and increasing the dose as needed), and establishing a schedule for taking the medication. These tasks will require some experimentation on the part of the parents, but with experience they will soon find the best recipes for their child, the ideal dose, and a workable schedule. Unfortunately, because there is presently no easy and available way of knowing with any precision the potency of any particular batch of marijuana, each newly prepared edible will have to be re-titrated, but with experience, caregivers will find this an increasingly less difficult task. It is also important to remember that cannabis is a very forgiving medicine; one would have to be considerably over the "ideal" dosage mark to cause any difficulty.

One way of minimizing what are usually minor therapeutic differences between one batch of cannabis and another is to try to use the same strain of marijuana every time an edible is prepared. At the same time, many patients who use marijuana as a medicine take advantage of the fact that there is a growing variety of available strains, each with slight differences in the percentages and ratios of the different therapeutic cannabinoids. This allows patients to empirically explore the different strains in an effort to identify the particular strain which appears to be the therapeutically most useful for their symptomatology.

The parents of autistic children carry a heavy burden. They are constantly challenged and frustrated by the child's inability to communicate, his impulsiveness, and his destructive and self-destructive behavior. They and other caregivers become emotionally drained and physically exhausted from the constant need for supervision. It is my hope that this paper will bring to the attention of many of these parents the possibility that there may be a new, if not officially or even medically approved, approach to their daunting challenge. While this approach may not work for all, it assuredly will do no harm.

MELATONIN THERAPY FOR SLEEP DISORDERS

BY DR. JAMES JAN

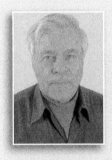

James E. Jan MD, FRCP(C)

Clinical Professor
Pediatric Neurology and Developmental Pediatrics
University of British Columbia
Senior Research Scientist Emeritus
Children's Hospital
Diagnostic Neurophysiology
4500 Oak Street
Vancouver, BC, Canada, V6H 3N1
jjan@cw.bc.ca

Dr. Jan is the author of over two hundred scientific articles and three books. As a child neurologist he worked with children who had various neurodevelopmental disabilities for more than forty years. In the early '90s he and his team introduced melatonin therapy for the sleep disorders of special needs children diagnosed with ASD, ADHD and various forms of intellectual deficits. This therapy is now used worldwide. Dr. Jan is semiretired now and no longer sees patients, but he teaches at the Children's Hospital and is involved in sleep research.

Melatonin (N-acetyl-5-ethoxytryptamine) is a small lipid and water soluble molecule which can readily enter all cells and bodily compartments. It is mainly derived from the pineal gland but it is also produced, in small amounts, in most tissues. Normally melatonin secretion into the bloodstream and spinal fluid begins in the evening, because darkness promotes its production and light inhibits it. Melatonin is thought to be present in all living organisms.

Research during the last fifty years, since its discovery, has shown that this hormone-like molecule has many important functions in the body. It plays a major role in sleep regulation, brain development, protection against toxins and it is a powerful antioxidant. It also synchronises metabolic activities and has shown beneficial effects on many diseases. Therefore, it is not surprising that there is a great interest in melatonin research among the scientific community.

Melatonin has been sold as an over-the-counter sleep aid since 1993 in the U.S. and since 2004 in Canada. It is synthesized commercially. Melatonin is produced from animal pineal glands is ineffective, dangerous, and fortunately not readily available. Melatonin products are sold in oral and sublingual tablets, capsules and in liquid forms. Some products, such as the sublingual tablets, capsules and liquid are called "fast-acting" because they act rapidly, but only promote sleep for three to four hours. Other, so-called "slow-release" products release melatonin slowly and promote sleep longer, for six to eight hours. These controlled-release tablets usually also contain fast-acting melatonin, therefore they are useful for treating both sleep onset and sleep maintenance difficulties. Melatonin is not a sleeping pill; in fact it is very different from hypnotic drugs. This natural sleep promoting substance is remarkably free from short- and long-term side effects, in contrast to hypnotics. Melatonin cannot be patented, because it is a naturally occurring substance, therefore any company may market it. Major pharmaceutical firms are not interested in investing money in researching it because, if they develop a better product, other companies can also sell it, and therefore the profits are limited. However, by modifying the basic formula, melatonin analogs have been developed, which are more expensive and do not appear to have an advantage over regular melatonin in sleep promotion. These analogs require prescriptions and cannot be sold over-the-counter.

History of melatonin therapy for sleep disorders

About twenty years ago our Melatonin Research Group at the Children's Hospital in Vancouver for the first time began using melatonin therapy for children with various neurodevelopmental disabilities and persistent sleep disturbances. Some children had severe intellectual deficits due to brain damage, autism spectrum disorders (ASDs), abnormal brain development, progressive neurological conditions and a variety of genetic disorders. Others had no intellectual disabilities but were diagnosed with attention-deficit/hyactivity disorder (ADHD) and anxiety disorders. For the most part, these sleep disturbances included difficulties falling asleep, frequent prolonged awakenings and early morning awakenings which were usually diagnosed as circadian rhythm sleep disorders. Early on we realized that children with severe neurodevelopmental problems responded similarly to melatonin therapy, whether their disturbed cognitive functioning was due to ASD, brain damage or maldevelopment of their brains. Therefore, their sleep disorders were not specific to their medical conditions but were related to their coexisting intellectual difficulties. It was puzzling as to why some children responded well to therapy whilst others did not but then it became clear that the treatment was only beneficial for those sleep disorders which were associated with low blood levels of melatonin or inappropriately timed pineal melatonin secretion. Frequent awakenings during the night were generally associated with low blood melatonin levels whereas difficulties falling asleep, without frequent awakenings, were most often related to delayed onset of pineal melatonin secretion. Early morning awakenings were sometimes due to low melatonin levels and, at other times, had neurological causes since the brain has different regulatory mechanisms for falling and staying asleep from those for waking up.

During the twenty years of our research we have not seen any significant short or long-term side effects or addictive properties and the effectiveness was not lost over time, as with hypnotics. Most importantly, better sleep was associated with improved health, behaviour and learning and in diminished parental stress.

Why do we need to sleep?

Research has shown that sleep is needed for metabolic restoration of the brain and cognitive development. Inadequate sleep predisposes children to poor health, such as infections, obesity, diabetes and heart disease; also to disturbed behaviour and numerous cognitive and memory difficulties. Healthy sleep is especially important for the brain development of young children because several years of markedly poor sleep may cause irreparable damage to their growing nervous systems. Complete sleep deprivation in animal experiments results in death within a couple of weeks. Loss of sleep is markedly disturbing; in fact, forced sleep deprivation is a known form of torture.

The human sleep-wake cycle parallels day and night changes and in this cyclic process, our environmental contact tells when to sleep. This partially explains why 70 to 80 percent of special needs children with marked cognitive problems, who have difficulties understanding environmental cues, experience persistent sleep problems. Children with anxiety or ADHD may understand that it is time for them to sleep, but their over-excited brain circuits do not give the required signals to initiate pineal melatonin secretion until later and, as a result, they have delayed sleep onset. Oral melatonin bypasses this delayed signalling and generally promotes sleep within thirty minutes.

Sleep Research in Children With ASD

Surveys show that the majority of children with ASD experience sometimes lifelong sleep disturbances which are most stressful for them, their caregivers, and the entire family. Usually these sleep difficulties are falling asleep, frequent awakenings and early morning awakenings, therefore, they are circadian rhythm sleep disturbances. Several studies have shown that melatonin therapy has a high success rate and the treatment is now accepted worldwide. In the past in several publications on melatonin treatment, we have included children with ASD. Then in 2007 our group published a carefully designed study of controlled release melatonin therapy for fifty children with severe developmental problems. Out of this group, sixteen children had ASD. All sixteen children responded, completely or partially, to melatonin therapy.

For children with ASD, melatonin was most effective for delayed sleep onset, but it also promoted longer sleep maintenance without any side effects. Better sleep was associated with parent-reported improvements in health, behaviour and learning. Occasionally a reduction in anxiety and self-stimulating mannerisms was also noted because melatonin has anti-anxiety properties. Sleep promotion techniques were generally ineffective in our 16 children before melatonin therapy but afterward they responded better to sleep hygiene.

Parental observations were the best method of diagnosing and following the children's sleep difficulties. Blood, saliva, and urine tests for melatonin levels were available, but they did not offer practical benefits since even a short melatonin trial was more informative. Sleep diaries, actigraphs, which measure movements, or video tapes, were useful in documenting sleep patterns, but polysomnography was almost never necessary.

Side Effects of Melatonin Therapy

The labelling of some over-the-counter products indicates that melatonin should not be given to children or to pregnant women. This warning is based on misinformation. In fact, over the years melatonin treatment in numerous studies has not caused a significant adverse effect in children.

Several years ago, a letter to a medical journal suggested that melatonin therapy might trigger seizures. This was an incorrect observation; in fact melatonin has anticonvulsant properties. It was also claimed that this therapy during puberty is dangerous, which was again incorrect because in contrast to animals, the sexual development and sexual behaviours of humans are not affected by melatonin.

Toxicity has not been observed either even with the ingestion of high doses, and taking melatonin during pregnancy has not caused malformations in the fetus in numerous animal studies. The reason for this high safety profile is likely because normally we produce our own melatonin throughout our lives. Vivid dreaming is commonly noted, but, to the vast majority of people taking melatonin, this is not a problem. This molecule has immunological benefits and we have commonly observed less frequent respiratory infections during therapy.

Suggestions for melatonin therapy

The following suggestions may be useful when contemplating melatonin therapy:

- Ideally, a thorough medical evaluation would be beneficial because children with ASD may also have sleep disorders which do not respond to melatonin therapy, for example sleep apnea.
- If possible, healthy sleep habits should be established first because mild sleep difficulties will respond without melatonin therapy.
- Recording the child's sleep pattern (going to bed, falling asleep, awakenings, and associated behaviours) in a detailed diary for one to two weeks before and during the initial treatment period is very useful because any change in sleep would become easier to notice.
- Melatonin is an over-the-counter medication, therefore a prescription is not required in the U.S. and Canada. Nevertheless, it is better when a health professional supervises the treatment.
- Fast-release melatonin is more useful when the child has difficulties falling asleep without frequent awakenings. Slow-(controlled-) release formulations are the best for multiple awakenings with or without sleep onset delay.
- The oral dose should be given about thirty minutes before the desired bed time, and not several hours earlier, which is impractical. Melatonin may be mixed with a spoonful of jam, pudding, or ice cream. Tablets should not be chewed because then the controlled-release melatonin is converted into fast-release. This is the reason why smaller tablets for children are better than the larger ones which are generally marketed for adults.
- There is no advantage in using liquid melatonin unless the child has swallowing difficulties.
- There are no dose formulas which fit everyone as melatonin is not a sleeping pill. Starting with 1 to 3 mg is the best and then small incremental changes can be made every couple of days. Parents know their own children well, so

they are in the best position to judge what the lowest and most optimal dose would be. Frequent awakenings are usually harder to treat than sleep onset delays and they often require higher doses, sometimes even up to 10 to 12 mg.

- Once the therapeutic threshold has been reached, additional doses do not result in deeper sleep. One cannot overdose a child into a toxic state, though large doses may cause temporary morning sleepiness.

- From time to time, when a child appears overly agitated, a larger dose may be given, or another dose could be administered one to two hours later. Repeating the dose in the middle of the night is only rarely helpful.

- Some children require melatonin replacement therapy for several months or years, others for life. Parents could stop the treatment every six to twelve months and, if the sleep problems recur, they could restart melatonin at the same dose. Melatonin can be stopped abruptly without causing any problems.

- In rare situations, when certain sleep centres of the brain are damaged, melatonin therapy is ineffective. When a child has early morning awakenings and melatonin does not fully help, a hypnotic drug is sometimes given as well. However, sleeping pills lose their effects with time.

- Melatonin may be administered during the day before medical tests (EEG, CT, MRI, and hearing evaluations) because it reduces the anxiety of children with ASD; therefore it makes them more co operative.

- Sleep hygiene should be continued, even when the melatonin therapy is successful.

- In our experience, when children are tired and sleepy, they are usually ready to go to bed and fall asleep. It is when they cannot fall asleep that they may exhibit difficult bedtime behaviours. In such situations, it might be wiser to treat them with melatonin first to correct their medical deficiency and then the difficult behaviours might diminish or even disappear. Certainly, behavioural therapies are more successful when the children are not exhausted.

MERIT APPROACH: INTEGRATING ABA WITH DEVELOPMENTAL MODELS

BY JENIFER CLARK

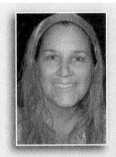

Jenifer Clark, MA, Ph.D. (c)

New York, NY
(212) 222-9818
clarkjenif@aol.com
MERIT-consulting.org
JeniferClark.com

Jenifer Clark has been working with children and families for over fifteen years. She received her master's in psychology from NYU and is completing her Ph.D. in clinical psychology at CUNY. She has worked as an ABA therapist and consultant since 1992. She specializes in working with children with autism and has taught atypical development at Hunter College. Currently she is the director of Boost!, an afterschool program for children with autism. This program focuses on teaching socialization and leisure skills to children on the spectrum, incorporating typical children as peers and social models. Ms. Clark is the co-founder and therapist for SibFun, a support group for siblings of children with special-needs. She consults at special needs and typical schools, and continues to consult with children and families.

Despite the wide base of empirical data that supports ABA in the treatment of autism, there are critics who express concerns over the impact that this treatment has on the emotional life of the child. Many argue that it is antithetical to design an intervention that would give a child with autism repeated experiences of having their distress ignored. Some are concerned about the impact these experiences have on a developing sense of self and the child's capacity to attach and increase relatedness. Parents can be put off by the data-driven nature of the ABA methodology. Many families have shared with me their stories of seeking to embrace a more developmental model, but feeling as if they are failing to offer their child much-needed remediation during a critical period.

It is clearly the case that children with autism struggle with the concept that it is worthwhile to communicate their needs to another person. This being the case there *are* significant detrimental effects that can evolve from repeatedly ignoring distress. If a child with autism is deprived of the experience of having their feeling states acknowledged—which is a precursor to acknowledging feeling states in others—how will they develop this capacity?

In response to these growing concerns, pediatric neurologists and developmental specialists are increasingly encouraging parents to use a blended intervention to treat their child's autism. They are recommending that parents set up a program for their child that incorporates ABA and other more developmentally based approaches. Many parents are at a loss for how to accomplish this integration, however. Therapists tend to be deeply committed to either one philosophy or the other, and there is considerable resistance to working cooperatively. Additionally, the dominant methodologies developed from two very different philosophies, and frequently contradict one another at times in terms of how the intervention should proceed and how to interpret the behavior of the child.

Clearly there is a tremendous need for a treatment model which attends to autism in its entirety: one which successfully integrates the incredibly effective remediation, repetition, and hierarchical teaching common to ABA with a developmental model that focuses on the equally important emotional development of the child. As ABA satisfies the need to remediate the core deficits of autism, *mentalization* emphasizes the need for a mutual acknowledgement of inner states. Mentalization (Fonagy et al, 2002) describes the process in which we attend to the thoughts and feelings of another. Mentalization-based therapies provide a way of conceptualizing our interactions with children with autism in a manner that consistently takes into account, and reflects back to them, their inner world.

An Integrated Model

I have developed a hybrid treatment approach called MERIT: Mentalization Enhanced Remediation—an Integrated Treatment. The MERIT model accomplishes this integration by continuing to emphasize the structured and hierarchical teaching that is a crucial component of remediation, while incorporating a mentalizing approach in all interactions with the child.

The three most important aspects of this model are providing mentalizing experiences to forge a relationship with the child, allowing mentalization to inform the treatment on a regular basis, and remediating the social-emotional areas that prevent the child from progressing in this area of development.

Forging the Relationship

In the initial phases of treatment, the therapist engages in mentalization in order to understand and forge a relationship with the child. As the therapist comes to understand how this child thinks, learns, and even copes with anxiety, all this information will influence how the therapist interacts with the child. This intimate relationship, which involves learning a child's likes and dislikes, as well as challenges and strengths, is in fact critical in using mentalization to treat autism.

It can be challenging to make sense of the inner life of a child with autism, and therefore mentalization plays a pivotal role in the treatment. We cannot relate firsthand to a child who experiences sounds as painful and sensory issues as completely preoccupying. And yet, this process of being understood is an undeniably crucial aspect of any development. A therapist must pose the question: How is this particular brain processing information? A therapist's job is to put him- or herself in a child's place, and to try to understand what it is the child is experiencing. A therapist must be able to determine the most constructive experiences, to help a child with autism learn and be able to relate. This understanding will be a powerful guide to the therapy, as well as a tremendous source of reinforcement and motivation for the child.

The Remediation

Traditional ABA programs that target areas such as verbal imitation, visual imitation, fine motor tasks, and expressive and receptive language skills are incorporated into the treatment. The way in which concepts are introduced, and the interactions before, during, and after each discrete trial, are profoundly influenced by the therapist-child relationship. This relationship is distinct from the relationship in some developmental programs in that the MERIT therapist will be directive. The MERIT therapist has an agenda, and that is to remediate the areas of core deficit exhibited by that particular child. The heterogeneous nature of autism means that although all children with autism can be helped by remediation, it is critical that individual differences be taken into consideration. Failure to do so can result in disengagement both from the work and, more importantly, from the therapist.

While engaged in their work, it is important that, despite their potentially limited capacity to understand language and gestures, the child feels understood. The therapist can increase communication through the use of language, gestures, and visuals. Additionally, the work itself should evolve in such a way that it reflects an understanding of the child. Even if the child has a limited ability initially to process the world around them, presumably they can take in the experience of being less frustrated than they had been in their previous interactions with others. They can then begin to trust that they can be successful. The nature of the relationship can be one of trust that nothing will be asked of this child that they cannot do (with some help). Ideally these interventions begin to remediate some of the areas of deficit that make it difficult to benefit from interactions with another or to process communication. The work builds upon itself. With each passing week the child develops more skills that allow him to better engage in social exchanges, but in the meantime the relationship, which is critical to the work, is continually growing.

Remediating Social-Emotional Capacities

Some of the areas of deficit particular to autism interfere with a child's ability to benefit fully from a mentalizing stance. *How can a child who can't perceive facial expressions benefit from his mother's warm smile? How can children with auditory processing deficits understand when they are being consoled? How can children who cannot attend to stimuli join their parents in reciprocal interactions?* These areas can be remediated to a measurable extent that will allow these children to gain more from formative interactive experiences.

Through remediation, children with autism can be taught to attend to the salient features in a social interaction, identify emotional states on faces, and participate in social reciprocations. Once these types of skills have been established, they will allow the child with autism to begin to participate more in the social world, which will in turn fuel their emotional development.

Conclusion

ABA and developmental models have proven success in treating children with autism. The future of autism treatment involves finding a way to integrate these proven methodologies that offers parents and treatment providers a clear and coherent philosophy regarding the treatment of children with autism. It is evident that there is a need for a treatment model that is well-integrated and cohesive, and at the same time inclusive and current with regard to what we know about the brain and neuroplasticity.

MERIT offers such an integration. MERIT takes into account the individual differences of the child as well as his unique learning style, and importance is placed on working with the family to enhance the child's outcome. Autistic children's success hinges on the remediation of so many compromised areas of functioning, and it is only when all of these core deficits are being addressed simultaneously, and in a way that fosters a connection to others, that a child can enjoy optimal success.

METHYL-B$_{12}$: MYTH OR MASTERPIECE

BY DR. JAMES NEUBRANDER

James A. Neubrander, MD, FAAEM

Comprehensive Neuroscience Center
100 Menlo Park, Suites 410 and 200
Edison, NJ 08837
(732) 906-9000; (732) 906-7888
www.drneubrander.com
www.neuro-center.com
www.IBRFinc.org

Dr. Neubrander trained in Pathology and Laboratory Medicine and is Board Certified in Environmental Medicine. He is the Medical Director of Autism Research for the International Brain Research Foundation and Medical Director of the Comprehensive Neuroscience Center in Edison, New Jersey. He serves on many scientific advisory boards dedicated to treating autism and neurodevelopmental disorders. He lectures many times each year at National and International Conferences and Physician Training Courses. His lectures are scientific, evidence-based, and emphasize newer treatments or modifications of established protocols that appear to enhance clinical outcomes beyond the results previously reported. He is the coauthor of several peer-reviewed articles, has been interviewed and filmed for many documentaries and television spots, has been referenced in many books written about autism, nutrition, and environmental medicine, and has been quoted innumerable times by scientists, researchers, clinicians, and lay persons, most notably for methylcobalamin, hyperbaric oxygen, and heavy metal detoxification.

Since the mid '90s, I was one of a handful of physicians who had been using the only two available forms of vitamin B$_{12}$, cyano-B$_{12}$ and hydroxy-B$_{12}$, to treat children with autism. We used these forms of B$_{12}$ because the majority of children with autism had an abnormal elevation of the organic acid known as FIGLU (formiminoglutamic acid). Though we believed we saw minor improvements by using B$_{12}$, we never saw anything remarkable. In the '80s and '90s, the Japanese had been studying the methyl form of B$_{12}$ for many disorders, none of which were autism. It was not until the late '90s that the methyl form finally became available in the United States, though it was not commonly used. In March of 2002, I became the first physician in the world to ever use the methyl form of B_{12} in a child with autism. Amazingly, the child showed many significant changes.

The second child I treated, who previously used three- to four-word utterances, began speaking in six- to eight-word sentences within two weeks. Not only was he now talking, he was also interacting with everyone. This included his shocked school bus driver whom he tried to kiss, and his even more shocked crossing guard whom he started hugging and talking to every day! Such social interactions, especially spontaneously initiated, were something that he never did prior to methyl-B_{12}. His parents jokingly said that things might have been better for them before they started the shots, because then they had a little peace and quiet in the house and not all his constant chatter!

Now, more than a million dose evaluations later, the single most predictable treatment I have seen to positively affect more than 90 percent of children on the spectrum is methyl-B_{12} injections if done according to the protocols I have continued to improve upon over the last seven years. Though shots are initially feared by most parents, they soon learn that the shots are painless, easy to administer, and give the greatest number of clinical responses when compared to oral, nasal, or transdermal routes of administration. Interestingly, prior to starting therapy, the majority of children who respond to methyl-B_{12} injections have high normal to high levels of B_{12} in their blood, rather than the low levels would be expected. The reason for this appears to be what I call "B_{12} diabetes." Just as blood sugar builds up in the plasma of a diabetic because it cannot get into the cell, B_{12} builds up in the plasma and does not get into the cell, possibly due to a transcobalamin transporter problem.

Methyl-B$_{12}$ is methylcobalamin. Every time you see the word "cobalamin," you can substitute the word "B_{12}." In the late 1920s, when vitamins were first discovered, they were called "*vital amines.*" Eventually the words were combined to form what we know today as "vitamin." When B_{12} was discovered, it was called the "cobalt vital amine" because a cobalt atom is found deep within the molecule. The name was later shortened to be called the "*cobalt vitamin,*" what we know today as "cobalamin." The cobalamins represent a *family* of cobalt containing vitamins. To better understand this, consider "cobalamin" to be the last name of a family, analogous to "the Smiths." The different types of B_{12} are analogous to the first names of each family member that identifies them from each other. For the Smiths, there could be Jennifer, Ashley, Megan, Michael, Matthew, or Jeremy.

For the Cobalamin family, the individual family members are named Methyl, Adenosyl, Hydroxy, Cyano, Glutathionyl, and Sulfito. They each have their own jobs and assignments to do. The two senior family members of the cobalamin family are methyl-B_{12} and adenosyl-B_{12}. Only these two forms have "coenzyme" properties that allow them to complete special assignments with specific enzymes found in the body, especially in the brain and mitochondria when we are discussing autism.

Methyl-B_{12}'s unique coenzyme activity unlocks the enzyme methionine synthase. Every time it is unlocked, methionine synthase transfers a methyl group to homocysteine allowing homocysteine to re-enter the methionine cycle. This reaction is vital for methyl groups to be passed from one molecule to the next, a process called transmethylation. For children with autism, the results of transmethylation are increased language, focus and attention, awareness, cognition, independence, socialization and interactive play, appropriate emotional responses, affection, eye contact, and improvements in gross and fine motor skills.

The science behind why methyl-B_{12} works for autism is sound. The folate cycle, methionine-homocysteine cycle, and homocysteine-glutathione pathway are intricately interwoven in a delicate balance that exists to create and then pass along methyl groups, and to create glutathione, the body's most important intracellular antioxidant. The folic acid cycle receives premethylated folic acid molecules from food, vitamins, or from a folic acid recycling process. Premethylated folic acid molecules are presented to the MTHFR (methylene tetra hydro folat) enzyme to become methylated folic acid. Methylated folic acid donates its methyl group to "naked B_{12}" for it to become methyl-B_{12}. Methyl-B_{12}, in the presence of methionine synthase, passes its methyl group to homocysteine which then becomes methylated (or re-methylated) homocysteine, also known as methionine. Methionine then adds an adenosyl molecule to become S-adenosylmethione (SAMe), the "universal methyl donor." It is SAMe's job to transfer the methyl group (transmethylation) to many different types of molecules in the brain to produce the clinical results previously discussed. Once the methyl group has been transferred, the remaining molecule, S-adenosylhomocysteine (SAH) still retains the adenosyl group. Unfortunately, SAH blocks further transmethylation until the adenosyl group is removed, a process that requires adequate zinc, and at times the removal of dairy. Once SAH loses the adenosyl group, what is left is "naked" (or parent) homocysteine, devoid of methyl of adenosyl groups.

Depending on various factors, "parent homocysteine" will proceed one of two ways.1 When oxidative stress is under control, homocysteine will enter the methionine-homocysteine cycle just described.2 However, when oxidative stress is high, homocysteine will be shunted down the homocysteine-glutathione pathway to create glutathione, the body's primary intracellular antioxidant. Oxidative stress is a condition where "wild unpaired electrons" cause significant tissue and cellular damage before they find a mate. Antioxidants provide such mates.

Jill James, Ph.D., demonstrated that children on the autism spectrum had lower values of active glutathione than controls. Richard Deth, Ph.D., found that methionine synthase is critical for a special dopamine receptor and normal brain function. Dr. Deth also documented that many substances damage or block methionine synthase activity, including mercury, the infamous agent found in vaccines containing thimerosal.

With this scientific background, one can begin to understand how the administration of injectable methyl-B_{12} works for children with autism from each of the three pathways previously described. In the folate cycle, the MTHFR enzyme is frequently mutated. This results in low production of the methyl groups needed to make methyl-B_{12}. By injecting methyl-B_{12}, we bypass the problem. In the methionine-homocysteine cycle, the addition of methyl-B_{12} allows more methyl groups to first be donated to SAMe and subsequently passed along to the crucial molecules in the brain that will reduce autistic symptoms. In the homocysteine-glutathione pathway, methyl-B_{12} has been shown to help restore the critical balance between methylation and transsulfuration.

Since March of 2002, I have treated thousands of children on the autism spectrum and have personally monitored over a million doses in my clinic. My research has included the clinical responsiveness to all forms of commercially available B_{12}: cyano-B_{12}, hydroxy-B_{12}, adenosyl-B_{12}, and methyl-B_{12}. It has investigated the clinical responsiveness from all routes of administration: oral, sublingual, transdermal, nasal, intravenous, intramuscular, suppository, and subcutaneous. It has evaluated the clinical responsiveness from shots varying from weekly to daily, from various stock concentrations, and from different pH values. It has evaluated the clinical responsiveness when B_{12} has been used in combination which other agents, most commonly folinic acid, glutathione, and/or N-acetylcysteine. It has investigated the clinical benefit and side effect patterns when used concurrently with TMG, SAMe, methionine, NAC, glutathione, B6, folic acid, folinic acid, 5-MTHF, DMG, ALA, etc. *In summary, from seven years of intense clinical research I cannot emphasize enough how much the right protocol matters. Which protocol is selected can make or break how effective the shots are for any given child.*

In my clinic, according to the protocols I have developed over the past seven years, I consistently find that the injectable form methyl-B$_{12}$ if far superior to any other route of administration when one considers the percentage of children who respond, the intensity of each response, and how many responses each child exhibits.

Key factors necessary to achieve maximum effectiveness are beyond the scope of this chapter. They include, but are not limited to the pH and concentration of the stock solution, the mcg/kg of the dose used, the frequency of the injections, the route of administration, and if given subcutaneously, the site of the injections, the evaluation tools used by the parents to report their findings, and the presence of selected key supplements reaching predetermined dosage ranges prior to implementing higher doses of methyl-B$_{12}$, or prior to increasing the frequency of the injections. The most common initiation protocol I use is a dose of 65 mcg/kg drawn from a stock solution of 25 mg/mL given at a ten-degree angle into the adipose tissue of the buttocks once every three days. A local anesthetic cream can be locally applied at the site of the injection.

As previously stated, the primary categories of improvement include increased language, focus and attention, awareness, cognition, independence, socialization and interactive play, appropriate emotional responses, affection, eye contact, and improvements in gross and fine motor skills. In my clinic, the frequency for at least some of these responses is 94 percent. The average number of responses is thirty to fifty out of a possible total of 135. Though the intensity of response can be very strong at times, the majority of parents report mild, mild-to-moderate, or moderate improvements. The positive effects build over 2½ to 4 years. Should the shots be discontinued prior to that amount of time, many children will regress. After 2½ to 4 years, many children can be weaned off their shots. 60 to 70 percent of children do better on daily shots, but only if certain key supplements are being taken at the recommended ranges provided in the Supplement Review Program as shown on my website.

Compounding pharmacies must make the injections. Depending on the pharmacy used, the shots usually range from $0.50 to $1.50 each. I only prescribe preservative-free shots in prefilled syringes rather than less expensive multi-dose vials that contain preservative. I do this because of two theoretical risks. First, injecting preservatives into children on the spectrum may exacerbate their inability to detoxify, something already known to be compromised in the majority of them because they have less glutathione than their peers. Second, even though alcohol swabs are to be used, the risk for Mycoplasma, bacterial, or viral contamination still exists, and I will not take that risk.

Best case anecdotal stories, including a section showing *Recovered Kids*, can be viewed in the video section of my website; www.drneubrander.com. One remarkable story is Caitlin's. Her mother was a speech pathologist who, while in training, refused to do a rotation to learn about autistic children because she wanted to have nothing to do with it. Unfortunately, when Caitlin was 2½ years old, Caitlin's mother was devastated when the doctor told her Caitlin was not just autistic, but severely so. Caitlin progressed very quickly from methyl-B$_{12}$ shots and fully recovered. Today, no one can tell she was ever autistic! Unfortunately, best case scenarios are unusual. The majority of patients show mild or moderate improvements which, as they follow my protocols for 2½ to 4 years, continue to improve.

Long-term use is safe as documented from pernicious anemia patients. Serious side effects do not occur. However, nuisance side effects are fairly common. The good news is that they usually pass within four to six months as the body adjusts to keep the good and delete the bad. Common side effects are hyperactivity, stimming, and mouthing objects. Occasionally sleep is disturbed though more often it improves. Side effects belong in two categories: positive-negative vs. negative-negative, and tolerable vs. intolerable. A common positive-negative side effect for young children is pinching or tantruming, as they become much more aware of what they want and ask for it in perfectly good "autism-ese." When you do not understand, they get upset and tantrum or pinch to get your attention so you will do what they want you to do. Now that they are much more aware of what they want, they also get upset and tantrum when you tell them to do something they don't want to do.

In summary, every child on the autism spectrum deserves a clinical trial of injectable methyl-B$_{12}$ because it has proven to be an effective treatment for the majority of children on the autism spectrum, if done correctly.

MITOCHONDRIAL DYSFUNCTION

BY DR. RICHARD E. FRYE

Richard E. Frye, MD, Ph.D.

Department of Pediatrics
Division of Child and Adolescent Neurology at the University
of Texas Health Science Center, and at The Children's Learning
Institute
7000 Fannin—UCT 2478
Houston, TX 77030
Richard.E.Frye@uth.tmc.edu

Dr. Richard E. Frye received his medical degree from Georgetown University. He completed his pediatric residency training at University of Miami and child neurology residency training at Children's Hospital Boston. Following residency Dr. Frye completed a fellowship in behavioral neurology and learning disabilities at Children's Hospital Boston. Dr. Frye completed a Ph.D. in physiology and biophysics at Georgetown University and a MS in biomedical science at Drexel University. Dr. Frye is board certified in Pediatrics and in Neurology with special competency in Child Neurology. Dr. Frye is also funded by the National Institutes of Health to study brain function in individuals with neurodevelopmental disorders. Dr. Frye is the medical-director of the University of Texas medically-based autism clinic. The purpose of this unique clinic is to diagnose and treat medical disorders associated with autism, such as mitochondrial disorders and subclinical electrical discharges, in order to optimize remediation and recovery.

Recent studies have suggested that autism may be linked to dysfunction of the mitochondria—the powerhouse of every cell in our body. In addition to a lack of production in cellular energy, mitochondrial dysfunction can affect both energy and non-energy producing metabolic systems since many metabolic systems feed their final biochemical products into mitochondrial pathways and/or derive their biochemical substrates from mitochondrial pathways. Furthermore, dysfunctional mitochondria can create reactive oxygen species that can be damaging to neighboring healthy tissues, as well as to non-mitochondrial cell function.

Those affected by mitochondrial dysfunction manifest nonspecific symptoms including developmental delay, loss of developmental milestones (i.e., regression), seizures, muscle weakness, gastrointestinal abnormalities and immune dysfunction. In general, mitochondrial dysfunction affects body systems that have high energy demands. Some of the same body systems that are dysfunctional in mitochondrial disorders are also dysfunctional in autism. In fact the clinical criteria of determining if a mitochondrial disorder is present depend upon the presence of many of the same symptoms that are common in children with autism. This indicates that at least a subset of children with autism reach criteria for a "probable" mitochondrial disorder even before biomedical testing is performed. By this line of reasoning, the multisystem dysfunction commonly seen in autism could be explained by underlying mitochondrial dysfunction. Consideration of this idea should be tempered with the fact that some high-energy organs commonly affected in individuals with mitochondrial disorders, such as the heart and the kidney, are not commonly found to be dysfunctional in autism.

Mitochondrial dysfunction is treated through three approaches: (1) precautions to prevent further mitochondrial dysfunction or metabolic decompensation; (2) vitamin supplements to support mitochondrial function; and (3) modification of the diet to optimize mitochondrial function.

Precautions

Individuals with mitochondrial dysfunction should avoid physiological stressors. Patients should avoid fasting, extreme cold or heat, sleep deprivation, dehydration, and illness. If an individual with mitochondrial dysfunction becomes sick, there should be aggressive control of fever and hydration. During illness an individual with mitochondrial dysfunction should be closely monitored and provided intravenous hydration with carbohydrates if necessary. Certain drugs and environmental toxins which depress mitochondrial function should be avoided. Common toxins which inhibit mitochondrial function including heavy metals, insecticides, cigarette smoke, and monosodium glutamate. Common drugs that inhibit mitochondrial function include acetaminophen, nonsteroidal anti-inflammatory drugs, alcohol, some antipsychotic, antidepressant, anticonvulsant, antidiabetic, antihyperlipidemic, antibiotic, and anesthetic drugs. Specific precautions are required for surgery and anesthesia.

Diet Modifications

Some patients respond to frequent meals high in complex carbohydrates. For some patients an overnight fast can be enough to destabilize mitochondrial function. Such patients can be treated with complex carbohydrates such as corn starch before bedtime while some can be awakened in the middle of the night for a snack while others may require a feeding tube to receive feeding overnight. Other patients respond to high-fat diets such as the ketogenic diet. Some patients respond to medium chain triglyceride oil supplementation since these fats do not require carnitine to be transported into the mitochondria.

Vitamin Supplementation

Vitamins may enhance mitochondrial enzyme function and may result in improved efficiency of energy generation. In addition, vitamins serve as antioxidants, which may slow the progression of the mitochondrial dysfunction. Standard supplementations for mitochondrial dysfunction include coenzyme Q10 (5-15 mg/kg/day), levocarnitine (30–100 mg/kg/day) and B vitamins. Typical B vitamins include thiamine (50–100 mg/day), riboflavin (100–400 mg/day), nicotinamide (50–100 mg/day), pyridoxine (200 mg/day) and cyanocobalamin (5–1,000 mcg/day). New coenzyme Q10 analogs, for example Ubiquinol, have better bioavailability than coenzyme Q10, providing the same effect at 1/10 to 1/20 of the dose. Acetyl-L-carnitine (250–1000 mg/day) is a natural constituent of the inner mitochondrial membrane. Biotin (5–10 mg/day) is an important cofactor for several mitochondrial enzymes, especially those that process fatty acids. Antioxidants useful for individuals with mitochondrial dysfunction include vitamins E (200–400 IU/day) and C (100–500 mg/day), lipoic acid (50–200 mg/day) and folic acid (1–10 mg/day).

History of Development

In 1962 two independent researchers linked dysfunctional mitochondria to medical disease. In the last thirty years, several dozen genetically-based mitochondrial disorders have been described—all of them rare. It is becoming increasingly recognized that mitochondrial dysfunction, as opposed to mitochondrial disease, most likely contributes to the development and progression of many common diseases such as Parkinson's disease or diabetes mellitus.

Although mitochondrial dysfunction in autism has only recently been more widely recognized, the first biochemical evidence of mitochondrial dysfunction was reported over twenty years ago. Dr. Mary Coleman from Georgetown University described an elevation in serum lactic acid in a subset of children diagnosed with autism. Over the past five years, others have confirmed elevations in lactic acid, as well as abnormalities in other metabolic markers of mitochondrial dysfunction in children with autism. One study from Portugal used traditional markers to screen children evaluated in their autism clinic for mitochondrial disorders. Children with abnormal markers underwent muscle biopsies to confirm a mitochondrial disorder. This population-based study estimated that between 4 to 7 percent of children with autism probably had mitochondrial disease in their population. However, other studies have shown that nontraditional serum markers of mitochondrial dysfunction are also elevated in children with autism. Thus, it is possible that studies that do not screen patients with nontraditional markers of mitochondrial dysfunction, such as the Portugal study, could be missing the diagnosis of mitochondrial disorders in some children. This raises the possibility that the estimated prevalence of mitochondrial disorders in children with autism has been underestimated. Clearly this is an important and evolving area of autism research that will lead to a better understanding and treatment of children with autism.

The success rate of treatment is very variable for several reasons. First, the efficacy of mitochondrial treatment, even for well-known mitochondrial disorders, has not been well studied. Second, the mitochondrial dysfunction identified in autism has not been well characterized and treatment for mitochondrial dysfunction in autism has not been well studied. Third, the benefit of treatment may not be obvious as treatment my simply prevent progression of symptoms rather than reverse symptoms. Fourth, any benefit from treatment may take several months to observe. In general, milder mitochondrial dysfunction responds better to treatment than more severe dysfunction and treatment initiated sooner in the course of the disorder will probably be more effective than treatment initiated after long standing mitochondrial dysfunction.

Most vitamins are well tolerated, even at high doses. Some children with autism may have behavioral side effects from some vitamin. Thus, it is important to start vitamins one at a time so that any side effects can be linked to a particular vitamin. Levocarnitine is linked to behavioral disturbances, especially in children with fatty acid abnormalities. Pyridoxine has been suggested to result in peripheral neuropathy at high doses. Children should be carefully monitored when the ketogenic diet is started as the diet can worsen the metabolic acidosis associated with mitochondrial dysfunction.

MUSIC THERAPY

BY THE AMERICAN MUSIC THERAPY ASSOCIATION

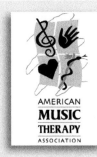

American Music Therapy Association

8455 Colesville Road, Suite 1000
Silver Spring, MD 20910
(301) 589-3300
Fax: (301)589-5175
info@musictherapy.org
www.musictherapy.org

Certification Board for Music Therapists
506 East Lancaster Avenue, Suite 102
Downingtown, PA 19335
(800) 765-2268 or (610) 269-8900
Fax: (610) 269-9232
info@cbmt.org
www.cbmt.org

If you are interested in locating a music therapist, please contact AMTA at findMT@ musictherapy.org or contact CBMT at info@cbmt.org. Both organizations will provide you with a free current list of board certified and qualified music therapists in your local area. Please provide the location in which you are looking and be sure to include your postal and e-mail address with your request.

What Is Music Therapy?

Music Therapy is the clinical and evidence-based use of music interventions to accomplish individualized goals within a therapeutic relationship by a credentialed professional who has completed an approved music therapy program. It is a well-established allied health profession that uses music therapeutically to address behavioral, social, psychological, communicative, physical, sensory-motor, and/or cognitive functioning. Music therapists are members of an interdisciplinary team of education or health care professionals who work collaboratively to address an individual's needs. For individuals with diagnoses on the autism spectrum, music therapy provides a unique variety of music experiences in a developmentally appropriate manner to effect changes in behavior and facilitate development of skills.

Recognized as a related service under the Individuals with Disabilities Education Act (IDEA), music therapy serves as an integral component in helping the child with autism attain educational goals identified by his/her Individualized Education Program (IEP) team, either through direct or consultant services. IDEA includes a definition of related services that the U.S. Department of Education notes is not exhaustive. In addition, in June 2000, the U.S. Department of Education issued a letter of policy clarification related to the use of music therapy. The letter reiterated the Department's continuing policy that "[i]f the IEP team determines that music therapy is an appropriate related service for a child, the team's determination must be reflected in the child's IEP, and the service must be provided at public expense . . ." [This interpretation stands with the 2006 regulations.]

How Can I Find a Board Certified Music Therapist?

Some music therapists work in school settings as a related service on a child's Individual Education Plan (IEP), either hired or contracted by a school district. Others have private practices or work for agencies that specialize in treatment for individuals with developmental disabilities. Some states fund music therapy services through Medicaid waivers or other state programs. Private health insurance reimbursement usually requires pre-approval on a case-by-case basis.

History of Development

The 20th century discipline of music therapy began after World War I and World War II, when community musicians of all types, both amateur and professional, went to Veterans hospitals around the country to play for the thousands of veterans suffering both physical and emotional trauma from the wars. The patients' notable physical and emotional responses to music led the doctors and nurses to request the hiring of musicians by the hospitals, formalizing the music interventions as therapy.

Music was used as a rehabilitative tool to improve respiratory function, increase attention, and boost morale. Interventions were also used to positively impact leisure skills, socialization, and physical and emotional function. It was soon evident that the military hospital musicians needed some prior training before entering the facility and so the demand grew for a college curriculum. The first music therapy degree program was founded at Michigan State University in 1944. In 1950, the first professional music therapy organization was founded. Since 1998 it has been known as The American Music Therapy Association (AMTA).

AMTA is committed to the advancement of education, training, professional standards, and research in support of the music therapy profession. The mission of the organization is to advance public knowledge of music therapy benefits and increase access to quality music therapy services. Currently, AMTA establishes criteria for the education and clinical training of music therapists. Members of AMTA adhere to a Code of Ethics and Standards of Clinical Practice in their delivery of music therapy services. Today, music therapists are employed in many different settings including general hospitals, schools, mental health agencies, rehabilitation centers, nursing homes, forensic settings, hospice programs, and private practice.

Music therapists must earn a bachelor's degree or higher in music therapy from one of over seventy American Music Therapy Association (AMTA) approved college and university programs; complete a minimum of 1,200 hours of clinical training; and pass a national examination administered by the Certification Board for Music Therapists (CBMT) to obtain the credential required for professional practice, Music Therapist-Board Certified (MT-BC).

With sixty years of clinical history in the U.S., music therapy currently receives national recognition in the following ways:

- The National Institutes of Health (NIH) National Center on Complementary and Alternative Medicine (NCCAM) website defines complementary and alternative medicine. Music therapy is included under Mind-Body Interventions.
- Music therapy is listed under the Healthcare Common Procedure Coding System (HCPCS) Code G0176 for billing Medicare in Partial Hospitalization Programs (PHP).
- Music therapy has a Procedure Code of 93.84 in the International Classification of Diseases-9th Revision Manual (ICD-9) used in reimbursement.
- Music therapy is listed on the U.S. General Services Administration (GSA) schedule under Professional and Allied Healthcare Staffing Services
- 621-047—Counseling Related Services (Includes: Community Counselor; Marriage/Family Counselor/Therapist; Mental Health Counselor; Rehabilitation Counselor; Social Worker (BS); Social Worker (MS); Music Therapist; Art Therapist and Dance Therapist (Registered DTR).

- Music therapists are eligible to apply for the National Provider Identifier system for billing under taxonomy code 225A00000X.
- Music therapy is a related service under IDEA and can be included on IEPs if found necessary for a child to benefit from his/her special education program.
- The Joint Commission and the Commission on Accreditation of Rehabilitation Facilities (CARF) recognize music therapists as qualified individuals who may provide services within accredited facilities.

Research Sample Overview

Trends regarding the level of evidence are emerging showing several positive trends; but, music therapy clinicians and scholars recognize the complexity and many unanswered questions regarding autism spectrum disorders. Research on specific music therapy interventions is part of an ongoing and growing body of evidence within the profession of music therapy. Research in published peer reviewed scholarly journals includes significant work in applied music therapy procedures as well as several systematic reviews examining, in aggregate, numerous studies on similar topics. Recommendations regarding assessment and referral criteria based on current research and clinical evidence are emerging.

Music therapy offers a particularly important interventions for individuals with autism spectrum disorders to engage and foster their capacity for flexibility, creativity, variability, and tolerance of change. These interventions tend to balance the more structured and behaviorally driven education required in school settings. One review protocol published in the Cochrane Collaborative of Systematic Reviews concluded music therapy was superior to "placebo" therapy with respect to verbal and gestural communicative skills (verbal: 2 RCTs, n = 20, SMD 0.36 CI 0.15 to 0.57; gestural: 2 RCTs, n = 20, SMD 0.50 CI 0.22 to 0.79).

The addition of music therapy interventions to a child's treatment program can have positive outcomes and may be an effective method for increasing joint attention skills in some children with autism. The Council for Exceptional Children (CEC) published an article examining the effectiveness and efficacy of various interventions and music therapy was one of the few professions listed as promising based upon the systematic reviews of research complied and listed herein.

An overall positive direction is noted in meta-analytic reviews of the literature on the subject of music therapy and autism in terms of an array of outcomes related to both therapeutic and specific educational goals. Variations for effect size occur within the broad category of the autism spectrum disorders and tend to reflect the idiosyncratic nature of the disorders between individuals. This is typical across disciplines.

Survey research indicates goal areas typically addressed by music therapists among persons with autism include language/communication, behavioral/psychosocial, cognitive, and musical, to perceptual/motor. Goal attainment was found to be high within one year, and parents and caregivers surveyed indicated subjects generalized skills/responses acquired in music therapy to non-music therapy environments.

Why Would a Person with Autism Need to See a Music Therapist?

The broad spectrum of autism calls for strategic approaches such as music therapy that can be tailored to the specific needs of each individual. Music Therapy provides a natural, enriching environment for addressing goals in areas such as communication, social skills, sensory issues, behavior, cognition, perceptual/motor skills, and self-reliance or self-determination. The therapist finds music experiences that strike a chord with a particular person, making personal connections and building trust. The constancy and predictability of a music therapy session allows the therapist to nourish the relationship and encourage cooperative participation, setting the occasion for maximizing the potential of each individual with autism while at the same time addressing deficits, behavior issues, and/or sensory issues that may have a negative impact on the person's life.

Research has shown that people with diagnoses on the autism spectrum often show a heightened interest and response to music, making it an excellent therapeutic tool to work with them. Because music is motivating and engaging, it may be used as a natural "reinforcer" for desired responses. By the same token, some individuals with autism may not indicate an interest in music, or may seem to have an aversion to music because of sensory issues or because of unfamiliar setting, people, or activities. Music therapy can assist these individuals gradually adapt to new situations and cope with sound sensitivities or individual differences in auditory processing.

What Does a Music Therapist Do for People with Autism?

After assessing the strengths and needs of each person, music therapists develop a treatment plan with goals and objectives and then provide the indicated treatment. Music therapists offer direct or consultative services both individually or in small groups, using a variety of music and techniques.

Music therapists:

- Involve individuals in singing, listening, moving, playing instruments, and creative experiences in a systematic, prescribed manner to influence change in targeted responses or behaviors.
- Create a musical, familiar environment that encourages positive interaction and allows people freedom to explore and express themselves.
- Utilize music that is preferred by and reinforcing to participants and is appropriate for ages, cultures, and environments in which they interact.
- Use the structure and multi-sensory stimulation (auditory, visual, and tactile) inherent in music to address multiple developmental issues simultaneously.
- Use the natural music setting to promote relatedness, relaxation, learning, and self-expression.
- Develop effective, customized strategies that increase self-reliance and independence.
- Develop effective goal directed treatment and strategies individuals and families can utilize on a daily basis. Through gradual fading of music therapy cues, music therapy supports generalization and transfer of learned skills, responses and behaviors to other environments and other people.
- The flexible nature of music therapy allows it to blend in with different theoretical approaches and models, so music therapists can work cooperatively with teams in various settings under a variety of treatment philosophies.

NEUROFEEDBACK (NEUROTHERAPY OR EEG BIOFEEDBACK)

BY DR. BETTY JARUSIEWICZ

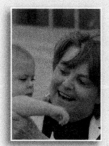

Betty Jarusiewicz, Ph.D., LCADC, ABPC

Atlantic Neurofeedback Center, LLC
222 Serpentine Drive
Bayville, NJ 08721
(732) 801-4505
bjarus@comcast.net

Dr. Jarusiewicz is the founder of Atlantic Counseling Center, PC, Atlantic Neurofeedback Center, LLC, and the Atlantic Research Institute. She produced the first controlled study of the efficacy of neurofeedback for individuals with autism spectrum disorder. Her work was published in the *Journal of Neurotherapy* and she provided the chapter on autism in the *Handbook of Neurofeedback*. She has produced research studies on the integration of Applied Behavior Analysis (ABA) with NFB, integration of chiropractic techniques with NFB, efficacy of NFB in developing REM sleep patterns, and efficacy of NFB for Cerebral Palsy. She along with Bob Paterson produced a radio show on AutismOne.org. She has given lectures regarding brain dysregulation in many venues. In the book *Healing Young Brains: The Neurotherapy Solution*, she was described as follows: "Betty Jarusiewicz, Ph.D., epitomizes the sensitivity and instincts found in the best therapist. She weaves an intricate and thoughtful therapeutic experience for her young patients, and they thrive under her care."

Neurofeedback is a brain learning strategy described by developers that enables persons to alter their brain waves. This technique helps to improve the brain to regulate all bodily functions by and including taking care of itself. When the brain is not functioning well, evidence generally shows up in one's electroencephalogram (EEG).[1] With appropriate software connected to the EEG a trained professional can train the various frequencies in the brain, such as delta (0–3 Hertz) which is associated with sleep, theta (4–7 Hz) which is associated with meditation, alpha (8–11 Hz) associated with daydreaming, low beta and SMR (Sensory Motor Rhythm) 12–15 Hz associated with light processing, and higher frequencies associated with more sophisticated processing needs. With the software, one can reward the frequencies desired and inhibit those causing dysregulation or nonfocusing. This brain training process is noninvasive (putting nothing into the body), but allowing the brain to be aware of it's functionality. When a trained professional assesses an individual it can be determined where the probable source may lie within the brain activity. This assessment process may include extensive analysis of brain activity, behaviors, and current environment.

A simple diagram showing a dysregulated brain with its irregular activity and the more efficient brain activity neurofeedback will develop is shown below:[2]

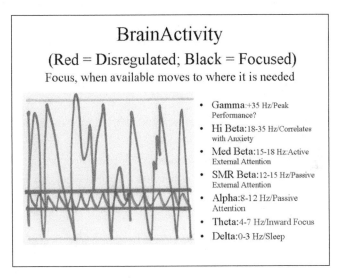

The distinguishing features of neurofeedback [3] are that it:
- Initiates learning at a neurological level
- The child witnesses his brain in action, thereby learning to control it
- Accelerates learning and modifies behavior more rapidly and efficiently (producing up to 4,000 reinforcements per hour)
- Develops brain abilities that translate to other life situations.

History of Development for the Treatment of ASD

Autogenic training, developed in Germany by J.H Schultz in the early twentieth century used verbal instructions to guide individuals to a more relaxed, controlled, physiological state. Temperature biofeedback, Galvanic skin response

(GSR), and electromyographic (EMG) by Galvani (early 1800s known response) were developed over time to respond to tension, spasms and muscle strength training (Kegel). In the 1970s a number of specific trainings were developed: breath training, (Hirai 1975) relaxation techniques by Miller for smoking, chronic headaches, or immune system insufficiency, Simonton for cancer, Bresler for stress management, Fehmi for learning attentional skills.[4]

Software programs added to EEGs began also in the 1970s: Sterman noting reduction in seizures and inhibition of excessive slow wave activity, Lubar noting a reduction in hyperactivity which was more effective than stimulant medication alone. These above programs are noted as SMR programs, using an eyes-open approach. Peniston and Kulkosky in the 1980s began work on an eyes-closed alpha theta program that enhanced meditation and mental imagery, which was useful for addiction, posttraumatic stress disorder, and peak performance work. Others, along with the above continued enhancing software, setting up protocols, and training practitioners.

Organizations developed to assist all interested parties in discussing and dissecting new developments. These included the Association for Applied Psychophysiology and Biofeedback (AAPB) founded in 1969 to focus on biofeedback and the International Society for Neuronal Regulation (ISNR) founded in 1995 to focus on neurotherapy training and research.

Sichel, Fehmi, and Goldstein[5] published a positive outcome with neurofeedback treatment in a mild case of autism in 1995. Others had been publishing research about behaviors that autism spectrum disorders share with other diagnoses such as: Hauri[6] (1981) insomnia, Kaiser and Othmer[7] (1995) attentional processes, Lantz and Sterman[8] (1992) epilepsy, Linden, Habib and Radojevic[9] (1996) attention deficit disorders and learning disabilities, Lubar and Shouse[10] (1976) seizure activity and hyperactivity, Swingle,[11] (1996) suppression of Theta in ADD/ADHD, Tansey[12] (1990) general therapeutic modality, and Thomas and Sattlberger[13] (1997) for chronic anxiety.

In 2002, Jarusiewicz published a pilot study[14] with matched control and ASD subjects showing the efficacy of neurofeedback for ASD children. *The Handbook of Neurofeedback*[15] describes many of the detailed research areas involving the approach, including a chapter on ASD. Coben and Padolsky (2007)[16] published another study specifically focused on ASD. Neurofeedback clinical and training associations such as EEG Spectrum International (www.eegspectrum.com), EEG Info (www.eeginfo.com), list ASD as one of the conditions that responds to neurofeedback, as well as many individual clinicians in practice reporting results on their websites. To find qualified professionals using neurofeedback use www.eeg-spectrum.com, www.eeginfo.com, www.isnr.org, and www.aapb.com.

An additional tool, quantitative EEG (qEEG) has been developed where the brain is analyzed thoroughly comparing the individual's brain to a typical baseline. A cap is used with as many as twenty-six electrodes to record samples of an ASD individual, and comparing results to typical databases, to ascertain differences been an individual and a norm. There is more research work required to establish if this analysis is thoroughly valid. Can we compare one person's brain to a typical database? Can the brain be simply analyzed? What types of analyses contribute to a clear understanding of brain activity? Various laboratories are providing databases and analyses include Sterman-Kaiser Imaging Laboratory, Q-Metrx, and other clinicians provide a qEEG analysis that may assist a clinician in determining protocol(s) for ASD. Also other types of brain analyses are being developed and used, including blood flow (hemoencephalography or HEG) analysis by Hershel Toomin,[17] SPECT (single photon emission computed tomography) scans analysis as described by Daniel Amen,[18] and informational-based brain mapping.[19]

One new interesting area of investigation has been mirror neurons. They have been said to assist the brain in mimicry, which is necessary in learning from others. Marco Iacoboni[20] describes some of the issues regarding this specific activity in the brain with autism. The Irlen Syndrome[21] is another area of investigation in brain activity related to seeing and reading.

Success Rate

Research comparing methods of success rates in still in its infancy. The deep questions behind this research must consider how one measures success in general. Is it in brain differences where various equipment and software may be utilized in measurement? Is it in behavior differences, where behavior checklists can be used? Who is to make the determination in differences, medical/alternative therapists, parents, schools, and/or individuals?

In a Dr. Jarusiewicz study in 2002[22] the Autism Treatment Evaluation Checklist (ATEC) [23] was used and showed a success rate of 26 percent total, with 29 percent for Speech, 33 percent for Socialization, 17 percent for Sensory, and 26 percent for Health, compared with a total of 3 percent, 0 in Speech, 7 percent in Socialization, 0 percent in Sensory, and 5 percent in Health over 4.5 months with twelve children trained and twelve wait-listed as controls. Dr. Coben [24] showed even greater success rates with his study.

A more medically based assessment process; Autism Diagnostic Observation Schedule (ADOS) has been developed by Catherine Lord [25], which intends to provide a "gold standard" of assessment for use particularly by researchers.

Most clinicians would state that most every person trained benefits in some or many ways. Benefits include: speech, attention, sleep, socialization, schoolwork, and seizures, if any.

One unique method in showing change involved drawings. Dr. Larry Hirsh-berg collected the following pictures showing the progress one child experienced:

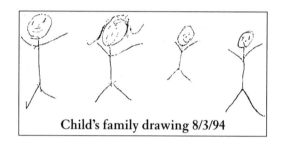

Child's family drawing 8/3/94

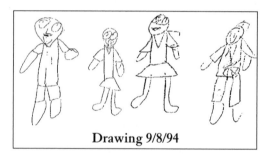

Drawing 9/8/94

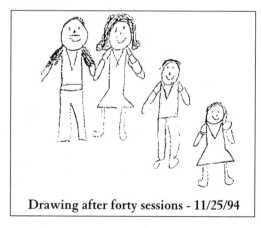

Drawing after forty sessions - 11/25/94

Cases

Dr. Jarusiewicz tells the history of Casey, who spoke not a word at five years of age. With neurofeedback and speech therapy Casey first began with animal sounds, including "moo" which to Dr. Betty sounded a little like Mom. Initially the school wanted to provide an assistive device so he would not have to learn to speak. But we asked for sufficient time to allow neurofeedback to work. With time and training Casey began to say "Mom" and both Dr. Betty and Casey's mom cried in the beginning when he used the term. When Casey began school, he had a full time aide to help him deal with school and other children. We remember though the day he said he wished to read aloud like the other students. Again we were moved by his growth. Needless to say, it did not take long for him to have his wish. By the third grade he was able to be successful at school without any aide. Today you would not even notice that he was considered significantly ASD in his early childhood or had any disabilities at all. As with most training, everything takes time.

Other cases include that of a young man (in his early twenties) who was not toilet trained. With neurofeedback he learned how to use the toilet and many other personal responsibilities of self-care, and is now adding to other life skills. A thirteen-year-old was brought in with uncontrolled behavior. This was particularly difficult as the mother has massive health issues of her own (problems with sight and walking). Within a few months this child was careful with others, particularly with his mother, had few problems at school and was able to function on a significantly higher level. Another teen was able to find meaningful work and make plans for college. It is important to recognize that everyone is different and will succeed with different approaches, but neurofeedback appears to be synergistic with many therapies.

Brain training often provides some results almost immediately, such as calming, better sleep, and better focus. Working with dieticians better diets (i.e., fewer carbohydrates and sugars, fewer meats) will help in most cases. Appropriate placement in schools is important, but most important is the parental understanding of and providing for the needs of this particular child. Sometimes as training progresses certain behaviors appear that look negative. But with an appropriate review it is often found that the child has "found" a new interest or idea, and may need help in using this new information.

A clinician when beginning to work with families of ASD individuals may provide a "Hints for all parents" [27] to lay out some groundwork regarding a training/treatment process. These include the following three major issues involving the child's behavior and what can be done for improvement beyond particular therapies:

1. Be aware of the food and drink and other materials that your child puts into his or her body:

    a. Contact a dietician who can help you determine level of carbohydrates, sugars, and types of protein, fruits, and vegetables your child can ingest without a problem.

    b. Eat as a family, preferably at the same time and the same food, and use that time for development of communication skills

2. Be aware of the skin discomforts and other environmental issues that may affect your child.

    a. Consider use of 100 percent cotton clothing

    b. Wash clothing in nonallergenic soaps (no dyes, no additives)

    c. Wash bed clothing in nonallergenic soaps

    d. Consider use of oatmeal baths to sooth skin

    e. Consider use of hats to shield child from sun and glare (if they will wear a hat)

    f. Be sure to use sun screen when outdoors

    g. Consider use of sensitive type toothpaste

3. Be aware of old coping behaviors that may need change as their brain is better able to sort out issues.

    a. Install appropriate schedules and requirements as possible now that your child can learn new behaviors. White boards throughout the home and school are useful with schedules and other hints

    b. Be consistent and always explain what you are trying to achieve

    c. Improve communication with your child

        i.   Listen longer, ask questions

        ii. Read with your child every evening. You may try reading faster.

        iii. Communicate around the dinner table each evening

        iv. Know that your child is capable beyond what you are seeing directly.

        v.   Ask for help

        vi. Get them into a socialization situation at all ages: schools, groups, activities

Risks:

To date we have not seen any major problem with side effects. Side effects may include extra activity, lower activity, or headaches. All of these can be reversed by the clinician with balancing protocols. We are using a technique that is noninvasive—that is, not putting anything in the brain or body, just interacting with the brain voltage and frequencies to train to a more efficient focus. It is important for the parent and clinician to work together to look at differences in the child. Sometimes the child will look as if they are regressing, but they may be developing new skills.

Contact Information:

Neurofeedback training for clinicians:

    www.eegspectrum.com

    www.eeginfo.com

    www.Stens-Biofeedback.com

    www.appliedneuroscience.com

Provider Listings

    www.isnr.org

    www.aapb.com

    www.eegspectrum.com

    www.eeginfo.com

NEUROIMMUNE DYSFUNCTION AND THE RATIONALE AND USE OF ANTIVIRAL THERAPY

BY DR. MICHAEL GOLDBERG

Michael J. Goldberg, MD, F.A.A.P
5620 Wilbur Avenue #318
Tarzana, CA 91356
(818) 343-1010
Fax: (818) 343-6585
office@neuroimmunedr.com
www.neuroimmunedr.com
www.nids.net

Dr. Michael J. Goldberg graduated from UCLA Medical School in 1972, after which he did his pediatric internship and residency at LAC + USC Medical Center, entering private practice in the San Fernando Valley in 1975. Since the early 1980s, his interest has focused on the development and treatment of immune dysregulation /neurocognitive disorders, including CFS/CFIDS and its particular connection to ADHD, in children and in adults. This interest has extended into the neurocognitive dysfunctional link between many children with autism/PDD and siblings or parents with ADHD and CFIDS.

He is actively pursuing collaboration with researchers to accelerate identification and potential new therapeutic modalities for these children. Dr. Goldberg is currently the founder and director of the neuroimmune dysfunction syndromes (NIDS) medical advisory board and research institute.

Author's note: If you believe your child truly has a disorder called "autism" this chapter does not apply to you. If your child was ever affectionate (which excludes a child from the diagnosis of "autism" per Dr. Kanner) and you believe your child might be suffering from a true medical disease, then please continue.

Background and Rationale

The Centers for Disease Control and Prevention now says that one child in every 110 has an autism spectrum disorder (ASD), which represents almost 1 percent of births in this country; including one in every seventy-one males. New rates are already quoting one child in ninety-one. No genetic or developmental disorder in the history of written medicine has ever come remotely close to 1 percent of children, much less greater. No genetic or behavioral syndrome with such profound symptoms can increase at the rates cited above without being in reality a true medical disease. Reviews of ASD medical research over the last decade (or more) clearly point to a disease-mediated neurological dysfunction (or encephalopathy) likely triggered by an immune system, neuroimmune dysfunction with a probable chronic viral infection or reactivation component.

I began my medical career as a general pediatrician. Once in private practice, it was not long before I started noticing parents and then their children coming in with unusual presentations that we were not taught about in medical school. In the late 1980s, through research, conferences and presentations, it became clear we were looking at a neuroimmune-mediated process, a disease process that was throwing off the brain, the nervous system, and overall physical function of the adults being discussed and the children presenting in my practice. Family histories of these children repeatedly showed a high link to allergies and other immune-mediated disorders (e.g., rheumatoid disease, thyroid dysfunction, multiple sclerosis [MS], lupus, irritable bowel syndrome, and chronic fatigue syndrome) within the family. Clinical patterns were very similar to children with allergies I had worked with since becoming a pediatrician, but there was now a large neurocognitive dysfunctional component, fatigue, and often "mono-like" symptoms, along with the "normal" allergies, immune problems, etc. This increase and change in patterns is consistent with the fact that all immune-mediated disorders (e.g., allergies, migraines, lupus, MS, Alzheimer's, leukemia, lymphomas, and diabetes) have increased dramatically in children and adults over the last twenty-five+ years. What was the rare, mixed ADD/ADHD child has now become the majority.

Open to ongoing debates about environmental factors, global warming, and the ozone layer, there can be no real debate that something has changed and is quite different than when we were all growing up. This is certainly not the environment we were programmed for 200 or 2000+ years ago. A simplistic way to understand the linkage of all of this is that many adults and children (now even infants) are starting not at the "neutral" of many years ago, but are being born in an already "immune-stressed" state. Then, whether an adult, adolescent, child, or infant, a combination of additional stresses—even simple allergies, rashes, eczema, congestion and/or infection are factors in many of these children—adds up to a point where our neuroimmune system becomes dysregulated and dysfunctional.

Unlike the idea of autism sixty years ago, most of these children today are linked by the concept of a dysfunctional neuroimmune system, open to the high probability of secondary infection with chronic viruses. It became obvious that these children have a hyperreactive immune system, explaining many food and environmental sensitivities and often outright allergies. The NeuroSPECT (*single photon emission computed tomography*) scans on these children consistently reveal reduced blood flow in areas of the brain, particularly the temporal lobes. This reduced flow is secondary to a neuroimmune shutdown (similar to how we all feel when fighting a cold or other illness) but continuing on an autoimmune course (it continues to be shut down in an unregulated manner). This is a disease process, not developmental or prewired genetically.

Assessment

Currently, when a child comes in to my office for evaluation, I begin by looking at his or her symptoms as a pediatrician, a medical physician. As I review their history and medical records, I try to determine if they have been injured during pregnancy or delivery, if there has been any brain injury or damage. If I cannot find physiological damage and the child presents in this dysfunctional state called "autism," I will begin a further workup. This usually includes blood work (focused on the immune system, viral markers, food allergies, and normal pediatric markers), and a NeuroSPECT scan (not routinely needed). I am looking for markers and data that suggest an autoimmune or viral profile. Testing being done now is primitive compared to research protocols we will look at to fully define the complexities of this immune and viral process, but, thankfully, there are general markers that at least help point to problems and help define therapies. While minimal blood work should include an immune panel (CD4, CD8, natural killer cells, B cells), viral titers, immunoglobulins, and general pediatric health screens, review and history alone are often only consistent with a disease process that can only be immune or viral in origin. If indicated, I may request neurological testing or other subspecialty evaluation such as a pediatric endocrinologist since some of the children show thyroid or growth issues, reflecting a classical autoimmune, endocrine issue. I will obtain a NeuroSPECT scan if needed.

Intervention

The first step in therapy should be to remove foods or other supplements that may trigger reactions or act as stimulants to their immune system. When asked about what is the healthiest thing to build up a child's immune system, my first response is "remove the negatives." That is the key to helping the immune system stop reacting inappropriately and is the first step to beginning to let the immune system and body repair themselves.

Dairy (bovine protein) is the number one allergen in the world. So the first step I will always take is to remove all milk and dairy products. Wheat/grains are the number two allergen in the world. It is very important to limit carbs. Berries, strawberries, cherries, and other red foods—these may hype up many children, possibly fire off the immune system (which then literally attacks the brain). From there it depends on the child and their food screen (as a guide, never an absolute). Some children do need to be off nuts (many) or citrus (some), which are number 3 and number 4 in the allergy groups. Most of these children should avoid nuts. Nuts are highly allergenic, and they contain arginine, which feeds herpes viruses (and is often in many of the supplements given to the children).

If a viral or fungal process is identified by blood work or suspected strongly from history and the patient's course, I will treat with an antiviral or antifungal medication. The "reactivated" or chronic viral activity generally seems to be herpes related when it comes to the central nervous system, particularly the temporal lobes. In medical school we are taught herpes viruses like to go to the temporal lobes of the brain. The idea of retroviruses playing a potential role merely heightens the medical magnitude of the problem. Within the herpes family, the main pathogens are probably HHV-6, HHV-7, and HHV-8 (consider higher-order herpes virus), not classical herpes simplex I or II. Whether variants of cytomegalovirus, Epstein-Barr virus, or mutated versions are present is open to ongoing clinical investigation.

I have found that children who have a history of fine or gross motor problems or a history of regressive behaviors or skills and/or an abnormal electroencephalogram (EEG) have a significant higher probability of a concurrent complex viral process. While open to further research, presumably when a virus—or now retrovirus—is present, I believe it is probably secondary to the immune dysfunctional state rather than the primary cause.

If there is evidence of a virus, with strict diet control initiated, I will then turn to an antiviral (antivirals will not work adequately if one is consuming foods or supplements irritating or creating ongoing dysfunction within the immune system). Antiviral choices at this time should be limited to known "safe" (when monitored) antivirals, which include acylovir (Zovirax), valacyclovir (Valtrex), and *famciclovir* (Famvir). While there are other stronger antivirals that might be considered in new trials, this author believes the key remains to help the immune system become healthy, and then it can, in theory, handle viruses and even retroviruses. I will re-stress that to have any chance of success, one must think of the role of the immune system as a critical ally, not be stimulating or trying to force manipulate it; and then one must dose at full, appropriate (but not over) therapeutic levels without starting and stopping blindly.

After diet eliminations (eliminate immune system stressors as much as possible), evaluation of an antiviral (usual), antifungal (sometimes), then I begin to look at applying a selective seratonin reuptake inhibitor (SSRI). This is not to treat a child for "depression" or to control behavior, but rather to attempt to address the temporal lobe hypoperfusion being seen on the NeuroSPECT scan.

Do one step at a time, change only one variable at a time, allowing time to analyze and observe if each step is truly working/helping. I have also learned over many years to first focus on physical changes (e.g., sharpness, alertness, brightness in the eyes, and general health), then to analyze, look, and focus on developmental and educational progress, as "rehabilitation" of a child, never training.

Like any other person, any biological organism, there are multiple variables affecting the mood, actions, and attitude of a child. None of us would have been able to learn if we were sent to school chronically ill, with a foggy brain, often painful headaches, and body aches. It's time to think of these children as what they are, pediatric patients who are very ill, often crying because they are in pain. This is not "behavioral." When functioning and feeling well, like other children, these children grow and develop, obviously brighter, happier, and ready to learn.

It is time to revert to medical school training, go back to pediatrics, and help support a child within our abilities. In the meantime, as a parent trust your instincts (pediatric principle 101: "listen to the mothers"), and believe in yourself and your child. Again, believe in your child: believe they were born with potentially normal, often above normal intelligence; believe they can be helped, that they can potentially recover. Then it is time to begin the right fight, a battle you, your child, and your family have a right to believe you can win.

NEUROPROTEK, FLAVONOIDS, AND ALLERGIES

BY DR. THEOHARIS THEOHARIDES

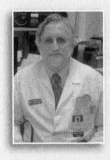

Theoharis C. Theoharides, MS, Ph.D., MD

Department of Pharmacology and Experimental Therapeutics
Tufts University School of Medicine
136 Harrison Avenue
Boston, MA 02111, USA
(617) 636-6866
Fax: 617-636-2456
www.mastcellmaster.com

Denise Hyman
Vice President for Customer Relations
Algonot, LLC
Box 294
5053 Ocean Boulevard, Sarasota, FL 34242
www.algonot.com
Phones (941) 346-9002
(800) ALGONOT (800-254-6668)
Fax: (941) 312-0872

Dr. Theoharis Theoharides is the Director of the Molecular Immunopharmacology and Drug Discovery Laboratory, as well as a Professor of Pharmacology, Biochemistry and Internal Medicine at Tufts University, Boston, MA. He received all his degrees from Yale University, is a member of 17 scientific societies and has published over 270 research papers and 2 textbooks. Dr. Theoharides is much more that just an eminent physician and pharmacologist; he goes a step further in posing new theories and defining the cutting edge of mast cell research. He was the first to show that mast cells can be stimulated by non-allergic triggers, such as stress hormones, to secrete inflammatory mediators selectively without histamine. Based on his discoveries, Dr. Theoharides proposed the novel concept that mast cells play a critical role in brain inflammation and autism. Dr. Theoharides extends his expertise beyond theory into practical options and offers hope for patients with diseases such as autism which, to date, have defied treatment.

NeuroProtek is a unique dietary formulation, which reduces patient gut and brain inflammation. NeuroProtek uses an exclusive combination of flavonoids, selected to reduce oxidative stress and inflammation both in the gut and the brain. Flavonoids are natural molecules found mostly in green plants and seeds. Unfortunately, our modern life diet contains progressively fewer flavonoids and those that are consumed are difficult to absorb because they do not dissolve in water. Under these conditions, the average person cannot consume enough to make a positive health difference.

The purpose of NeuroProtek is to maximize the anti-inflammatory effects of flavonoids while also overcoming any absorption obstacles, There are approximately 3,000 flavonoids. Of those, three are used in NeuroProtek: luteolin, quercetin, and the quercetin glycoside rutin, which are obtained from chamomile (>98 percent pure). To increase their absorbability, these flavonoids were mixed in unrefined olive kernel oil imported from Greece. Chondroitin sulfate was also included in the formulation to correct intestinal barrier damage. There are NO preservatives and NO dyes.

NeuroProtek is formulated in a softgel capsules. The capsules must be taken with food in a dose of two capsules taken twice per day. It may take six to twelve months before measurable benefits are observed. NeuroProtek does not require a prescription. Dr. Theoharides is the recipient of U.S. patents No. 6,624,148; 6,689,748; 6,984,667; 7,115,278 and EPO 1365777, which cover methods and compositions of mast cell blockers in neuroinflammatory conditions, as well as U.S. Patent application 10/811,825 covering diagnosis and treatment of austim spectrum disorder (ASD). All patents have been assigned to Theta Biomedical Consulting and Development Co., Inc. (Brookline, MA, U.S.A.). The name NeuroProtek has been trademarked in the U.S.A. with U.S. registration No. 3225924 and has also been assigned to Theta Biomedical Consulting and Development Co., Inc. (Brookline, MA, U.S.A.)

History of Development

www.autismedia.org/media3.html

Gut-Blood-Brain Barrier Disruption, Mast Cells and Brain Inflammation

Autism treatment has been elusive. In the majority of cases, the cause of autism is unknown. Although some possible autism susceptibility genes have been identified, no single or group of genes can explain the disturbing rise in the incidence of autism from two children out of every 100,000 only twenty years ago, to one out of every 110 children presently. To date, research has focused on the behavioral and neurologic manifestations of autism spectrum disorders instead of what led to them.

In the development of NeuroProtek, the researchers hypothesized that autism starts when the protective *gut-blood and blood-brain barriers* break down either during pregnancy or early in life. Such a barrier disruption allows neurotoxic molecules to reach the brain ultimately resulting in inflammation and defective nerve processing. This premise is supported by the fact that many autistic patients have antibodies against brain proteins, which implies that immune cells reached the brain through a leaky blood-brain barrier.

Recent research has also shown that mast cells, immune cells typically known for causing allergic reactions, can also be activated by environmental, infectious, and stress triggers and lead to disruption of the blood-brain-barriers. One such mast cell trigger, neurotensin, is frequently found at high levels in the serum of young children with autism.

Blood-brain-barrier disruption in autistic children is also evidenced by the fact that their serum contains a number of autoantibodies against brain components. Mast cell activation during pregnancy or perinatally, in response to allergic or non-immune triggers, could disrupt the gut-blood-brain barriers and permit neurotoxic molecules to enter the brain and result in brain inflammation. Mast cell activation could be particularly critical during gestation, since mast cell-derived mediators might act epigenetically to alter the expression of autism susceptibility genes.

Mast Cells and Autism

The possible association between autism and mast cells was first investigated because many symptoms that characterize patients with autism are also present in patients with mastocytosis, a spectrum of disorders that involve proliferation and activation of mast cells in the skin (urticaria pigmentosa, UP) and other organs. The Mastocytosis Society, Inc. (www.tmsforacure.org) together with the American Academy of Allergy, Asthma and Immunology recently produced a video, entitled *"Mast Cell Activation Symptomatology"* (available to physicians and patients), which highlights the fact that allergies may be only one aspect of mast cell activation. Preliminary research results indicate that the prevalence of autism in mastocytosis patients is ten-fold higher (1/10 children) than the general population.

Allergic Symptomatology and Autism

The observation that most children with autism have either a family or personal history of immune or allergic disorders prompted the proposal that autism may be a "neuroimmune" disorder. There have been numerous studies and papers that support this proposal. One study investigated infants born in California between 1995 and 1999 and reported that maternal asthma and allergies during the second trimester of pregnancy were correlated with a greater than two-fold elevated risk of autism in their children. In another study, 30 percent of autistic children had a family history of allergies as compared to 2.5 percent age-matched "neurologic controls." A more recent study reported that immune allergic response, represented by the frequency of atopic dermatitis, asthma and rhinitis was increased in 70 percent of Asperger patients compared to 7 percent in age-matched healthy controls.

A recent preliminary report of 362 children with autism in Italy also indicated that the strongest association of autism is with history of allergies. In a National Survey of Children's Health, parents of autistic children reported symptoms of allergies more often than those of other children, with food allergies being the most prevalent complaint. Another study reported an increased prevalence of non-IgE mediated food allergy in the autism group compared to normal controls. It is also interesting that a recent study conducted in Germany reported an independent association between atopic eczema and attention-deficit hyperactivity disorder (ADHD), which has considerable phenotypic overlap with autism.

The link between allergic symptomatology and autism is also supported by the observation that in many cases, autistic symptoms worsen when a patient's allergic symptoms flare up. However, even in these symptomatic cases allergy tests, such as skin prick or (RAST), are often negative. These circumstances suggest a non-allergic trigger of mast cells.

Environmental and Stress Mast Cell Triggers

Mast cells are critical for allergic reactions, but are also important in regulating immunity and inflammation. Mast cells are located close to blood vessels both in the gut and in the brain. Functional mast cell-neuron interactions occur in these locations increasing both intestinal and brain permeability. This may help to explain the intestinal and neurologic complaints of autistic patients. Many substances originating in the environment, intestine or brain can trigger mast cell secretion. These triggers include: bacterial and viral antigens; environmental toxins such as polychlorinated biphenyl (PCB) and mercury; and neuropeptides such as neurotensin and corticotropin-releasing hormone (CRH). CRH is typically secreted under stress, which stimulates selective release of vascular endothelial growth factor (VEGF).

The ability of viruses to trigger mast cell activation is an important consideration in their contribution to autism pathogenesis. A number of rotaviruses have been isolated from asymptomatic neonates and could activate mast cells at that age. Once activated, mast cells secrete numerous vasoactive, neurosensitizing and proinflammatory substances that are relevant to autism including interleukin-6 (IL-6). IL-6 can disrupt the gut-blood-brain barriers as well as promote the development of Th 17 cells which are critical for the development of autoimmune diseases. In this context, it is crucial to note that high IL-6 gene expression was found in autistic patients. This finding was also associated with increased levels of serum neurotensin, IL-6 and IL-17.

Why the chosen flavonoids?

Flavonoids are naturally occurring compounds mostly found in green plants and seeds. Whether taken as pills, tablets, or hard capsules, all flavonoids are difficult to absorb in powder form. and are extensively metabolized to inactive ingredients in the liver. In fact, less than 10 percent of orally ingested flavonoids are absorbed. In addition, very few flavonoids are beneficial; instead, many others such as morin have no anti-inflammatory activity, while pycnogenol is weakly active (as compared to luteolin or quercetin) but could cause liver toxicity. As an additional consideration, the most common source of the flavonoid quercetin is fava beans, which can induce hemolytic anemia (destruction of all the blood cells) in those 15 percent of people of Mediterranean origin, such as Greeks, Italians, Jews, and North Africans, who lack the enzyme glucose-6-phosphate dehydrogenase (G6PD).

Quercetin, and its closely structurally related flavonoids rutin and luteolin, have potent antioxidant and anti-inflammatory actions. Quercetin and luteolin can also inhibit the release of histamine and prostaglandin D_2 (PGD_2), as well as the proinflammatory molecules IL-6, IL-8, and tumor necrosis factor (TNF) from human cultured mast cells. Moreover, quercetin inhibits mast cell activation stimulated by IL-1, and mast cell-dependent stimulation of activated T cells involved in autoimmune diseases. Luteolin also inhibits IL-6 release from microglia cells, as well as IL-1- mediated release of IL-6 and IL-8 from astrocytes. Quercetin also inhibited and reversed acute stress-induced autistic-like behavior and the associated reduced brain glutathione levels in mice.

However, there are about 3,000 flavonoids in nature and many impure flavonoids are sold under such names as "bioflavonoids," "citrus flavonoids," "soy flavonoids," or "pycnogenol." Unfortunately, such preparations *do not* specify either the source or the purity of the flavonoids. This problem is even worse given that many autistic patients could have reactions to the impurities, fillers, or dyes. The selection of specific beneficial flavonoids, as well as the source, purity and absorbability of those flavonoids were taken into consideration in order to develop the most beneficial product with the least amount of associated risk, NeuroProtek.

Success Rate

Though to date the trials of NeuroProtek are limited, the results are very promising. In the initial trial ten children (ages three to eight) diagnosed with autism were orally administered a total of four NeuroProtek capsules per day for a period of four to six months. At the end of the trial period a significant improvement of core autism symptoms, such as poor communication skills and social interactions, was observed by the parents of the patients. In the best case outcome, two children (one boy and one girl, ages four and six years old, respectively), who prior to treatment were unable to speak, could not identify words, would get upset when asked to repeat a task, and would break into "wing flapping movements," after treatment were able to answer simple questions, could make words with block letters, and would allow the researcher to hold them.

Given the encouraging outcome of trials to date, applications for randomized, double-blind, placebo-controlled clinical trials have been submitted by Dr. Theoharides to Autism Speaks, the National Institutes of Health, and the Department of Defense.

Risks/Side Effects

The NeuroProtek formulation has received a *Certificate of Free Sale* from the Food and Drug Administration (FDA). This certification ensures the amount, purity, source and manufacture of the ingredients in a facility inspected by the FDA and fulfilling Good Manufacturing Practices (GMP).

Quercetin and its related flavonoids rutin and luteolin are safe because they are purified from chamomile, to avoid the problems associated with fava beans mentioned above, and are highly pure (>98 percent).

There are no side effects known; however, this formulation (as well as any flavonoids) must be used with caution with drugs that are heavily metabolized by the liver as it may affect the resulting blood levels of such compounds.

OCCUPATIONAL THERAPY AND SENSORY INTEGRATION

BY MARKUS JARROW

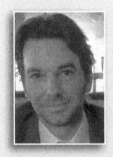

Markus Jarrow, OTR/L, C/NDT

Clinical Director
The SMILE Center | The Sensory Motor Integration + Language
Enrichment Center
171 Madison Avenue 5th Floor
New York, NY 10016
(212) 400-0383
markus@smileny.org
www.smileny.org

Markus Jarrow received his BA in Occupational Therapy from Sargent College of Boston University in 1997. Markus has more than twelve years of experience in pediatrics, specializing in the evaluation and treatment of children with autism spectrum disorders, sensory integration dysfunction, and neuromuscular disorders. Markus has extensive training in Sensory Integration, Neuro-Developmental Treatment, and DIR/Floortime methodologies. His approach to treatment draws from the fundamentals of these three models in a comprehensive style that addresses the whole child. Markus co-founded The SMILE Center | The Sensory Motor Integration and Language Enrichment Center in 2009, a state-of-the-art pediatric treatment facility in New York City.

W hy does my child spin? Why does my child refuse so many foods? Why does my son scream every time I try to put a coat or hat on him? Why does my daughter always hum and look out of the corner of her eyes?

Occupational therapists can provide valuable insight, both practical and neurological, to help families better understand many of the questions they struggle with when raising a child with an autism spectrum disorder. Occupational therapy and sensory integration (SI) can be very effective treatment approaches for children with ASD. In order to understand how sensory integrative treatment can be effective, it is important to understand the basics of sensory integration theory and dysfunction. This chapter will provide you with a brief overview.

What is Occupational Therapy?

Occupational Therapy is a broad profession that shares a common goal of utilizing functional and purposeful activities, or occupations, to increase an individual's functional independence. In the scope of treatment of children with autism spectrum disorders, occupational therapy can be very effective in improving functional fine and gross motor skills, postural control and movement patterns, motor planning, self-help skills, hand-eye coordination, and visual perceptual and spatial skills. However, perhaps most significant is the impact that a sensory integration treatment approach can have on a child's sensory processing skills. After all, if a child cannot maintain an optimal level of arousal and appropriately integrate sensory information, his or her ability to learn and acquire new skills will be greatly comprised. A child who relies of self-stimulatory or self-regulatory behaviors to control their arousal level, or tune out adverse stimuli, is a child less available for engagement, learning, and skill acquisition. Therefore, with this population in particular, sensory integration is one of the primary frames of reference utilized by occupational therapists.

History of Sensory Integration

Sensory integration is a theory and treatment approach originally developed by the late occupational therapist, Dr. A. Jean Ayres, Ph.D., OTR in the 1960s. She defined sensory integration as the ability to organize sensory information for use by the many parts of the nervous system, in order to work together to promote effective interactions with the environment. Sensory integration had evolved over the years, but much of the original theory remains. It is a dynamic and child-directed treatment approach based on specific principles, treatment techniques, and equipment. It is a problem-solving and individualized approach that requires ongoing analysis and assessment in order to monitor changes in the child and adapt the treatment accordingly. A trained occupational therapist utilizes a wide range of techniques and strategies in order to help a child achieve and maintain an optimal level of arousal. It is in this state that adaptive responses can be made to incoming sensory information. This in turn, enables them to become more confident, successful, and interactive explorers of their worlds.

While Dr. Ayers's treatment and research pertained primarily to the vestibular, proprioceptive, and tactile systems, toward the end of her life, she began to look much more closely at the important roles of the auditory and visual systems. Unfortunately for all of us, she was unable to conclude her work as she lost her life to cancer. More recently, several occupational therapists have made great strides in further identifying the important roles of the auditory and visual systems. Two therapists in particular turned their research and experience into very effective and practical treatment modalities and protocols: Therapeutic Listening and Astronaut Training.

What to Expect From Sensory Integration Therapy

Typically a child will first be evaluated by an occupational therapist trained in sensory integration. This process may include a variety questionnaires and evaluation tools including the Sensory Integration and Praxis Test (SIPT). The evaluation will also consist of interviewing with the caregivers as well as further clinical observations of the child in order to obtain insight into their sensory profile and needs. The entire process may take anywhere from a few hours to a few lengthy visits over the span of several sessions. Following a thorough assessment, a treatment plan will be formulated and a recommendation will be made regarding the frequency and duration of the child's treatment.

Sensory integrative treatment is best implemented in a therapy gym outfitted with a wide variety of specific equipment and adaptable environments. These treatment facilities are referred to as sensory gyms. Therapists, however, have found creative solutions to providing treatment with limited space and materials, such as in schools and in the home. Treatment should only be carried out by a clinician trained in sensory integration and should involve the parents/caregivers, as carryover into the home is critical. No matter how effective the clinician is, he or she may only have an hour or two a week with the child. It is therefore essential that a home program be implemented. This may include simple modifications to the home, adaptations to the child's routines, toys, clothing, etc. as well as specific, scheduled treatment strategies to be carried out in the home and/ or school. This is referred to as a sensory diet. This piece is critical in ensuring optimal progress.

In treatment, you may see your child flying and spinning through space on suspended equipment. You may see her climbing over or under enormous padded obstacles, up rope ladders, or through suspended tunnels. She may zip by you on a scooter board with headphones on, holding tight to a bungee cord, or jump from a platform into a crash mat or ball pit. She may be laying on her side, rhythmically spinning to the sounds of outer space.

Treatment with another child may appear completely different . . . at least initially. You may see him sitting with the clinician in a dimly lit room, wearing a weighted vest, covered in heavy blankets, attending to an activity. You may see him gently rocking on a swing with the clinician cradling him from behind, or slowly rolling over a soft surface to a rhythmical hum of the therapist. SI treatment can appear very different from one child to the next, as it is individualized to each child's unique sensory needs. While an experienced clinician can make treatment simply look fun and playful, rest assured, careful clinical reasoning is behind every move.

The cost of an evaluation can range from a few hundred dollars to a couple thousand dollars. Private treatment ranges greatly from less than one hundred to two hundred dollars or more per one-hour session. Sessions can be as short as thirty minutes; however, the nature of the treatment tends to lend itself to longer sessions. Occupational therapy evaluations and treatment are typically covered, to some extent, by local school systems as well as Early Intervention programs for children less than three years of age.

Occupational therapists can work with children with ASD in a variety of settings. In schools, treatment often carries over to the classroom as the primary focus is improving function in school related tasks and environments. In a private practice, sensory gym, or outpatient setting, the OT typically has access to more therapy equipment and can address issues related more to the home and community, as the parents are generally more present.

What is Sensory Integration and Sensory Integration Dysfunction?

In order for a child to appropriately move through space and interact with their world in an alert, regulated, and effective manner, they must take in an extraordinary amount of sensory information, unconsciously interpret it, and then make appropriate adaptive responses on a rapid and continuous basis. This is an incredibly complex process that relies on an intricate network of sensory systems functioning appropriately and simultaneously. It is called sensory integration. It's an amazing process that most of us take for granted; it just happens and we never think twice about it. However, for many of the children with ASD, this is not the case.

For a child with sensory integration dysfunction, the seemingly simple task of walking across a classroom, putting on a T-shirt, finding a toy in a closet, listening to mom on a busy street corner, walking barefoot on a beach, skipping down the sidewalk, or playing in a swing in the park may be perceived as overly challenging, seemingly impossible or even terrifying. Sensory integration dysfunction can impact every aspect of development including: social-emotional, behavioral, attention and regulation, gross and fine motor, postural, adaptive and self-help, visual motor, visual spatial/perceptual, speech and language, and academic. Our ability to appropriately meet the many challenges faced in our daily lives is a result of the integration and proper "wiring" of five major sensory systems: vestibular, proprioceptive, tactile, auditory, and visual.

The vestibular system is located in the inner ear and is the integral system that responds to gravitational forces and changes in the head's position in space. It is the sense that tells you when you're right side up or upside down, and is responsible for helping with balance and spatial orientation. The vestibular system is also responsible for proving a stable basis for visual function, even when the head is moving through space. Also, for example, when an object is getting larger in your visual field, your vestibular confirms that you are not moving, thus indicating that the object is coming toward you. The appropriate response can then be made, whether it's to move out of the way, catch it, etc.

Movement is a component of almost everything that we do; so vestibular function applies to almost every interaction we have with the world. It's the sense that, when overstimulated, makes one feel seasick and carsick. It's the sense that thrill seekers try to satiate with roller coasters, bungee jumping, and skydiving. Because of its role in movement and space, it works hand in hand with the auditory and visual systems in order to provide us with a sense of our three-dimensional spatial envelope, compelling us to move, explore, and understand. This collaborative system is referred to as the vestibular-visual-auditory triad.

Without this functioning triad, it would be impossible to appropriately process movement, space, time, and sequencing. When we enter a new restaurant for the first time, we immediately take in a sense of the room's size, relative shape, and arrangement of its contents. After navigating the delicate environment and casually taking a seat, we understand the quiet clinging of pots is coming from the open kitchen behind us and to the left; the gentle humming sound is coming from overhead ceiling fans; and the waitress walking slowly from across the room will be within a respectful distance in seven or eight seconds; the necessity to kindly request a glass of water in a suitable volume level for the environment. None of these seemingly simple processes that we take for granted would have been possible without appropriate integration of the vestibular-visual-auditory triad. This same analysis can be reapplied to countless scenarios, in countless environments, on countless different levels.

"Without a properly functioning vestibular system, sights and sounds in the environment do not make sense—they are only isolated pieces of information disconnected from the meaningful whole. It is the integration of the sensory information that holds the key to finding the meaning in the world. Because movement is part of everything we do in life, it could be said that the vestibular system supports all behavior and acquisition of skills, as well as helping to balance the stream of sensory information that constantly bombards the system." (Astronaut Training: A Sound Activated Vestibular-Visual Protocol for Moving, Looking and Listening; Kawar, Frick & Frick, 2005)

The proprioceptive system is a network of sensors throughout our muscles and joints that work together to create an internal body map. It is through proprioceptive awareness that we know the position of our body, even when we cannot see it. It is through intact proprioception that we can navigate a dark, familiar environment, or reach and grab something behind us without looking. It is also the sense that grades our pressure, allowing us to use the appropriate force when picking up a brick, versus a thin paper cup of water.

Input to the proprioceptive system through deep pressure, and much more significantly, resistive muscle activation, or "heavy work," enhances serotonin release and can be very grounding and organizing. This is why some people stomp their feet or clench their fists when they are angry or overwhelmed. This is why others chew on hard plastic pen caps when their attention wanes in a lecture. It is difficult to feel secure in oneself or in one's environment without a secure sense of body scheme. The proprioceptive system collaborates extensively with the closely associated tactile system. Together, they provide us with the critical sense of body awareness.

The tactile system is made up of the largest organ of our body, the skin. It is the system that provides us with the sense of touch for pleasure, pain, discrimination, and protection. Being that the tactile system is our exterior boundary, it is critical that it appropriately processes the wide variety of elements and touch sensations that surround us. If dysfunctional, pleasurable touch can instead be misinterpreted as noxious, or potentially dangerous sensations can go unregistered and become damaging.

Each of these systems must function properly and collaboratively in order to support appropriate sensory integration. A typical sensory system processes a wide variety and range of intensity of information, and makes the necessary filtrations in order for a person to function comfortably and without conscious effort. However, with many children with autism spectrum disorders, we find that one or more of these systems does not function properly. Any of the sensory systems can be hyper-responsive (sensory avoiding) or hypo-responsive (sensory seeking) to incoming information.

This can be easily demonstrated with an example of the tactile system. A hyper-responsive tactile system (sensory avoiding) is generally associated with a high level of arousal. This child is typically in varying states of fight or flight and is therefore less available for engagement and learning. She may avoid messy play and unfamiliar textures at all cost, may hold objects in her finger tips, avoiding contact with palms, may need to remove tags from shirts and only wear soft old clothes, may avoid standing close to peers and other people, may resist cuddling and affection even from parents and family members, may present with poor body awareness, stiff movement patterns, delayed motor planning, and difficulty with fine motor skills. This girl may tend to be inflexible and rigid in her ways, in an effort to attempt to control a world that she perceives as threatening.

A hypo-responsive tactile system (sensory seeking) is generally associated with a low level of arousal. This child may typically appear "tuned out" and is therefore also less available. In order to obtain input to raise his arousal, he may gravitate to messy and unfamiliar textures in an effort to better process his body and the things around them, may not seem to notice or mind when socks or clothing are twisted in uncomfortable ways or when sticky food is on his hands or face, may frequently bump into others or play excessively rough without ill intentions, and may present with poor body awareness and poorly graded, ballistic movement patterns, delayed motor planning, and difficulty with fine motor skills. This boy may tend to be disorganized in his ways, as he has difficulty making sense of his world.

Sensory issues can often be mistaken for behavioral problems. If a child has vestibular and visual issues, which impact his perception of his position in space, he may have great difficulty sitting upright in a chair without falling from time to time. To avoid falls or embarrassment, he may fidget to better process his body, or get out of his seat often. He, in turn, will present as a child who "won't" stay seated. Another child with severe tactile defensiveness may be terrified to stand in line next to his peers due to the fear of being touched. To protect himself, he stands away from the group with his back against the wall or casually wanders out of reach. He again, will present like a child who "won't" stay in line. With children with sensory integration dysfunction, it is important to remember that these behaviors may be nothing more than effective coping mechanisms. When the underlying sensory issues are addressed, the behavior may disappear all together.

What is Sensory Integration Therapy?

Sensory integration is a complex treatment approach. A breakdown of a few of the basic principles can help to provide a general understanding. We, as humans, need a wide variety of sensory and motor experiences to develop and sustain typical nervous system function. Much like plants need a full spectrum of light to grow and flower to their potential, we respond strongly to sensory information. Consider the devastating effects of prolonged sensory deprivation. Consider the positive effects of gently rocking a baby or tightly hugging a friend in need. Within the range of typically functioning systems, we find some variance. One "typical" adult may ride roller coasters every Saturday afternoon. Another may gasp at the sight of one. With a little encouragement, perhaps, she hops on and keeps her eyes closed. These two people are quite different, yet fall within a range where they experience a variety of rich sensory movement experiences. Children with ASD sometimes present with a much greater range. For whatever reasons, their nervous systems are wired differently.

Children inherently attempt to provide themselves with what they need and avoid what they are frightened by. They constantly listen to their bodies and try to regulate themselves. By listening to what their bodies tell us, we can help them to make a great deal of positive change. A therapist can provide them with calculated input that is stronger and more effective in reaching the threshold of the system the child is trying to stimulate. In turn, the child may begin to process the input more appropriately and therefore need less of it over time, demonstrating fewer sensory seeking or self-stimulatory behaviors. Children demonstrate self-stimulating behaviors for a reason. It is our responsibility to determine why.

The child who avoids sensory input faces another challenge. They develop compensatory strategies to protect themselves, and seldom subject themselves to the sensory information. Therapists utilize various strategies to help desensitize the child. This is never done through repeated exposure of the noxious experience. It often involves looking carefully at the stimuli and the relationships of the supporting sensory system. The clinician can then systematically address them in order to support sensory integration. For example, a defensive tactile system may better process touch following appropriate input to the proprioceptive system. A vestibular system may better process movement following appropriate input to the auditory or proprioceptive system.

Consider this example:

One young girl may spin around for hours and never get dizzy. Another young boy may fearfully cling to his mother when she tries to put him in a swing at the park, or even just picks him up. These ranges pose a problem. The first child appears hypo-responsive (sensory seeking) and unable to provide herself with strong enough movement input to satiate her vestibular system. This compels her to spin, climb, run, jump, and crash. After all, if you were hungry, wouldn't you eat something? The second child, on the other hand, appears hyper-responsive (sensory avoiding) and avoids movement at all cost. If you had arachnophobia would you pet a tarantula? His vestibular system, however, still requires and craves input despite his interpreted fear. So almost instinctually, he has discovered that by looking out of the far corners of his eyes, by looking at spinning objects, or by closely following long linear edges visually, he can stimulate his vestibular system.

These two children are significantly impacted by this relatively simple sensory dysfunction and have developed effective coping mechanisms. However, the vestibular system works closely together with other systems to support many functions, so the ramifications may increase and broaden over time if left unaddressed. Both of these children are less available for engagement and learning.

The first child can only provide herself with so much movement input, due to human limitations. A trained therapist on the other hand, can make informed clinical decisions after assessment, and assist the child in obtaining calculated rotation and movement experiences in all planes that provide strong and organizing input to every receptor of the vestibular system. This may be followed with further resistive activities that activate her core muscles to provide additional grounding and organizing information. The movements can provide the vestibular system with its threshold of input, allowing it to better process movement and support more refined motor skills. It can also result in a substantial period of time to follow in which she seeks less movement and is more available to the world around her. Due to the plasticity of our nervous systems, this input can decrease over time as the system becomes rewired, or integrated.

Based on the profile of the second child, he likely presents with poor tactile and proprioceptive processing. This is commonly associated with low muscle tone and poor postural control. This typically results in decreased body awareness and motor planning, with one of the end functional outcomes being a fear of moving through space. If this child does not perceive his body properly when seated or walking, he most certainly will not feel safe when placed in a swing and pushed three feet off of the ground. A trained therapist will identify these patterns and recognize the need to address his tactile and proprioceptive systems, despite the fact that the initial red flag went off when mom reported an issue that appear to be related to his vestibular system. All involved systems will be addressed in treatment.

Specific brushing/deep pressure strategies and resistive activities that connect him to the support surface can be very effective in improving body awareness. A child needs to feel connected to the ground before they can feel free in space. Core muscle activation can improve alignment and postural control and help lay the foundation for the introduction of new, controlled movement experiences. A careful sequence of movement may now be explored, paired with continued body awareness work. All activities are paired with his passions and interests. He ideally gains ownership of his body in space and begins to freely explore on his own. The timid, fearful child can now become a confident explorer.

This example provides a little insight into the SI treatment approach. These principles can be applied to a variety of issues involving all of the sensory systems. Sensory integrative treatment can effectively help to change a child's "wiring." It is the clinician's goal to provide the child with the tools necessary to create their own ideas and develop more naturally and spontaneously in a world that they can make sense of and feel safe in.

PARENT SUPPORT

BY DR. LAUREN TOBING-PUENTE

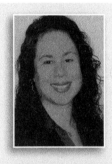

Lauren Tobing-Puente, Ph.D.

361 East 19th Street
New York, NY 10003
(917) 838-9274
services@drtobingpuente.com
www.drtobingpuente.com

Dr. Lauren Tobing-Puente is a NYS Licensed Psychologist with many years of clinical experience with children and families, specializing in autism-spectrum disorders (ASDs). She received her Ph.D. in Clinical Psychology from Fordham University, with a specialization in child and family therapy. As a Developmental Individual Differences and Relationship-based (DIR) model Certificate Candidate (Level II), Dr. Tobing-Puente uses the DIR approach both in her private practice and as the Clinical Coordinator of the Rebecca School, one of the largest DIR schools worldwide.

Dr. Tobing-Puente has expertise in the assessment and treatment of children, and in providing support groups for siblings and parents. She has worked with parents of children with special needs in a variety of school, home, community-based, and hospital settings, and has used a variety of psychotherapeutic, developmental, and behavioral treatment approaches. Her research studies on the experiences of parents of children with ASDs have been presented at national conferences and have been published by reputable scientific journals.

The following is a brief overview of the role of parent support in the treatment of children with autism spectrum disorders (ASD). This chapter provides an understanding of the need for parent support, focuses on the impact on caregivers raising children with ASDs, and the various supports available to them, so that they can be most effective in their parenting, in their implementation of the child's treatment program, and in other aspects of their lives. This overview is based on both the research literature and on the author's wealth of clinical experience in this area.

Impact of Parenting a Child with an Autism Spectrum Disorder

Parents of children with ASDs are impacted by their children's challenges in many ways, including emotionally, financially, with respect to their marriages and partnerships, and their everyday routines. Regarding the emotional impact, much research has shown that mothers of children with ASDs consistently report very high levels of child-related parenting stress (parenting stress related to the child), with parenting stress scores ranging from the 95th to 98th percentiles.[1] Parenting stress has been found at greater levels for parents of children with ASDs than for parents of children with normal development[2] and parents of children with other special needs.[3] Parents of children with ASDs also have reported more general psychological distress than parents of children with other special needs, including depression[4] and anxiety. Likewise, parents with higher levels of parenting stress have reported higher levels of psychological distress.[5]

Many parents of these children report high levels of guilt and/or self-blame regarding their children's diagnoses, despite no evidence in the scientific literature that parents' behaviors play a role. Years of clinical work with parents have indicated that without the identification of the exact cause(s) of ASDs, many parents reflect on things they did or did not do during pregnancy or infancy, resulting in blaming themselves and experiencing guilt related to their child's diagnosis.

Parenting satisfaction (how satisfied one is in the parenting role) and parenting efficacy (how competent one feels as a parent) are impacted for parents of children with ASDs. Mothers of children with ASDs have reported lower parenting satisfaction and parenting efficacy than parents of children with normal development.[6] Parents' sense of their child's attachment to them is also often impacted, due to the difficulties children with ASDs have forming relationships. Such is often the case for parents of children who look at their parents less often, who initiate affection with them with less frequency (or do not accept affection), and/or show significant difficulties being soothed by their parents when they are upset. This results in the self perception by parents that they are less effective in the role of a nurturing parent and a decrease in satisfaction in the caregiver role. Lower levels of parenting satisfaction are associated with higher levels of psychological distress for mothers of children with ASDs.[5]

Raising a child with an ASD impacts family's everyday routines in many ways. Any family dynamic is disrupted when a crisis is introduced particularly in the form of illness, or developmental challenges. Parents of children with ASDs consistently report much less "free time" available, related to the amount of time necessary to participate in their children's therapies at home and after school hours. As a result, there is often limited time and/or energy for parents to spend on themselves, for both necessary tasks (e.g., trips to the supermarket) and leisure activities (e.g., going out for dinner; exercise). Parents of children with ASDs often report a significant impact on their relationships with friends and family members. Such parents often report isolation from those who have supported them in the past. This can occur both as a result of others spending less time with them due to their discomfort around or limited understanding of children with ASDs, or from parents having limited time to maintain their connections.

The impact of raising a child with ASD on parents' marriages and partnerships has been a focus in recent years. Lower relationship satisfaction scores have been found for couples raising children with ASD than for couples with children without developmental disorders.[2] For parents who do find occasional time for themselves or with their partner, child care is often an issue. Children with ASDs have specific needs that the average babysitter is not skilled to manage.

Support for Parents of Children with ASDs

Support for parents of children with ASDs is a critical component of their children's treatment. Just as is the case with any responsibility humans have, their ability to carry it out depends on their resources, and their physical and emotional states. For example, people are less likely to perform well on a test when they are more fatigued or feeling anxious or sad. Likewise, parents' ability to take part in their child's treatment is a function of how well they themselves are functioning. With the high levels of parenting stress and psychological symptoms that parents of children with ASD often experience, many parents find it difficult to fully take part in their children's treatment, especially in the context of typical family responsibilities (e.g., career, homework, housework, etc.). Support can help parents manage these challenges.

Parents of children with ASDs benefit from a range of supports that vary in terms of their focus and setting. The following are ways that parents of children with ASD can be supported in order to decrease symptoms of distress and, in turn, be increasingly available for involvement in their children's treatment. The supports described are not exhaustive, and their effectiveness may differ depending on how they are delivered and on the individual characteristics of the parent who receives them. Just as children's treatment protocols are individually tailored to meet their needs, so should the support provided to their parents. The quality of support may be more important than the quantity, as parents reporting higher satisfaction with their social supports, but not a greater number of social supports reported lower levels of psychological distress.[5]

Developing a Sense of Parental Mastery

One of the initial sources of support parents receive is often from the therapists who work with their children. Support is provided by enhancing the parents' understanding of the nature of their children's challenges and their progress, and teaching parents strategies that work best for their children. It is quite helpful having regular access to and communication with one or more professionals that clearly understand the child's challenges and the best ways of helping them succeed.

Parents' ability to take part in their children's treatment, including their sense of mastery over its components and carrying over strategies into their daily routine are critical factors for children's progress. From the Developmental Individual-Differences and Relationship-based (DIR) perspective,[7] parents are recommended to play a primary role in the development of children with ASDs. Support from the therapists working with one's child can significantly help parents in this way and can have a positive impact on parents' sense of competence and their satisfaction with parenting.

Parents often benefit from individual support that focuses on their own specific issues related to themselves and their child. Individual counseling with a mental health clinician allows opportunities for focusing on parents' own experiences and developing coping strategies that can help them manage their parenting stress and any symptoms of psychological distress. Here, they can specifically address their struggles in order to become more effective in their parenting role and feel increased contentment overall. Self-care is imperative for parents so that they are available to their child to help them develop the key components for social, emotional, and intellectual development, including the ability to focus and attend, engage, interact, and use ideas creatively and logically.[7] Marriage counseling with a mental health clinician who has a background in families of children with ASDs is often helpful for addressing issues within the marriage. Support for the siblings of children with ASDs is also important for addressing the impact on the entire family.

Enhancing Social Connections

Parents of children with ASDs also find support in settings in which they can interact with parents of children with similar challenges. Parent support groups, often led by a mental health clinician, are provided regularly by many schools and local organizations. Such groups provide opportunities for parents to share their experiences, discuss ways of helping their children (e.g., by sharing information on treatment protocols and behavioral strategies) and caring for themselves. With the guidance of mental health clinicians, parents can receive psychoeducation about the latest research on ASDs and treatment and strategies that can help their children and themselves. Education regarding what is known about the cause(s) of ASDs is often crucial for parents who experience guilt and self-blame. Listening to others who have had similar experiences helps parents feel a sense of community, contrasting their experience of isolation from others.

Modern technology has provided parents with other options for informal support. This is often helpful for parents who aren't able to attend support groups (e.g., due to scheduling or babysitting difficulties). Message boards and listservs for parents of children with ASDs have become very popular in recent years. Benefits of message boards and listservs include their convenience and accessibility, without the challenges of scheduling of face-to-face support groups. This can be especially helpful for parents who live in remote areas. However, online technology does not afford the personal contact of support groups or provide the same opportunity to develop true relationships with other parents. Another concern with online technology is how the content is monitored. Without consistent moderation by a clinician, it is difficult to ensure that the content is appropriate and factual.

Financial Support

Financial support is often a vital aspect of support for parents and their children, as parents often report stress related to financial strain. There is often an enormous financial toll of diagnostic second opinions, follow-up appointments, and additional therapies for their children as all of these services may not be provided by schools or covered by insurance companies. Parents are often unaware of the financial resources that may be available to them, such as the Medicaid waiver program or Supplemental Security Income (SSI) that can provide eligibility for certain therapies or services (e.g., respite care) or a monthly stipend to assist in their child's care. Parents can contact their child's service coordinator, social worker, or an agency that advocates on behalf of families confronting ASD, and provides information about entitlements and resources.

In summary, parents of children with ASDs experience high levels of parenting stress, psychological distress (e.g., depression, anxiety, guilt), marital strain, and social isolation. Parents should be as much the focus in treatment as the children themselves, as their well-being is critical to their ability to be a part of their children's therapy. The optimal functioning of the parents is essential if the treatment strategies are to be successfully implemented. These families require access to a variety of supports, including communication with children's treatment providers, individual and group counseling, and advice regarding financial management and entitlement benefits.

46

PERSONAL SERVICE CANINES: WILDERWOOD IS CHANGING LIVES ONE DOG AT A TIME

by Tiffany Denyer

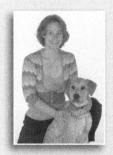

Tiffany Denyer, RN

Wilderwood Service Dogs
1319 Tuckaleechee Trail
Maryville, TN 37803-4353
wilderwood@charter.net
www.wilderwood.org

Tiffany Denyer, Founder and Executive Director of Wilderwood Service Dogs, holds a BSN with a specialty in psychiatric care. For thirteen years, she has worked as a psychiatric nurse with all age groups. She holds certification in Service Dog Training, High School Assistance Dog Programming, and has been working with canines all her life. Tiffany is a forerunner in her field, and one of only five practitioners in the nation to provide service dogs to individuals with brain disorders. Her work with service dogs and children with autism is groundbreaking as children are improving at a speed unseen in the medical and therapy communities. Her work is currently undergoing a five year research study by Maryville College in Maryville, Tennessee, documenting the improvements in these children.

Wilderwood Service Dogs provides service dogs for all neurological disorders, including Alzheimer's, Parkinson's, post-traumatic stress disorder, and children on the autism spectrum. The changes occurring in these individuals are dramatic after the placement of a dog. Children that once were nonverbal are now verbal. Children that haven't slept a complete night in years are now sleeping through the entire night. Children who once suffered from oftentimes traumatic stimming behaviors, no longer stim. Children who have suffered from pica issues have seen those issues improve to the point where they no longer exist. Parents who once feared for their children's lives because they were flight risks no longer worry. Families that had all but given up attending church, or restaurants, or events, together as a family unit, have regained the ability to worship and eat together again. And all of these changes are because of the impact of one four-legged, furry, floppy-eared, slobbery, kissing dog. Amazing!

Wilderwood Service Dogs provides service dogs for all neurological disorders, including Parkinson's, Alzheimer's, post-traumatic syndrome, children on the autism spectrum and more. Because autism is affecting one in every seventy boys and one in every three hundred girls today, according to the Autism Society of America, most of our service dogs are going to children with autism. Our clients, generally, come to us at the point that the medical and therapy communities have expressed to the parents that though they may see some improvements in their children, they won't see improvements come in leaps and bounds. Our work of placing service dogs with children with autism has had remarkable results. We see children that have been nonverbal for years, begin to talk. We have seen children that stimmed so badly that they would hurt themselves or others, stop the behavior completely via the gentle interruption of the dog. Wilderwood's clients with pica issues, the eating of nonfood items, will completely stop the behavior. Children who have extreme sensory and anxiety issues, which would not allow them to sit still for five minutes, are now able to sit in a classroom for hours as a result of being tethered to their service dog. All of these improvements are a direct result of the introduction of a service dog into their daily lives.

Wilderwood was founded by Tiffany Denyer, a licensed and registered psychiatric nurse. Because of her nursing background and her experience with dogs, she believed that she could make a difference for these clients who suffer from neurological disorders. Tiffany studied in California under Dr. Bonnie Bergin, the world's first service dog trainer for the physically handicapped, and founder of the first accredited university in canine studies. After her education, Tiffany returned to East Tennessee in order to merge her understanding and training as a nurse with her understanding and training of dogs. What has transpired is nothing short of creating miracles. Most of Wilderwood's clients families have all but lost hope that their lives would represent anything close to normal ever again. Wilderwood has succeeded in changing that outcome, "one dog at a time." Wilderwood's staff, under the careful vigil of Tiffany has the knowledge and skill to know exactly what kind of dogs these families need. When families are asked why they chose Wilderwood over other service dog organizations, the number one answer is "when we spoke with Tiffany about our situation and our needs, it was like she had been living in our living room. She got it!" Wilderwood knows and understands their client's lives and the special needs of their children.

Wilderwood trains all of its service dogs for the specific needs of each of their children. No two children on the autism spectrum are alike, and none of our dogs are trained the same. They all are versed in the basic service dog commands; however, each family takes home a dog that has been trained to meet their individual needs.

The best way to discuss our success rate is to discuss the research study that is being conducted by Maryville College in Maryville, Tennessee. Maryville College is conducting a five-year study of the impact that our service dogs are having on the lives of these children and their families. The study is currently at the half way mark and the results have been unprecedented. Not only are these children improving quickly, in some cases in a matter of weeks, the improvements continue to get better long after the dog is taken home! One of our favorite stories is about a young boy named David. David was deathly afraid of dogs, eliciting screams of fear if one was seen through the car window. David was going through puberty and the accompanying med changes were resulting in extreme behavioral issues. These issues continued to escalate until David was hospitalized and restrained because he was a threat to himself and others. His parents no longer took him on family vacations or included him in any family activities because his behavior had gotten so violent. Despite many warnings, David's parents brought David to Wilderwood to get a service dog. David was tethered to his dog, Levi, on the second day and his life has not been the same since. David no longer has violent outbursts. He no longer is a flight risk. He has improved so much that his dad was able to take him on a camping trip, just he and David, and enjoy an experience that most father and sons take for granted. David's dad was able to set up the tent without worrying about David wandering off. They were able to enjoy the experiences of a camping weekend, all because of a service dog named Levi. David's parents believe that had it not been for Levi, he would still be in the hospital and would not be a part of their family's daily life.

Adding a dog to a family is certainly an adjustment. Adding a *service dog* to your family is life changing. Service dogs are with their partners 24/7 and go wherever their partners go. It takes a commitment to provide for the extra needs of this new family member. Service Dogs must be worked as service dogs and not allowed to become family pets and this, at times, can be difficult for other family members to understand or endorse. Parents must consistently use the service dog to interrupt their child's inappropriate behavior. Service dogs will quit working in as few as three weeks if their skills are not used adequately. At first this can be overwhelming for parents who are already stretched and exhausted. However, when parents succeed in their efforts, we see miracles occur of these children.

Most families have found that in the past they have used whatever techniques and tools they could to survive. For example some of our families have children that are severe flight risks, and their children put themselves and others in terrifying situations on a daily basis. These parents learn to hold onto their children with a "death grip" to keep them safe. We have seen a child held so tightly that her little arm was actually "burned" by the gripping mother because that was the only tool her mom had to keep her from running into a street and into the path of a car. This same little girl walked through a store for the first time, just like any other young twelve–year-old girl, once she was safely tethered to her loving service dog! This change took place within the first week of getting her new service dog. How liberating must it have felt to this child to get to walk through a store only attached to her new best friend? How awesome it was for mom that she could feel confident that her daughter wasn't going to bolt and hurt herself or others? What a miracle!

For more information on Wilderwood, please visit our website at www. wilderwood.org. You may call Deanna Hall, Public Relations Director, at (865) 379-2188 if you would be interested in finding out more about the organization or would like for someone to come and speak about Wilderwood and how we are changing lives one dog at a time. If you would like specific information about whether a dog would be of help to your child or family member suffering from a neurological disorder, please call Tiffany Denyer directly at (865) 660-0095.

We at Wilderwood Service Dogs are humbled and honored to be a part of the miracles occurring in the lives of our families. We believe and know that dogs have an ability to communicate on a level with these children in a way we often don't understand, but have proof that it works! We know that these dogs allow our clients to have control over something in a world where oftentimes they can't even control the movements of their own body. Wilderwood's clients tell their dog to sit, or come, or to bring them something in "language" we do not always understand but inevitably their dog will sit, come or bring it! The dog's response is immediate and for those affected by neurological issues, getting immediate feed-back is paramount to their learning processes. Only a dog can be around 24/7 and provide this immediate feedback day in and day out. Their service dog becomes a constant in a world that is every changing and difficult to manage.

Service Dogs are not only are impacting their partners, but their affect is far -reaching. For children that take their dogs to school, teachers are reporting that everyone in the classroom is positively impacted. Families that have quit going together to church, restaurants or sporting events, are now able to enjoy life as a family unit once again. Parents that have endured dirty looks because their child is seen as "needing a spanking" or they are "bad parents," are no longer ostracized because there is a visible understanding that there is a disability when the service dog is present. Best of all, children that once were shunned because they were seen as "different," are now being approached by other children and adults and treated as special because they have a dog. Wilderwood's service dogs are opening experiences and opportunities that once seemed impossible. Our client's lives have been dramatically changed because of a furry, four legged animal, with sloppy kisses, which loves unconditionally and sees them as perfect, just the way they are!

47

PHARMACEUTICAL MEDICATION MANAGEMENT: THE WHY, WHEN, AND WHAT

BY DR. MARK FREILICH

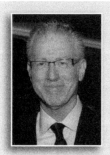

Mark Freilich, MD

Total Kids Developmental Pediatric Resources
New York City
(212) 787-2148
info@totalkidsny.com
www.totalkidsny.com

Dr. Mark Freilich is a developmental pediatrician and founder/
medical director of Total Kids Developmental Pediatric Resources.
Total Kids provides a holistic, dynamic and integrated approach to
evaluation and management of children with differences and variations in development
and learning. The Total Kids approach takes into account every child's and family's unique
and individual areas of strengths and needs. The Total Kids approach is not limited to an
office-based evaluation. It involves observation in venues where the child actually functions
on a day-to-day basis.

When dealing with your child with an autism spectrum disorder, or any other
developmental, medical, or behavioral issue, you must remember that you
are in the driver's seat. You will most definitely need a good GPS system—a team
of specialists who will become your co-navigators or partners in the process.

During your journey, you will more than likely contemplate whether the road
called pharmaceutical medication management will need to be taken. Addressing
a variety of behavioral and regulatory manifestations can often be a bumpy, curvy,

and not easily navigated road. This chapter will attempt to set guidelines to clarify the why, when, and what of pharmaceutical medication management.

The need to implement medication management depends on the underlying etiology, the severity of manifestations, the effect it is having on the child's and family's life in a variety of venues, and the effect other treatment modalities are having on reducing or ameliorating the symptoms.

Medication management is often the treatment of last resort. It is reserved for situations in which all other treatments have been implemented but have not produced the desired outcomes. On the other hand, medication management may be considered as a first line of treatment, when it is deemed that all other therapeutic options will not be able to achieve their maximal impact without having medication on board. Medication as a first line of action may allow the child to become more available to the positive effects of the various other treatment approaches that have been deemed appropriate. This can lead to a reduction in or the eventual elimination of medication.

When implementing pharmacologic medication management, ongoing evaluation and monitoring is essential. Practical management goals in medication management include: determining the medication that can best impact the targeted symptoms; finding a medication that produces the least number of side effects; and determining the lowest effective dosage (often a point of balance between maximal positive effect and minimal ill effect). This will require a slow titration process, with frequent communication between you and the prescribing physician. The process of determining the appropriate medication and the appropriate dosage cannot be completed overnight. The process will, at first, require weekly office visits (or at least weekly telephone communication) with the prescribing physician. If, at any point before finding the "optimal" dosage, the physician hands you a prescription and tells you that the plan is to administer the medication and return in a month's time, please consider another medication manager. Your medication manager should ideally be a developmental pediatrician, pediatric psychiatrist, or a neuropharmacologist. Your general pediatrician should be used only if he or she feels confident in having enough experience with the medication management process, or if no other more qualified physicians are available in your area.

The question of when you should seek advice in regard to the need for medication management needs to be addressed. Signs that would alert you to the need for medication management include:

- Your child's safety is being questioned

- Increased episodes of physical aggression toward self and others
- Episodes of physical or verbal aggression are prolonged and not responsive to other intervention techniques
- Uncontrolled temper tantrums
- Fear that your child will hurt you or other members of your family or support team
- Increase in repetitive or stereotypic behaviors despite other interventions being in place
- Increase in anxiety, impulsivity, and inattention despite other interventions being in place

There is no one specific medication to treat the core deficits or various manifestations of autism spectrum disorder. Medication, however, can be helpful in decreasing some of the symptoms of this spectrum disorder. You will need to have a great deal of patience, as you may go through a lengthy trial-and-error process. You must determine, with the help of your "team," the symptoms you are hoping to decrease or ameliorate by the use of a specific medication. Manifestations that may be helped by various pharmacologic agents include:

- Attention/distractibility/focus
- Repetitive/stereotypic behaviors
- Depression
- Anxiety
- Severe irritability
- Aggression/self-injurious behaviors
- Mood stabilization

There are a variety of categories of medications that can be used when targeting a specific symptom:

Stimulants:

A class of medications used to treat ADHD and narcolepsy by increasing alertness and wakefulness.

Antidepressants:

A class of medications used to treat depression, anxieties, and obsessive behaviors.

Mood Stabilizers:

A class of medications used to reduce volatile behavior and emotional outbursts, as well as sudden and unpredictable mood shifts.

Anti-Anxiety Medications:

A class of medications used to reduce symptoms of fear and anxiety.

Antipsychotics:

A class of medications used to treat the symptoms of psychosis (loss of contact with reality). They can also be used to stabilize mood and reduce hyperactivity, tics, and self-injurious behaviors.

Anticonvulsants:

A class of medications generally used to treat severe disorders. Many children with autism develop seizure activity at some point in their lives. They may be needed to control seizure activity. They do not cure the condition. They also can be used to treat mood stabilization and other problems..

Miscellaneous psychoactive pharmaceuticals:

Can be used for sleep, bedwetting, and other problems.

In the medication management process, try not to "cocktail." Cocktailing is the addition of one or more medications to the current mix in an attempt to fine-tune the outcome or counteract side effects. It is preferable to make a real effort to find one medication that has an impact on key symptoms you have targeted, with the least number of side effects. Adding one or more medications can place you and your child on a hamster wheel. Adding new medications to counteract unwanted side effects, or overreaching in the hope that you will be able to totally eliminate a particular symptom, should not be the driving force.

Remember that at this point in time, there are no miracle cures. You need to choose the intervention pathways (be it medication management or other approaches) that will reduce symptom manifestation. Ultimately, your goal is to clear the way and allow your child to make the journey towards increased communication skills, improved relatedness, and maximized social capabilities.

PHYSICAL THERAPY

BY MEGHAN COLLINS

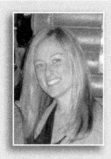

Meghan Collins, MPT

Rebecca School
40 E. 30th Street
New York, NY 10016
mcollins@rebeccaschool.org

Born and raised in New York. Graduated from the University of Scranton, 2005. Started working with children on the autism spectrum shortly after graduating. Currently, Physical Therapy Supervisor at Rebecca School. I want to thank my parents, Pat and Gene, for being a constant source of support and love.

Movement is a cornerstone for successfully functioning in one's environment and developing a sense of self. It is a sensation that a typically-developing individual becomes aware of and learns to modulate and control through various experiences. Multiple sensory systems, including the vestibular, proprioceptive, visual, and tactile, impact how a person perceives they are interacting with their environment. As babies, we practice interacting with our environment through both repetitive and spontaneous movement and a sense of where our bodies are in space develops. After we develop a sense of our bodies and where they are in space, movement is typically task-specific.

Motor development is an integrated experience between internal physiological development and the external environment. Richard Schmidt took Piaget's theory of scheme formation and related it to movement. Four things that impact the schema formation of motor learning, according to Schmidt, are the initial conditions of the movement, the response parameters for the motor program, sensory consequences of the movement, and the movement outcome. Motor learning is "a set of [internal] processes associated with practice or experience leading to relatively permanent changes in the capability for responding."

The World Confederation for Physical Therapy defines physical therapy as "a health care profession that provides treatment to individuals to develop, maintain and restore maximum movement and function throughout life. This includes providing treatment in circumstances where movement and function are threatened by aging, injury, disease or environmental factors."

Physical therapy with children on the autism spectrum may look very different from the physical therapy you or I may seek out. While we may have experienced some physical impairment that has impacted our ability to function successfully in our environment and need help in restoring, for those with autism, physical therapy can be used for a variety of developmental purposes. Children with autism typically have difficulties processing and integrating sensory information, including movement. For example, they may have low muscle tone, or have a tough time with coordination and sports. These issues can not only interfere with basic day-to-day functioning but can have an impact on social and physical development.

Younger children with autism often exhibit significant delays in reaching developmental milestones. Therefore the earliest forms of physical therapy may include working on skills such as sitting, rolling, crawling, standing, and walking. As the children get older, they may receive physical therapy to address concerns regarding muscle strength, endurance, balance, coordination, motor planning, ball skills, and various forms of locomotion.

Core muscle weakness and low muscle tone are common issues that need to be addressed during physical therapy with children on the autism spectrum. Core muscle strength and tone impact many aspects of movement and motor control such as postural control, balance, and coordination. Postural control is the ability to maintain the position required to perform other movements or tasks. When a person has poor core muscle strength and postural control, it makes it difficult to perform or participate in activities away from their body or outside their base of support such as throwing or kicking a ball. A common therapeutic intervention used is maintaining upright in various positions (sitting and lying on back, front, or side) and planes (frontal, sagittal, or transverse) on a therapy ball. The child may need support from the therapist to maintain a desired posture. They may also be able to perform another activity simultaneously increasing the difficulty of the task and challenging their ability to adapt or modify their posture accordingly. Core muscle strength and postural control are essential is general play, such as riding a tricycle or bicycle, or scooter.

Another common issue addressed during physical therapy is praxis or motor planning. This is an individual's ability to formulate a plan, organize their body appropriately, and execute the plan. The first step in praxis is ideation, formulating an idea or plan, and is the cognitive part of the process. Children with autism often have difficulty with ideation as it is thought to be largely related to integrate the sensory information they are receiving from their own body and environment. Next is the subconscious organization or development of a plan of how they are going to accomplish the task at hand. Lastly, the plan gets executed, which is the physical or motoric part of the process. The amount of thought and effort a typically-developing individual puts into learning a novel skill may be the same amount of thought and effort a child with autism has when learning how to run, skip, or hop. Creating, constructing, and executing an obstacle course play or negotiating playground equipment are common ways a child may work on their motor planning skills during a physical therapy session.

Overall muscle strength and endurance may be addressed during community walks or stair climbing. Limited range of motion or muscle flexibility may be addressed by traditional stretching or massage. Aerobic fitness may be a concern as weight-gain and lethargy are common side effects of various medications children on the autism spectrum may take. Traditional exercise may be performed during therapy sessions, such as push-ups, sit-ups, or jumping jacks, to improve aerobic capacity. Successfully moving through a classroom or hallway requires good body awareness, visual spatial ability, modulation and coordination. Balance activities may include negotiating stairs with and without support from the railing or wall, walking across a balance beam, standing one foot, hopping, moving onto, off of, or across uneven or moveable surfaces, and roller-skating.

Another very useful tool often used in physical therapy is ball play. Ball skills require knowing where one's limbs are in relation to the rest of their body and modulation of force. One should be able to orient one's body in order to send or receive a ball. Ball skills include overhand and underhand throwing, kicking, and catching. When evaluating child's ability to throw a ball, a physical therapy will typically evaluate the fluidity of movement, the ability of the child to hit the target (overshooting or undershooting), repeated misses of the target in the same direction, or stepping with the opposite foot. When kicking a ball, a physical therapists will typically evaluate the fluidity of movement, appropriate ball contact, coordinated knee bending, the ability of the child to hit the target (overshooting or undershooting), or repeated misses of the target in the same direction. When catching a ball or receiving it after a kick, a physical therapist may evaluate the ability of the child to follow the trajectory of the ball as it approaches them, correct orientation of the body with regard to the ball's height, direction, or force, and hand placement (e.g., are their hands open and ready, are they closing their hand too soon or too late, are their hands rigid or stiff.) If a child is having difficulty catching a medium-size ball, balloons serve as good substitutes until the child becomes more familiar with the task.

A child receiving physical therapy will improve their gross motor function which is an important aspect of socialization, allowing the child to participate in general play, physical education, or sports. The key to a successful physical therapy session is making the activities during the session motivating for the child. Ultimately kids just want to have fun!

PPAR AGONISTS (ACTOS)

BY DR. MICHAEL ELICE

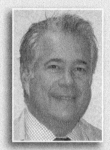

Michael Elice, MD

Autism Associates of New York
77 Froehlich Farm Boulevard
Woodbury, New York 11797
info@autismny.com
(516) 921-3456

Dr. Elice is a board-certified pediatrician and has been in practice for thirty years. Dr. Elice is a graduate of Syracuse University and the Chicago Medical School. He completed his pediatric residency at the North Shore University Hospital in Manhasset, NY. He has academic teaching positions and is on the staff of North Shore University Hospital and Schneider Children's Hospital. He is an associate professor of pediatrics at the New York University Medical School and the Albert Einstein School of Medicine. He is on the medical advisory board of the New York Families for Autistic Children (NYFAC) and is a member of the National Autism Association New York Metro Chapter. He has lectured at Defeat Autism Now! Conferences around the country.

There are times in modern medicine when a single patient can enlighten our understanding of a disease or disease process and can serve as an impetus for further discovery. Thus, it is becoming accepted that autism is a complex neurodevelopmental disorder. Although the specific causes remain to be determined, there is strong evidence that genetic, environmental, inflammatory, immunological and metabolic factors play a prominent role in this disease.

Cytokines are small proteins that direct the movement of circulating white blood cells to sites of inflammation or injury. Originally studied because of their role in inflammation, cytokines and their receptors are now known to play a crucial part in a wide range of diseases with prominent inflammatory components. For example, elevated levels of cytokines in the joints of patients with rheumatoid arthritis coincide with movement of monocytes and T cells into the synovial tissues. Inflammation is also a key factor in asthma, in which cytokines recruit eosinophils, or white blood cells that respond to allergies, to the lung. Psoriasis is another example of cytokine-mediated cell recruitment and inflammation. Multiple sclerosis is an example of how cytokines can influence the progression and severity of an autoimmune disease.

Altered immune responses in children with autism spectrum disorders (ASDs) have been well documented. In 1976, Stubbs published that five of thirteen autistic children had no detectable rubella antibodies despite prior immunization. (1). An additional study by Stubbs showed that certain white blood cells known as monocytes and T lymphocytes were functioning abnormally. (2) In children with ASD, there is a preponderance of helper 2 (Th2) T cells over the helper 1 (Th1) T cells. This finding was confirmed at the Cincinnati Children's Hospital Medical Center. (3) In 2005 the study of children with ASD had their cytokines compared to control patients. In all, the Th2 cytokines were significantly higher than the Th1, demonstrating an abnormal autoimmune and /or inflammatory response.

Peroxisome proliferators-activated receptors (PPARs) are a class of nuclear transcription factors that are activated by fatty acids and their derivatives. They were discovered by early electron microscopists in the 1950s. Christian de Duve, in Brussels, Belgium, subsequently isolated these structures, demonstrated hydrogen peroxide generation and renamed them peroxisomes.(4) By the 1990s, PPARs were identified and shown to be transcription factors. They were found to control a number of genes, most of which have little or nothing to do with peroxisomes. PPAR-γ is important both in fat cell metabolism and modulating cellular responsiveness to insulin. Hence, the connection with diabetes. They were subsequently found to regulate T-cell responsiveness and to suppress macrophage and microglia activation. Both of these actions are relevant to multiple sclerosis and other neurodegenerative diseases as well.

The discovery that insulin sensitizing thiazolidinediones (TZDs), specific PPAR-gamma (PPAR-γ) agonists, have antiproliferative, anti-inflammatory, and immunomodulatory effects has led to the evaluation of their potential use in the treatment of diabetic complications and inflammatory, proliferative diseases in noninsulin-resistant, normal glycemic individuals (5). In addition to improving insulin resistance, currently approved TZDs have been shown to improve psoriasis, ulcerative colitis, other autoimmune, atopic, inflammatory, and neurodegenerative diseases (e.g. asthma, atopic dermatitis and multiple sclerosis, Alzheimer's disease, Parkinson's disease) These discoveries pave the way for the development of drugs for treating metabolic diseases for which therapy is presently insufficient or nonexistent.

The anti-inflammatory effects on neural cells include suppression of cytokines and enzymes involved in free radical production including NOS (nitric oxide synthases) and COX-2 (cyclooxygenase-2). (6) Some PPAR agonists have been proven to be blood-brain barrier permeable, suggesting direct effects on brain physiology. Pioglitazone, known as Actos, and rosiglitazone, known as Avandia, activate PPAR-γ, which suppresses T cell, macrophage, and microglial, immune responses. If the suppression of these immune responses is of potential benefit for inflammatory diseases of the brain, then pioglitazone should provide therapeutic benefit in multiple sclerosis and other autoimmune disease entities. These drugs were originally designed as antidiabetic drugs due to their insulin sensitizing effects and have been in clinical use for many years. The clinical safety of Actos has been established by clinical studies worldwide, in which over 4,500 subjects have been treated. Since FDA approval, Actos has been widely prescribed to several million patients. The adverse effects associated with PPAR-γ agonists are generally mild and transient. Those effects returned to their baseline upon withdrawal from, or completion of the studies. (7). Since the recent studies with PPAR-γ drugs in animal models of neurological conditions and diseases have led to clinical testing of these drugs in Alzheimer's disease and multiple sclerosis, they make promising candidates for a therapeutic approach to influence the clinical course of autism spectrum disorders.

In a clinical practice dedicated to treating children on the autism spectrum with over 3,000 patients, Marvin Boris, MD and Michael Elice, MD, are treating patients with Actos in the attempt to improve their immune status. The age of patients ranged from two years and older. The diagnosis of autism was established by pediatric neurologists, developmental pediatricians, and /or psychiatrists meeting the DSM-IV criteria prior to being seen in their practice. (8) All the children had been receiving behavioral and educational therapies. These included speech, occupational and physical therapy, applied behavior analysis (ABA) and auditory integration training (AIT). The children also received biomedical interventions for at least one year from the group.

The main hypothesis is that treatment of autistic children with Actos that is currently FDA approved for treatment of type 2 diabetes, but which also shows important anti-inflammatory and cytoprotective effects on neural cells, will provide clinical benefit associated with a change in serum cytokine levels. In order to determine if Actos is safe and tolerable to autistic children, monthly exams, measurements of blood for liver enzymes, standard chemistries, and glucose and insulin levels are performed. Effects on disease are assessed by evaluation of the aberrant behavior checklist (ABC) as recommended by the American Society of Psychiatry. Modification of inflammatory markers in the autistic patients was accomplished by measurement of serum cytokine levels and reactive oxygen species, and by isolation and characterization of serum T cells.

In over five hundred patients prescribed Actos, as an off-label treatment conducted in this private practice setting, Boris and Elice have shown improved cognitive function and improved receptive and expressive language as well as increased spontaneous language, decreased hyperactivity, decreased lethargy, decreased stereotypical behavior (stimming), better eye contact, and socialization.

Blood plasma samples from autistic children treated off-label with Actos for up to six months were analyzed for nine different cytokine levels by ELISA (enzyme-linked immunosorbent assay) assay and compared to values from non-treated patients. For eight of nine cytokines, Actos reduced plasma levels. Patients showed improved behavior described by treating physicians and parents with no adverse effects. This suggests that Actos is safe in autistic children and can influence inflammatory responses, which could moderate clinical symptoms.

50

QIGONG: MASSAGE FOR YOUNG CHILDREN WITH AUTISM

BY DR. LOUISA SILVA

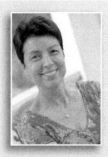

Louisa Silva MD, M.P.H.

Visiting Professor
Teaching Research Institute
Western Oregon University
www.qsti.org

Dr. Louisa Silva is a doctor of Western medicine, Chinese medicine, and Public Health. She is currently on the faculty at Teaching Research Institute, Western Oregon University, where for the last ten years, she has led the research investigating a qigong massage program for young children with autism, and developed and validated a curriculum and training materials for parents and early intervention staff to deliver the program in the home and preschool. She is the Director of the Qigong Sensory Training Institute, a nonprofit corporation dedicated to early intervention, treatment, training, and research for young children with autism. Her most recent book is *Helping your Child with Autism: A Home Program from Chinese Medicine*.

The Qigong Sensory Training Home Program: A Parent-Delivered Massage Intervention from Chinese Medicine.

Over the past nine years, a five-month, parent-delivered massage intervention has been proven in scientific studies to lessen the severity of autism and improve sensory and self-regulation problems in young children with autism. Known as the Qigong Sensory Training Home Program, and based on principles of Chinese medicine, research documenting its effectiveness has been published in both Eastern and Western scientific journals.

In this intervention, parents are trained to give their child a daily fifteen-minute massage that is tuned to their child's particular physical reactions to touch on different parts of their body. Within a few months, the children relax, open up, and participate more in home and school life. As sensory sensitivities disappear, behavior and tantrums improve. As key symptoms of autism disappear—e.g. avoiding eye contact, not being curious about social encounters—social and language learning increases.

The intervention allows the knowledge of Chinese medicine, combined with the power of parent touch, to give parents a way to help children to be more comfortable in their own skin. The key to a successful outcome for the child is a parent who is able to get the massage into the child's daily routine and keep it there for a minimum of four months. When this happens, the massage starts a healing and balancing process that continues as long as the massage is given daily.

The intervention, known as *qigong massage* was first developed in Italy by Dr. Anita Cignolini. Originally, it was a dual intervention, taught to parents, and delivered by a Chinese medicine trained physician. Subsequent research in the U.S. at the Teaching Research Institute, Western Oregon University, adapted and modified the intervention for delivery by parents at home with support from trained Early Intervention staff.

At the present time, research has been done on two levels of intensity of the intervention: 1) The QST Home program, a home program involving seven hours of training and support for parents, and 2) The QST Dual program which involves parent training and support, as well as twenty supplementary treatments for the child, given by trained professionals. Preliminary research comparing the two, shows that parents with mildly and moderately affected children do the best with the QST Home program, whereas parents of children with severe autism who are severely stressed by their child's autism, benefit more from the QST Dual program. For those parents who do not have access to training and support, the massage is fully documented in a training book and DVD that is available at www.qsti.org.

Research is ongoing, and although all research has been done in the under-six age range, anecdotal reports from parents who have treated their older children indicate that it can be beneficial in older children as well.

Success rate

This program is equally effective in low-functioning as in high-functioning children. By five months of treatment, data shows: parent stress decreased by 32 percent, autistic behavior decreased by 26 percent, sensory and self-regulation problems decreased by 28 percent, and overall autism decreased by 18 percent. Parents continuing the massage for another year or two, report continued improvements in their children's growth and development.

Best-case scenario

Anthony was a five-year-old boy with severe autism. He was very irritable, had frequent and long tantrums, very little language, and required twenty-four-hour care. He was in diapers, slept very little and irregularly. He only ate about five foods and he had terrible constipation. Any small change in his routine would provoke a severe tantrum, and it was nearly impossible to take him to the store or to visit relatives. His parents were sleep deprived and exhausted. Even though he was in a special pre-school with a one-on-one aide, he didn't seem to be making progress.

The first week of the massage, his mother noticed that he had several large, dark green, stinky bowel movements. After that, his constipation got better, and he started to eat more and different foods. Within three weeks of starting the massage, he began to sleep regularly at night. His mother noticed that he would turn and face her when she spoke to him. She took him grocery shopping for the first time, and it was not a problem! Within another three weeks, he was fully toilet trained.

Five weeks into treatment, he fell down in the parking lot and skinned his knee and cried. His mother was astonished, as he had never shown any reaction to pain before. After that, when his little sister cried, he would become concerned; he became much more interested in her. His language started to improve and he made his wants and needs known.

All of a sudden, he started to move into the terrible two's. Every time his mother asked him to do something, he said "No!" But she remembered that learning to say "No" was in his next stage of development, so she recognized this as progress. Within a few weeks, she could talk him through the "Nos." By the end of the five-month intervention, he had put on seventeen months of language development.

Now, two years later, his parents are still doing the massage every night, and he is in regular school without an aide. He is up to grade level in his language and social skills. His mother says he will always be quirky, but she no longer worries that he will not be able to take care of himself.

A different scenario

There is such a variability in children with autism, and all children don't progress at the same rate or start from the same starting point. Here is an example of a very severely affected child who improved considerably, was much more comfortable by five months, but still had a long way to go. Jamie was a child with very severe autism. He had a severely deformed head, and had worn a helmet for nine months to try to correct it. He ate a very limited diet, and was very constipated. He had severe tantrums, and did not fall asleep at night. Often he was awake most of the night. He was not toilet trained, and had no receptive or expressive language. Within the first week of massage, he slept through the night. After several weeks, he began to toilet train. By two months, his tantrums had abated. At the end of five months, he would turn his head when his mother spoke to him, and could understand simple directions, but had not yet started to speak. His mother felt that the massage had helped his physical problems significantly, but wanted more language for him. We instructed her to continue the massage for at least another year.

We think that the true worst-case scenarios are those where the parents are not able to do the massage regularly. In those cases, their children do not get the benefit. There are many reasons why parents might not be able to give the massage regularly—reasons of physical and emotional illness, reasons of massive additional stressors, and reasons where the personal beliefs of the parents are against the idea that Chinese massage can benefit autism. In our experience, however, the great majority of parents have been able to successfully learn the massage, get it into their child's routine, and continue it for months or years at a time.

Contact information and resources

More information about the QST Home Program book and DVD is available on the website at www.qsti.org. Parents and Early Intervention staff who are interested in bringing a training workshop to their area can contact the website to make arrangements.

51

RELATIONSHIP DEVELOPMENT INTERVENTION

BY LAURA HYNES

Laura Hynes, LMSW; RDI Program Certified Consultant

Extraordinary Minds, Inc.
308 Forest Avenue
Staten Island, New York 10301
(347) 564-8451
L.Hynes@yahoo.com
www.extraordinaryminds.org
RDIconnect.com

Laura Hynes graduated from Stony Brook University with a Bachelor of Arts in Psychology and a minor in Child and Family Studies in 2001. She obtained a Masters in Social Work in 2005 from New York University and is a licensed social worker in the State of New York. In 2008, Laura became certified in Relationship Development Intervention She is the president and founder of Extraordinary Minds, Inc., where she currently provides RDI services to families.

Relationship Development Intervention is a unique approach to treating autism spectrum disorders. Developed by Dr. Steven Gutstein, RDI is based on the most recent research in autism spectrum disorders (ASD), neurology, and developmental psychology. The RDI theory is based on providing individuals with ASD opportunities to attain a better quality of life than what is typically expected for them. It is a parent-based approach, whereby trained consultants teach parents how to change the way they are communicating and interacting with their child to improve the child's dynamic intelligence.

> "Give a man a fish and you feed him for a day. Teach a man to fish and you feed him for a lifetime."
>
> —Chinese Proverb

To best understand dynamic intelligence, one must understand static intelligence. Most individuals with ASD are quite proficient in static areas. Think of static intelligence as anything that has a right or wrong answer, that is unchanging and always produces the same outcome. Labeling, requesting, social scripts, academics, following directions, and memorization are all examples of static skills, and likely what a child with ASD is adept at.

Think about dynamic intelligence as the ability to manage situations that present themselves with elements of uncertainty. Examples of dynamic skills include the ability to problem solve, share experiences with others, curiosity, empathy, and taking another's perspective. All these things are uncertain, in that there is no right or wrong answer, and no way to predict what specific outcome will occur. This type of intelligence is what is most often lacking in individuals with ASD.

There are other interventions for ASD that focus primarily on strengthening static skills; increasing language, teaching scripts to navigate social situations or following a schedule Challenge yourself to think of these types of skills as compensatory for deficits in dynamic thinking.

- Is increasing one's vocabulary improving the ability to share experiences and communicate with other people?
- Is teaching a child a social script for the playground preparing them for what to do when they don't get the response they were taught to expect?
- Is creating a picture schedule teaching a person to be flexible and manage the real world, where unexpected things happen all the time?

"One can imagine training or therapies that are designed to teach the various parts of the brain to work together in a more coordinated way, to make them function as a team rather than individual players."
—Marcel Just, MD

Years ago, the scientific community believed that the brain was unable to change. The only way we knew how to teach individuals with ASD was to give them the skills to compensate for their brain's difficulty managing uncertainty. We know now that the brain is an experience dependent organ; it changes and grows based on the types of learning experiences it is exposed to on a day to day basis. It is not only possible but critical to begin addressing and remediating the deficits of ASD instead of merely working around them.

"Children's cognitive development is an apprenticeship—it occurs through guided participation in a social activity with companions who support and stretch children's learning."

—Barbara Rogoff

Neurotypical individuals begin thinking dynamically very early in life. The relationship between parent and child is critical for the development of active thinkers and communicators. This parent-child relationship is referred to as the guided participation relationship. Guided participation is found cross-culturally, in every society, since the beginning of time. Children act as cognitive apprentices to the more skilled and competent adults, learning from their guides, who provide them with ongoing challenges and the support necessary for them to be successful. Guides balance teaching various skills with a more important goal, providing the foundations for active thinking, learning, and cognitive growth.

Consider a young child raking leaves with his father. The father is not teaching his child to rake the leaves in a way that he would expect the child to go out and independently do this the following weekend. The father is teaching his child the goals beneath the goal; the foundations for learning. The child is learning how to collaborate with his father, how to flexibly manage problems and come up with solutions, and how to anticipate and communicate to one another about what they are doing.

Unfortunately, when ASD is added to the guided participation relationship, the child provides the parent with poor social and emotional feedback, leaving the parent with inadequate information and opportunity to provide the child with opportunities to learn in a dynamic way. This is where RDI becomes so valuable.

"There is no greater reward than serving as a catalyst for another person's journey towards fulfilling their true potential."

—Dr. Steven Gutstein

Dr. Gutstein, developer of the RDI program, looked closely at the guided participation relationship between typically developing children and their parents and how parents provide their children with opportunities for dynamic growth. He was able to identify where the breakdown in this relationship occurs with children with ASD. But more importantly, the RDI program is designed to reestablish the guided participation relationship, thereby improving the child's ability to function in a dynamic, everchanging world.

Through his extensive research on autism and the guided participation relationship in autism, Dr. Gutstein systemized several core areas of dynamic intelligence that are lacking in individuals with ASD. These elements of dynamic thinking are incorporated into guided participation objectives that make up the dynamic intelligence curriculum.

Parents often yearn for their child to establish peer relationships. Peer relationships, as all relationships, require the ability to collaborate, where partners are able to coordinate their actions, thoughts, and ideas to reach a common goal. Parents and professionals alike want nothing more than for the child with ASD to go out on the playground and make up a game with a peer. This type of collaborating requires a more basic understanding of social reciprocity called coregulation that is typically lacking in individuals with ASD.

Co-regulation is the most basic form of interaction and communication. It is simply, when one person takes an action in response to their partner's action. There is no end goal or task involved. It is purely about the process of being in the moment with the other person. Oftentimes, individuals with ASD are either, passive and prompt dependent or controlling and rigid. To establish co-regulation with a passive partner, the parent must help the child to understand that he or she can bring something to the interaction without being told what to do. To establish co-regulation with a controlling child, the parent must provide the child with an authentic role that allows the child to provide suggestions for enhancement without the usual controlling features. Co-regulation can be established. As the individual with ASD understands and participates in basic social reciprocity, many new opportunities for interacting and communicating occur.

There are two types of communication, instrumental and experience sharing communication. Instrumental communication is used to obtain something and a specific response is expected. Examples of this would be requesting a toy, asking a question or providing a direction. Once the desired object is received, the question answered, or the direction taken there is no longer a need to communicate with the other person.

Experience sharing communication, by nature, does not require a specific response. When you express what you like or dislike, what you are feeling or describing about your day, you will expect a relevant but not right or wrong response. Think about all the things that have to be considered in order to successfully have a conversation. We must interpret the other person's language, his or her non-verbal communication; gestures, facial expressions, intonation change, pauses and innuendo; and do it simultaneously.

The value of language in the human experience is to communicate and share experiences with others. In the RDI program, parents look at what type of communication they are using with their child. Is it mostly instrumental; asking questions or providing directions or is it mostly experience sharing; commenting, sharing preferences and ideas? Parents are taught to increase their experience sharing language and decrease their instrumental language. By providing the child with ASD language that does not require a specific response, parents are teaching the child the true value of language, to share with others.

The RDI program also teaches parents to create an environment conducive to the development of broadband communication. By incorporating more nonverbal communication, into every day experiences parents create a need for the child to look, monitor, and become a more active communicator. Likewise it is important to avoid the skill of eye contact and provide reasons to look, a pathway to melding communication and language into its most human dynamic form.

By utilizing nonverbal and broadband communication, parents are also increasing the child's opportunities to reference. Social referencing, the ability to access information from a guide when wary or unsure, is in place by twelve months of age in typically developing children. Individuals with ASD have great difficulty using social referencing to manage uncertainty. When faced with a situation that is uncertain, they will often respond with fight or flight, melt down, or withdrawal. Referencing, often a deficit, is a better option. The goal is to allow the child to discover that there is value is looking to their more competent guides for information, to "borrow" their perspective when they are unsure as to how to process information. The RDI program teaches parents how to create moments of productive uncertainty that create just enough curiosity without being so uncertain that the child feels anxious. The productive part of productive uncertainty will vary for every individual. For example, parents can create productive uncertainty by merely stopping while walking together. Some individuals however will require a more deliberate or extreme approach to productive uncertainty such as pulling a hammer out of washing machine while doing laundry together.

By teaching the child the value in looking to more competent guides for help processing information, we are actually teaching them how to become more effective problem solvers. In this regard it must be remembered that one must have a healthy dependence on a more competent guide to learn how to effectively and competently navigate a dynamic, ever changing world. This leads to true independence.

The RDI program teaches parents the value in helping their child to become more active thinkers and problem solvers. There are many ways to do this on a day-to-day basis, but the first is to look at areas where they may be overcompensating, perhaps doing things for their child that he or she is likely capable of doing. To create feeling of competence in the child, the child needs to have opportunities to be successful at thinking, considering and problem solving. Take a simple everyday example of a child who wants a drink. Mom holds the juice and places the cup in front of the child, upside down. By just waiting and not providing the solution to "turn over your cup", Mom has created an uncertain moment where she is asking the child to monitor his environment, think about and consider the situation and take some kind of action to fix it. If the child is not able to figure out what it is Mom is asking of him, Mom can use a statement such as "I don't think I can pour the juice yet," or "Your cup is upside down!" This type of statement is stating the problem rather than the solution, allowing the child the opportunity to think and problem solve on his own. The RDI program teaches parents how to identify opportunities and create dozens of moments such as these throughout their day.

> **"If there is anything that we wish to change in the child, we should first examine it and see whether it is not something that could better be changed in ourselves."**
>
> **—C. G. Jung**

The RDI program is broken down into systematic and workable objectives. Because it is a parent based intervention, parents work on their own objectives prior to the assignment of any objectives for the child. As parents move through their own objectives and as they change their behavior, many child objectives are inadvertently addressed. Thus early on, from the very beginning observable improvements in the child's dynamic abilities are often noticed early on.

RDI begins with an in depth look at the parent's readiness to begin the work of reestablishing the guided participation relationship. Parents work collaboratively with their consultant to develop short and long term goals for themselves, the child with ASD as well as siblings, they examine and modify current schedules to create more quality time for guided participation, they work to improve their limit setting abilities and identify and modify areas where they may be over-compensating for the child.

Once parents are demonstrating readiness to learn how to guide their child, a dynamic assessment is done. The Relationship Development Assessment looks at the state of the guided participation relationship and consists of parents and child engaging in predetermined activities provided by the consultant. Based on the information gathered during the RDA, objectives are assigned.

As parents adopt guided participation as their primary mode of parenting and become competent guides, they begin using the dynamic intelligence curriculum for their child. The dynamic intelligence curriculum is comprised of over a thousand dynamic, developmental objectives that follow the continuum of typical development. The RDI program thus provides parents and children with a second chance at getting back on developmental track with mastery of small, manageable and observable objectives and goals.

Face to face meetings between parents, consultant, and child occur regularly, usually once or twice per month. During these meetings assignments are broken down, plans for work at home through role play and demonstration occur. Parents leave their meeting with an assignment to complete at home with their child based on what particular parent or child objective is being addressed between sessions. They provide the consultant with video journals and other forms of communication demonstrating how they are working on their current assignment and how they are actively analyzing and evaluating the work they are doing with their child. From the very beginning of the RDI program, parents are taking the responsibility to think about and consider their successes and breakdowns with their child and eventually to guide their child without the support of a consultant.

The RDI program is a unique and invaluable resource to families. It values parents as the most important influence in their child's life. Parents are provided the skills and direction to become successfully reconnected with their child. Knowing that their child's growth is due to their own guidance and nurturing empowers parents to persevere through difficult times and look to the future with hope.

RESPEN-A

BY DR. FRED STARR

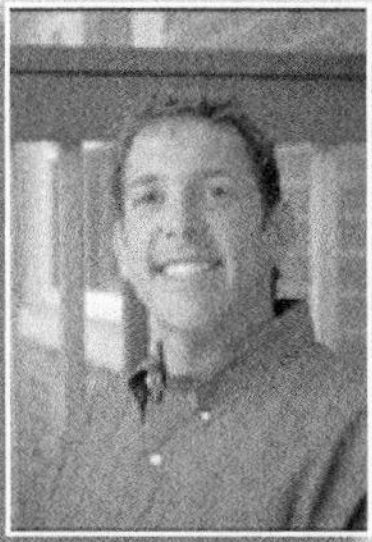

Fred S. Starr, M.D., FAACAP, BCIA-EEG

Medical Director
5 Starr Psychiatry & Neurofeedback
1503 17th Avenue South
Nashville, TN 37212
(615) 292-1664
www.5starrpsych.com

Dr. Fred Starr is the medical director of 5 Starr Psychiatry & Neurofeedback, president of The Tennessee Chapter of The American Academy of Child and Adolescent Psychiatry, and an active contributor to the Middle Tennessee Autism Foundation. Dr. Starr helps his patients by treating the underlying problems causing their symptoms, thus reducing or eliminating their need for conventional psychiatric medications. Recognizing the interaction between the external environment and its connection to a person's mind, body, and soul he is able to effectively treat mental illness. He has extensive experience and success in treating ADD, AHDD, Alzheimer's, Autism, and minor brain damage. He has completed specialized training in hyperbaric oxygen therapy, and eye movement desensitization and reprocessing therapy, and is board certified in quantitative electroencephalography and neurofeedback. Dr. Starr founded the Anna Starr Foundation after suffering the tragic death of his six-year-old daughter Anna due to complications of epilepsy. The Anna Starr Foundation exists to treat and study new treatments for this debilitating disorder. He lives in Hawaii, has two sons, and enjoys yoga and windsurfing in his spare time.

The theory behind Respen-A was developed by Elaine DeLack, R.N (E.D), a private researcher based in Stanwood, Washington. She is the founder and CEO of MedDEV, Inc., developer and patent applicant of Respen-A, a proprietary formulation of transdermal reserpine. Quantitative electroencephalograms (qEEGs) has been conducted by Dr Starr on autistic children treated with Respen-A over a three-week period. Fred S. Starr, MD, FAACAP, BCIA-EEG, is a child and adolescent psychiatrist based in Nashville, Tennessee.

History of Respen-A development for the treatment of ASD

The theory behind the medication, Respen-A, stems from the epidural anesthesia procedure given to women during childbirth. In the United States it is reported that almost 90 percent of women receive an epidural during pregnancy.

DeLack contends that it is the actual labor inducing drugs such as oxytocin (Pitocin) given in concurrence with the epidural, that can cause autism. Oxytocin is known to be involved in social behavior, bonding and language development, which are the main deficit areas of autism and ASD. The hypothalamic neurohypophysial system (HNS), which is implicated in autism, is responsible for the production of the naturally occurring neurotransmitter oxytocin. When oxytocin brain levels reach a threshold, growth of the HNS, and brain development stops.

The Pitocin given during childbirth, crosses the placenta into the infant's system, and is metabolized by the infant's liver cytochrome P-450 enzyme known as CYP 3A4. Bupivacaine, and ropicacaine, which are local anesthetics found in epidurals, are also metabolized in part by CYP 3A4, and thus compete with pitocin, which leads to increased levels of oxytocin in the infant. This buildup of pitocin affects the HNS, and causes premature inhibition of brain development in the infant, resulting in an increased risk of autism. It is also reported that females produce more CYP 3A4 enzymes than males, which might explain why boys are at greater risk of autism than girls.

Another hypothesis is with the enzyme monoamine oxidase-A (MAO-A), which is usually found in high levels in infants, and diminishes with age. MAO-A metabolizes the neurotransmitter serotonin, in addition to norepinephrine, and histamine. As MAO-A levels decrease, serotonin levels increase, this can cause impairments in the brain in the areas associated with communication, speech, emotion and bonding. Prior research has revealed that reserpine increases the activity of MAO-A twofold within seventy-two hours of the first dose [16] Respen-A is a proprietary homeopathic 4X dilution of reserpine in glycerin administered via a transdermal disc. The pattern of qEEGs performed on a pilot study of five patients taking Respen-A; depict a marked decrease in abnormal brain activity. QEEGs provide a good indication of two and three dimensions of a person's brain.

Success rate of Respen-A

The potential success with patients taking Respen-A is tremendous. Increased MAO-A activity, will reduce the risk associated with Pitocin and epidurals from childbirth. This will in turn reduce the incidence rates of ASD, meaning new cases developed over time. QEEGs will be able to depict the decrease in abnormal brain activity, especially in the temporal lobe (as shown in Dr. Starr's clinical findings), with the best-case scenario meaning improved auditory and semantics processing, thus enabling the ASD child, to communicate better. The temporal lobe is responsible for long-term memory, comprehension, naming, and other language functions.

Risk and/or side-effects of Respen-A

A main side effect of Respen-A would involve decreased levels of serotonin, which can lead to increased motor activity, and hyperactivity in patients. This is especially true in patients taking antidepressants together with Respen-A. In this case, the dosage levels can be modified and decreased. The worst-case scenario would mean decreased levels of serotonin, which can potentially decrease release of hypothalamic corticotropin-releasing hormone (CRH), decreases adrenocorti-cotropic hornone (ACTH) secretion, which can possibly lead to an even greater diminished response to stress than otherwise seen in ASD patients. Patients on Respen-A also require supplemental daily calcium, as it will decrease calcium levels.

THE SCERTS MODEL

by Dr. Barry Prizant, Dr. Amy Wetherby, Emily Rubin, and Amy Laurent

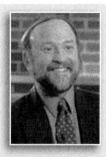

Barry M. Prizant, Ph.D., CCC-SLP

Adjunct Professor
Center for the Study of Human Development
Brown University, Providence, RI

Director
Childhood Communication Services, Cranston, RI

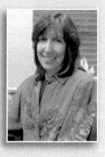

Amy M. Wetherby, Ph.D., CCC-SLP

Professor, Department of Clinical Sciences

Laurel Schendel Professor,
Department of Communication Disorders

Director, Autism Institute in the College of Medicine
Florida State University, Tallahassee, Florida.

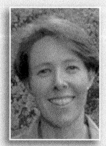

Emily Rubin, MS, CCC-SLP

Lecturer, Yale University School of Medicine
New Haven, CT

Director, Communication Crossroads
Carmel, CA

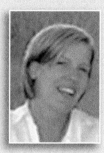

Amy C. Laurent, EdM, OTR/L

Adjunct Faculty
Department of Communication Disorders
University of Rhode Island, Kingston, RI

Adjunct Faculty
Department of Communication Sciences and Disorders
Emerson College, Boston, MA

Private Practice Affiliate, Communication Crossroads, North
Kingstown, RI

For further information on the SCERTS Collaborators, the SCERTS Model, or for contact information, go to www.SCERTS.com.

What is SCERTS?

SCERTS is an innovative, research-based educational model for working with children with autism spectrum disorder (ASD) and their families. It provides specific guidelines for helping an individual with ASD to become a competent and confident social communicator, while preventing problem behaviors that interfere with learning and the development of relationships. It also is designed to help families, educators and therapists work cooperatively as a team, in a carefully coordinated manner, to maximize progress in supporting that individual.

The acronym "SCERTS" refers to the model's focus on:

"SC" - Social Communication—the development of spontaneous, functional communication, emotional expression and secure and trusting relationships with children and adults;

"ER" - Emotional Regulation—the development of the ability to maintain a well-regulated emotional state to cope with everyday stress, and to be most available for learning and interacting;

"TS"—Transactional Support—the development and implementation of supports to help partners be highly responsive to an individual's needs and interests, modify and adapt the environment, and provide tools to enhance learning (e.g., picture communication, written schedules, and sensory supports). Specific plans are also developed to provide educational and emotional support to families, and to foster teamwork among professionals.

Who developed SCERTS?

Currently, the SCERTS Model collaborators include the transdisciplinary team of Barry Prizant, Amy Wetherby, Emily Rubin, and Amy Laurent, who have training in Speech-Language Pathology, Special Education, Behavioral and Developmental Psychology, Occupational Therapy and Family-Centered Practice. The SCERTS Collaborators have more than 100 years experience in university, hospital, clinical and educational settings, and are actively involved in clinical work, research, and educational consultation. The collaborators have published extensively in scholarly journals and volumes on ASD and related disabilities. A comprehensive two-volume manual (Prizant, Wetherby, Rubin, Laurent & Rydell, 2006) provides detailed guidance for assessment and intervention efforts using the SCERTS model, and an electronic scoring system (SCERTS Easy-Score, 2010) allows teams to enter data resulting in graphing and tracking of progress over time.

How did the SCERTS Model evolve?

The SCERTS Model is derived from an integration of more than three decades of empirical and clinical work and is consistent with recommended tenets of evidence-based practice espoused by researchers and clinical scholars focusing on autism spectrum disorders (ASD) and related disabilities (National Research Council, 2001). SCERTS was developed in response to encouragement and feedback from researchers and clinicians in the field of ASD, as well as from parents who were familiar with our work and desired an alternative framework to educational approaches currently available. More specifically, the developmental, social-pragmatic focus of the model has been the hallmark of our research and published work over the past three decades and has been influenced by other developmentally-based social communication intervention models outside of the field of ASD. The model reflects and integrates our empirical research and clinical investigation in understanding conventional and unconventional communication in ASD, including communicative functions and intentions of behavior and is philosophically consistent with tenets of recent work in positive behavior support. The model is also based upon our work addressing the relationships among communication, social-emotional development and emotion regulation and incorporates developmental research and practice addressing social-emotional factors, arousal modulation, and emotional regulation.

The SCERTS Model integrates person-centered philosophies in practice. For example, as in our previous work, the model draws from the contemporary research on the learning style of individuals with ASD. This is reflected, for instance, in the SCERTS Model's emphasis on the use of visual supports throughout the natural routines of a child's day. In addition, the SCERTS Assessment process addresses individual differences in the core deficit areas of communication and social-emotional development, and examines relative strengths and motivations for an individual as well as the challenges and needs of the individual. The SCERTS Model views learning and development as transactional and collaborative, therefore the assessment process also includes documentation of interpersonal support and learning support provided by typical partners including educators, therapists and family members.

Finally, the family-centered philosophy espoused in the model has been influenced by our work on the impact of disabilities on the family, and our application of family-centered research and practice, both within and outside the ASD literature. Based upon this description, it is evident that the SCERTS Model is consistent with and/or has been directly influenced by the contemporary evidence-based practices and education/intervention approaches both within and outside of the field of ASD. We believe, however, that the SCERTS model offers an important and novel contribution to available educational approaches by establishing clear priorities in the areas of social communication, emotion regulation, and transactional support in a manner that addresses the complex interdependencies among these most crucial areas. The model thus reflects a new conceptualization of education/intervention that most closely addresses the core deficits observed in ASD and therefore represents an example of what we believe to be the "next generation" of intervention approaches for ASD.

Priorities and Practices in the SCERTS Model

The SCERTS model targets the most significant challenges identified by research that are faced by individual's with ASD and their families, Social Communication, Emotional Regulation and Transactional Support. The scope and sequence of developmental targets is derived from descriptive group research studies representing core challenges in ASD. Additionally, targets are selected based on research indicating that they are predictive of gains in language acquisition, social adaptive functioning, and academic achievement. Determination of priorities occurs through family-professional partnerships (family-centered care), and by prioritizing the abilities and supports that will lead to the most positive long-term outcomes as indicated by the most comprehensive reviews of intervention research (National Research Council, 2001). As such, it provides family members and educational teams with a plan for implementing a comprehensive and evidence-based program that will improve quality of life individuals with ASD and their families.

The SCERTS Model is not an exclusive approach, in that it provides a framework in which practices and strategies from other approaches may be integrated. It is a lifespan model that can be used from initial diagnosis, throughout the school years, and beyond. It can be adapted to meet the unique demands of different social settings for younger and older individuals with ASD including home, school, community, and ultimately vocational settings. The SCERTS Model provides a flexible curriculum that is developmentally informed but also allows for individualization of goals and objectives based on an individual's developmental abilities, family priorities and functional needs. As such, it can be used with individuals across a wide range of ages and developmental abilities, including nonverbal, minimally verbal and highly verbal individuals. As noted, detailed guidance for implementing the SCERTS Model is provided in a two-volume comprehensive manual (Prizant, Wetherby, Rubin, Rydell & Laurent, 2006).

The SCERTS Model includes a well-coordinated, systematic assessment to program planning process (SAP-SCERTS Assessment Process) that provides quantitative data and qualitative data resulting in a developmental profile. This information, along with caregiver input, are used to help a team select and prioritize goals and objectives, measure the individual's progress through ongoing tracking, and determine the necessary supports to be used by the individual's partners across social settings (educators, peers, and family members). There also is a systematic activity planning process that ensures that the highest priority goals and objectives are addressed in everyday activities and routines throughout the day. The assessment process utilizes observational checklists and caregiver questionnaires and ensures that:

- functional, meaningful, and developmentally-appropriate goals and objectives are selected
- individual differences learning style, interests, and motivations are respected
- the culture and lifestyle of the family are understood and respected
- the individual is engaged in meaningful and functional activities throughout the day
- supports are developed and used consistently across partners, activities, and environments
- an individual's progress is systematically charted over time
- program quality is measured frequently to assure accountability

In the domain of Social Communication, the SCERTS Model emphasizes the importance of child- initiated communication in natural as well as semi-structured activities for a broad range of purposes such as requesting, protesting, sharing attention, sharing emotion, and sharing experiences. As children mature, these purposes expand to include the importance of considering one's listener's perspective when initiating, taking turns in conversation, selecting topics, and repairing communicative breakdowns. Goals for the individual are identified in the curriculum components of join attention and symbol use and target both verbal and non-verbal forms of communication. The scope and sequence of goals covers a broad developmental range from early gestures to sophisticated conversational discourse. Families and educators work together to identify and develop strategies to successfully support an individual's active participation and communication in meaningful daily activities.

In the domain of Emotional Regulation, a plan to support an individual's emotional regulation is developed based on an individual's developmental profile and needs. Goals for the individual are developed in the curriculum components of Self-Regulation (an individual's ability to regulate independently) and Mutual Regulation (regulation that occurs with the support of partners). The plan may include sensory-motor (e.g., regularly scheduled exercise and "regulating" breaks and supports), and language-based strategies (e.g., visual schedules, ER choice boards) and a plan used by all partners to modify learning environments. Partners also become expert at reading an individual's signals of emotional dysregulation (which may include problem behaviors such as protests and refusals) and respond with appropriate support as needed. Such support may include offering sensory input, simplifying difficult tasks, providing information through the use of visual supports, as well as emotional support such as verbal reassurance or encouragement. The goal of ER support is to maximize attention and learning by supporting a well-regulated state and to prevent escalation into more problematic behavior.

In the domain of Transactional Support, goals for partners are developed in the curriculum areas of Interpersonal Support and Learning Supports. In Interpersonal support, we measure how all team members are being responsive to an individual's behaviors, and are modifying their own behavior such as simplifying language, providing appropriate modeling and supporting an individual's independence. Based on this analysis, appropriate changes in interpersonal support strategies allow all partners to be "on the same page." In Learning Support, we examine how all partners are designing activities to support active participation and are using augmentative, visual and organizational supports, and modifying activities and learning environments.

Appropriate modifications and additions in learning supports are made based on this analysis to best support social communication, emotional regulation and learning.

For example, when enhancing smooth transitions with individuals who are pre-symbolic, partners would be encouraged to use objects or photographs to depict upcoming activities. Likewise, when enhancing smooth transition with those at later stages of development, partners would be encouraged to use graphics or the written word to outline the daily schedule as well as steps within each task. Partners would also be encouraged to modify activities and learning environments according to the individual's strengths and needs. Examples of these supports include adjusting the social complexity based upon the individual individual's needs, adjusting the task demands to ensure the individual feels successful, and infusing motivating and meaningful topics to ensure the individual's active engagement in activities. Additionally, plans are developed to provide educational and emotional support to families, and support among professionals.

How does SCERTS compare to other approaches?

The SCERTS curriculum provides a systematic method that ensures that specific skills and appropriate supports, stated as educational objectives, are selected and applied in a consistent manner across an individual's day. This process allows families and educational teams to draw from a wide range of effective practices that are available, and to build upon their current knowledge and abilities in providing an effective program. One of the most unique qualities of SCERTS is that it is a team-based model that can incorporate practices from other approaches including contemporary ABA (e.g., Pivotal Response Therapy, LEAP), TEACCH, Floortime, RDI, Hanen, and Social Stories. The SCERTS Model differs most notably from the focus of "traditional" ABA, an approach that typically targets responses in adult directed Discrete Trials, by promoting initiated communication in everyday activities, by drawing extensively from research on child and human development, and by integrating knowledge and practice from a variety of disciplines.

Implementation and Research in the SCERTS Model

As of this writing, the SCERTS Model manuals have been available for only four years, yet practice and research in the SCERTS Model has expanded both nationally and internationally. School systems and agencies across the U.S. and Canada, and in New Zealand, Australia, and Europe are using the SCERTS Model as the framework for guiding educational and clinical practice for individuals with ASD and related disabilities. The SCERTS Model manuals have been translated into Japanese and will be published in 2010. Clinical and educational data supports the effectiveness of practices in the SCERTS Model within agencies and schools, and longitudinal research following large samples of children is currently in progress in both the U.S. and Canada. It is expected that results of this research will be forthcoming in the next one to three years. Introductory and Advanced trainings are provided on a regular basis in East and West Coast training institutes, and at many other locations nationally and internationally.

SENSORY-BASED ANTECEDENT INTERVENTIONS

BY GINNY VAN RIE AND DR. L. JUANE HEFLIN

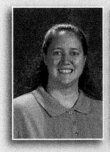
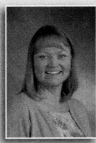

Ginny L. Van Rie, M.Ed. and **L. Juane Heflin,** Ph. D.

gvanrie1@student.gsu.edu
jheflin@gsu.edu

Georgia State University
Educational Psychology and Special
Education
PO Box 3979
Atlanta, GA 30302-3970
(404) 413-8333

Ms. Van Rie is a certified special educator who has taught children with ASD and extremely challenging behavior for over nine years. As a lead teacher, she helps other teachers intervene positively and proactively to minimize maladaptive behavior and support student achievement. Her goal is to create an environment to match the learning and behavioral needs of each individual student with ASD. She was honored as the "Outstanding Doctoral Student of the Year" in Special Education at Georgia State University in 2009. Dr. Heflin has over twenty-five years of experience learning about and advocating for individuals with ASD and coordinates the autism program at Georgia State University. She co-edits the journal, *Focus on Autism and Other Developmental Disabilities* and coauthored the book, *Students with Autism Spectrum Disorders: Effective Instructional Practices*, published by Prentice Hall in 2007 (second edition available in 2011). Both Ms. Van Rie and Dr. Heflin have been recognized as "Heroes for Autism" by the Greater Georgia Chapter of the Autism Society of America.

Researchers have provided copious evidence that modifying antecedent events (those that occur prior to instruction) can have a strong positive effect on student engagement and success.

In some situations, the antecedent variables that occasion student resistance are predictable, such as giving the student a large amount of work to do (Sweeney & LeBlanc, 1995). For many of those with ASD, the antecedent conditions are uniquely individual, as was the case of a child who interacted willingly unless his shirt was wet or his toys had been moved, at which point he became aggressive (Napolitano, Tessing, McAdam, Dunleavy & Cifuni, 2006). Banda and Kubina (2006) discovered that asking two or three conversational questions that the adolescent answered willingly (e.g., "Did you watch football yesterday?"), prior to asking him to empty his backpack, arrange his daily schedule, and go to his locker resulted in quicker transitions and less resistance. Reinhartsen, Garfinkle, and Wolery (2002) documented that allowing children to choose the toy they wanted to play with resulted in higher levels of appropriate engagement as compared to when teachers gave children a preferred toy. Other antecedent interventions that have been used to increase adaptive behavior and reduce what others thought to be problem behaviors in individuals with ASD include the use of Power Cards (Keeling, Myles, Gagnon, & Simpson, 2003), alternative seating (Schilling & Schwartz, 2004), and self-operated auditory prompts (Taber, Seltzer, Heflin, & Alberto, 1999). The National Autism Center (2009a, p. 43) determined that sufficient empirical validation existed to identify antecedent interventions as "Established Treatments." However, none of the variations cited in the *National Standards Report* relate to sensory-based interventions.

It is well documented that individuals with ASD process sensory stimuli differently than individuals with typical development and those with other disabilities (e.g., Ben-Sasson et al., 2007; Crane, Goddard, & Pring, 2009; Ermer, & Dunn, 1998; Harrison, & Hare; 2004; Rogers, Hepburn & Wehner, 2003; Tomcheck & Dunn, 2007). These differences in sensory processing result in reduced availability for instruction that inhibits learning. Sensory-based antecedent interventions support the attainment of optimal levels of arousal to promote the acquisition of skills necessary for independent functioning.

Primary Developers

The theory of optimal arousal, introduced by Lueba (1955) and extended by Zentall and Zentall (1983) is based on the premise that all organisms have an optimal level of arousal and engage in behaviors either to increase or decrease stimulation in order reach those optimal levels. Dunn (1997) stated that individuals could be both hypo- and hyper-responsive to sensory stimuli and that an individual's response to the same sensory stimuli can change over time. She developed a conceptual model of sensory processing in which individuals respond to sensory stimuli based on their sensory receptor thresholds. Individual could have high thresholds and not register sensory input or need to seek additional sensory input to trigger their sensory thresholds. In contrast, individuals could have low sensory thresholds and be overly responsive to sensory stimuli or try to avoid sensory stimuli because the stimulation makes them uncomfortable (Dunn, 2001).

Success rate (including a "Best case" anecdote)

Van Rie and Heflin (2009) conducted a study to determine which form of sensory-based antecedent interventions would establish optimal levels of arousal as measured by correct responses on instructional tasks. Consistent with Dunn's (1997) premise, the type of sensory-based intervention needed to match the arousal level of the child in order to produce a level of arousal that facilitated learning. In the study, each child participated in five minutes of antecedent sensory-based activities prior to instructional tasks. The sensory-based interventions consisted of bouncing on an exercise ball and swinging in a suspended swing. Use of a rigorous research methodology, including analysis via an alternating treatment design with replication, resulted in the ability to draw conclusions about the effects of the interventions. The two students who were over-aroused in the classroom setting, Tony and Al, gave a greater number of correct responses after they spent five minutes swinging in a slow linear manner. Carl, who was under-aroused in the school environment, performed better on the instructional tasks after he spent five minutes bouncing on the exercise ball. These results can be interpreted not only to substantiate the variability of sensory processing difficulties present in the diverse population of individuals with ASD, but also to implicate the need to evaluate each individual's sensory processing patterns in order to select the most appropriate sensory interventions.

Risk and/or side-effects (including a "Worst case" anecdote)

Given the frequency with which sensory-based interventions are used (Heflin & Alaimo 2007; Hess, Morrier, Heflin, & Ivey, 2008; Schreibman, 2005) and a lack of reported adverse effects, there is little risk in using sensory-based antecedent interventions. As documented by Van Rie and Heflin (2009), the critical factor is choosing the appropriate sensory activity to facilitate rather than inhibit learning. The greatest risk manifests in using arousing activities (e.g., bouncing, jumping, running) for children who already are over-aroused or using calming activities (e.g., slow swinging, slow rocking, relaxation) for students who already are under-aroused. In these cases, the levels of arousal would deviate further from those which are needed for optimal arousal. A worst case anecdote is illustrated when Troy, who was over-stimulated in the classroom, was invited to bounce on the exercise ball prior to instruction. Using a Pairwise Data Overlap calculation (Parker & Vannest, in press) the effect size for bouncing was .52, indicating the intervention did not support Troy's learning. In contrast, the effect size was 0.97 for swinging, indicating that the intervention which modulated his level of arousal to optimal was highly effective for enabling Troy to respond correctly on his instructional tasks.

Contact information for developers/practitioners/clinics/etc.

Many practitioners and parents can intuitively determine if a child is over- or under-aroused. If a formal measure is needed, The Sensory Profile (Dunn, 1999), which includes the Short Sensory Profile (McIntosh, Miller, Shyu, & Dunn, 1999) can be used to identify sensory processing challenges. The measure is available from Pearson Assessments

A number of authors have described alerting and calming activities that can be used to affect levels of arousal. Readers are referred to the texts by Heflin and Alaimo (2007), Myles, Cook, Miller, Rinner, and Robbins (2000), and Yack, Aquilla, and Sutton (2002).

Documentation of the effects of an intervention is critical to determining whether or not an appropriate intervention is being used. Resources that describe the process of creating and analyzing graphed data to allow decisions to be made about continued use of an intervention include texts by Heflin and Alaimo (2007), Alberto and Troutman (2009b), and the guide entitled "Evidence-Based Practice: Autism in the Schools" created by the National Autism Center and available free online (www.nationalautismcenter.org).

55

SENSORY GYM: EMERGE AND SEE

BY AMANDA FRIEDMAN AND ALISON BERKLEY

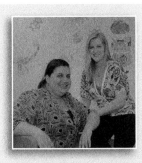

Amanda Friedman

amanda@emergeandseeonline.com
(914) 494-9888

Alison Berkley
alison@emergeandseeonline.com
(917) 312-6600

Emerge and See is located within Watch Me Grow; a sensory gym providing OT, PT, and Speech services
361 East 19th Street @ 1st Avenue, New York, NY 10003

Emerge & See evolved from an after-school social group into a full-fledged and burgeoning business. Alison and Amanda started as coworkers and grew into business partners due to their like-minded philosophies and multi-faceted approaches to education. Realizing their dream, they grew out of the classroom and into the sensory gym setting. They firmly hold the understanding that there is a dire need for a new vision of education and a new form of engagement with those on the spectrum. The services offered expanded to meet the needs spoken of by so many parents and professionals in the community. A true embodiment of academic instruction as well as balanced and structured play therapy; Emerge & See continually meets students' greatest capacity for learning without ceiling and nurtures strong developmental foundations. Inevitably, this duo cemented their own personal and professional belief that every child can learn and every idea is a bright idea!

Academic Learning within a Sensory Gym Setting

Description and Procedures

Emerge & See is an educational center housed within a sensory gym for children diagnosed with autism spectrum and sensory processing disorders, emotional needs, learning disabilities, and other developmental differences. Emerge & See provides a collaborative approach and individualized, comprehensive educational program capitalizing on sensory integration techniques to support maximal learning and regulatory opportunities. Their mission statement is:

To incorporate love of learning, trust of self and the community, and respect into a fun and developmentally sound educational program for students with developmental and emotional differences. Services include but are not limited to

- 1:1 educational tutoring in Math, English, Fine and gross motor skills, and communication (verbal, non verbal, gesturing, eye contact, PECS, etc).
- Dyad pairings of students with siblings or other clients to establish social integration abilities, communication skills, and build relationships that will be meaningful and long term in one another's lives. Activities include games, paired writing and art sessions, imaginative play, sensory based play, and practice of social experiences.
- Social groups will provide coping skills, affective understanding and learning how to initiate interactions with adults and more specifically with peers to have long-lasting relationships in their lives.

The owners, Amanda Friedman and Alison Berkley have a combined fifteen years experience in the field of special needs with diverse backgrounds. The established location of Emerge & See at Watch Me Grow Sensory Gym in Manhattan is a viable business providing therapies (Speech, OT, PT) which mesh well with the services they offer. Emerge & See is driven to customize programs for clients to support them not only throughout their educational experience but at home and within their families, communities and potentially their work force.

The Therapy—Academic Learning within a Sensory Gym Setting

Teaching students academics has traditionally occurred within a classroom setting in large groups with brief periods of recess granting the freedom of energy release, regulation and socializing with peers. We are presenting a pairing of structured academic learning within a sensory gym setting so immediate access to motivating equipment and play is readily available. Educational concepts can be embedded into physical activities utilizing equipment which meets students' different sensory profiles and students can experience learning in a way that empowers them and gives them an outlet for their individual learning styles. Recent educational trends have seen less and less time allotted for such necessary integrative time in schools. Occupational Therapists have long understood the need for physical activity to stimulate students' arousal levels prior to academic and fine motor activities. The brain is constantly hungry for input and when the body is satiated so is the mind. We must encourage children to play and learn from instinct and social settings. Play is an open doorway into engaging with students with ASD and the start of a teaching relationship with them. "Play then is the highest expression of human development in childhood, for it alone is the free expression of what is in the child's soul. It is the purest and most spiritual product of the child, and at the same time it is a type and copy of human life at all stages and in all relations. . . . For to one who has insight into human nature, the trend of the whole future life of the child is revealed in his freely chosen play." (Froeble, Chief Writings on Education p. 50–51) To best access clear and untainted connectivity in learning the body must be awake for the mind to perform its best! Play and movement are vital to students understanding of their physical and internal selves within their immediate environments and their ability to project into future scenarios, imaginative play, and abstract thinking. In building off of these primal sensory needs, the door to academic learning is opened in a positive way that nurtures a desire to learn and a sense of security in both physicality and intellect.

There are two main types of sensory play most children crave; manipulation of self and objects and release of emotion and energy. Often children on the autism spectrum feel very out of control; much of their lives are dictated by rigorous schedules of therapy, doctors, and evaluations, compounded by language difficulties, anxiety-based rituals, and sensory/emotional dysregulation. Manipulating their own bodies, toys, and sensory-based materials (bubbles, water, shaving cream, etc.) they are able to see an immediate correlation of their independent actions to a tangible and concrete change in the world. This creates a sense of security and confidence that lends itself to healthy learning. The latter form of play is vital to reducing stress, over-excitement, confusion, and typical childhood energy! "For the first few years a child has no skill in the manipulation of his senses, and the channels of enjoyment of sense experience and intellectual experiment, which are open to every adult, are not at his disposal as avenues for the discharge of energy. If, therefore, he is to save himself from fretfulness and misery, he is compelled to allow a great deal of his energy to express itself instead through muscular activity." (p 62 *Play in Childhood*, Margaret Lowenfeld 1969) Thereby, students thrive when learning is interwoven with physical release. Many academic foundations can be taught to children who may not be ready for "in seat" work, however, they harbor a capacity for learning that is unique to their own sensory and learning styles. We must begin to cater to students not only for their fundamental deficits, but amplify their ever present, yet often splintered *abilities* as well. Challenging students to reach their maximum success is not defined by our standard views of education, but rather what they need to function within their families and communities. Teaching students within a sensory gym setting lends itself to great joy, trust between teacher and student, and generalization with peers and activities found outside a typical classroom.

History of treatment

While sensory integration is addressed intensely by occupational therapists it is often neglected by teachers. The use of a sensory gym for the sole purpose of teaching academics and foundational problem-solving skills is truly "cutting edge" and there is a new vision of what defines functional and appropriate education. Sensory Integration has been known and defined for decades with clear connections to cognitive improvements. "Essentially, the theory holds that disordered sensory integration accounts for some aspects of learning disorders and that enhancing sensory integration will make academic learning easier for those children whose problem lies in that domain. Sensory integration, or the ability to organize sensory information for use, can be improved through controlling its input to active brain mechanisms. . . . Sensory integrative processes result in perception and other types of synthesis of sensory data that enable man to interact effectively with the environment. Disorders of perception have been reasonably well established as concomitants of early academic problems." (Ayres, 1972 p. 1) "It is a provisional theory with continued modifications anticipated as research and clinical knowledge help it evolve." (Ayres, 1986 p. 9)

Success Rate (Best Case)

While case studies over the past fifty years have made distinct connections between sensory regulation and academic/cognitive growth, valid research studies still have yet to be published supporting the concrete success rate of sensory integration as a tool for educational progress. Albeit, teachers, parents, caregivers, and therapists universally agree that visual-spatial activities and specifically targeted movement-based exercises aid students in academic readiness, foundational understanding of concepts needed for educational improvement, and overall emotional, physical, and developmental well being.

Risks and Side effects (Worst Case)

Students must be closely supervised on sensory gym equipment and staff must be appropriately trained in securing swings, balance beams, and other obstacle course materials. It is important to have a good relationship with therapists in the gym who can aid in advising on students regulation profiles (vestibular vs. proprioceptive preferences). It is important to note if students have seizure disorders or require adaptive equipment such as helmets, knee pads, etc. Clear limits and routines must be established so students understand when it is time to "work" and "take a break." This of course depends on the students' ability to communicate and understand rules for behavior and safety

56

SEQUENTIAL HOMEOPATHY: THE HOUSTON HOMEOPATHY METHOD

BY CINDY GRIFFIN AND LINDYL LANHAM

Cindy L. Griffin, DSH-P, DIHom., BME, BCIM, DCNT, FBIH

Homeopathy Center of Houston
7670 Woodway Drive, Suite 340
Houston, TX 77063
(713) 366-8700
www.HomeopathyHouston.com
Info@HomeopathyHouston.com

Ms. Griffin is President/Co-Founder of Homeopathy Center of Houston, and Regent and Instructor of Homeopathic Clinical Studies for Houston School of Homeopathy in Houston, Texas. Trained in sequential and classical homeopathy, and biomedical approaches to autism, she is a regular conference speaker at Autism One, National Autism Conference, and has spoken at international conferences in Australia and Canada. She has authored a four-year curriculum on Sequential Homeopathy, as well as many magazine articles on autism, homeopathic self-care for flu, vaccine injury, women's health, and sits on the editorial board of the Journal of the American Association of Integrative Medicine. She is Board Certified in Integrative Medicine by the American Association of Integrative Medicine. Many children have recovered from autism under her oversight, including her own son, who recovered from Asperger's syndrome with the Houston Homeopathy Method. She and Lindyl Lanham have created the only sequential homeopathic method for autism based on the vaccine injury/biomedical/gut-brain model of autism.

Affiliations and Certifications:
- Board Certified in Integrative Medicine, AAIM
- Diplomate of College of Natural Therapies, AAIM
- Editorial Board Member, JAAIM
- Board Member, Texas Health Freedom Coalition Steering Committee
- Member Texas Complementary and Alternative Medicine Association
- Fellow of the British Institute of Homeopathy

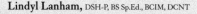

Lindyl Lanham, DSH-P, BS Sp.Ed., BCIM, DCNT

Homeopathy Center of Houston
7670 Woodway Drive, Suite 340
Houston, TX 77063
(713) 366-8700
www.HomeopathyHouston.com
Info@HomeopathyHouston.com

Ms. Lanham is Vice President/Co-Founder of Homeopathy Center of Houston, and primary creator of the Houston Homeopathy Method of Sequential Homeopathy for Autism and ASDs. Their method is the original and only sequential homeopathic method worldwide to be designed around the vaccine injury/biomedical/gut-brain model of autism. She has coauthored a number of articles that have appeared in several autism magazines including *The Autism File*, and *The Autism Perspective* and has been interviewed numerous times for VoiceAmerica and Autism One Radio, among others. She is a regular speaker at Autism One, has spoken at the National Autism Conference, as well as the MINDD conference in Australia and the NuPath conference on homeopathy and autism in Canada. Lindyl worked with autistic children as early as 1972, and continues to focus on autism as her primary specialty. She has seen many children with autism fully recover using the Houston Homeopathy Method under her direction and direct consultation. She is board certified in Integrative Medicine, and is the mother of a son recovered from Tourette's syndrome with the Houston Homeopathy Method and natural medicine.

Affiliations and Certifications:
* Bachelor of Science in Special Education
* Board Certified in Integrative Medicine, AAIM
* Diplomate of College of Natural Therapies, AAIM

S tanding on the shoulders of giants, the Houston Homeopathy Method incorporates the best applications of homeopathic remedies into a cohesive, comprehensive and effective complex method gaining improvements and even full recoveries in children with autism. Sequential homeopathy provides the infrastructure of the approach, clearing the damage of physical, chemical, medical and emotional traumas. Working in reverse chronological order, these traumas are addressed by the use of well-researched, and often bio-medically confirmed, homeopathic remedies appropriate to each event.

References to the Law of Similars can be found in ancient Egyptian papyrus and Greek medical documents, but Samuel Hahnemann, M. D. (1775–1843), is the genius behind modern day homeopathy. His multiple editions of *The Organon* still today provide the guidelines for classical, constitutional or sequential home-opathy.

For over two centuries, homeopathic medical treatment has brought about recovery from acute and chronic health issues for millions of people worldwide in a rapid, gentle and permanent way. Until the 1920s homeopathy accounted for approximately 25 percent of all medicine practiced in the United States. Its renowned use has been long acknowledged throughout the world as a major medical therapeutic approach. In many European communities homeopathy is recognized alongside conventional medicine as an alternative mainstream medical approach.

Homeopathy is founded upon the Law of Similars, *Similia similibus curentur*, or "like cures like" (Gk. *hómoios* = similar to and *páthos* = suffering.) Dr. Hahnemann observed from his experiments with cinchona bark, used as a treatment for malaria, that the effects he experienced from ingesting the bark were similar to the symptoms of malaria. He therefore reasoned that, as a fundamental healing principle, homeopathic remedies must be able to produce symptoms in healthy individuals similar to those of the disease. Upon further experimentation, he realized that by inducing a similar "artificial disease" through the use of a tiny and diluted amount of a substance (a homeopathic remedy) that recovery would follow. For example, peeling an onion causes the eyes to burn, sting, itch and water. These same symptoms are relieved by the use of homeopathic *Allium cepa* (red onion) during a cold or allergy attack.

Over time, Hahnemann discovered that smaller amounts achieved greater therapeutic benefit, and that diluted amounts of substances actually were the most therapeutic while doing no harm. Most homeopathic remedies today, made from minerals as well as botanical and biological sources, are considered "micro-doses" or "nano-doses" of the source substance and are made in pharmaceutical laboratories under current international standards called current Good Manufacturing Practices (cGMP.)

Most homeopaths believe:

- Healing = wholeness.
- True healing is self-healing—living creatures naturally seek balance and health
- Homeopathy's role is to augment the rebalancing and healing process

However, while there are as many ways of practicing as there are homeopaths, two diverse philosophies in the homeopathic world stand out: classical and sequential.

Classical homeopathy focuses primarily on the "Totality of Symptoms" and finding the single remedy that most completely covers all of the client's symptom-pictures. The classically trained homeopath goes into great depth exploring the mental as well as the physical symptoms and searching extensively for the one remedy that appears to envelop not only the greatest number of symptoms but also the greatest number of characteristics composing the client's constitution. The chosen remedy should address the predominate symptoms as well as predominant characteristics and should be prescribed according to minimal dosing laws.

While being first classically trained, the sequential homeopath not only looks at the client symptom-picture, but also at a detailed history of traumatic events. Strongly influenced by the work of Constantine Hering M. D. (1800–1880), the "father of American homeopathy," and author of "Hering's Laws of Direction of Cure," sequential homeopaths focus primarily on the etiology by close examination of the client's history believing that illness occurs when the immune system is compromised or stressed by traumatic events and is no longer functioning optimally. The immune system is charged with resisting and responding to invaders and impacts from physical, chemical and emotional traumas. However, eventually these traumas can weaken the resistance and bring about physiological changes in the body's regulation resulting in illness. Sequential homeopathy uses homeopathic remedies to allow the body to "return to the scene of the crime" and address the damage left behind, harness the resources of the immune system to resist and destroy the offenders in a reverse chronological sequence, allowing the restoration of equilibrium and true health. Employing the natural balancing mechanisms of elimination, respiration, and inflammation (heat which will kill bacteria or viruses) the body will return to homeostasis (balance). Once balance is restored, the body can then reestablish wholeness (self-healing).

With its basis in the sequential therapy work of Jean Elmiger, MD, broadened by an updated view of the use of isopathy (the use of a homeopathic remedy made from an actual pathogen or chemical toxin in order to aid the natural detoxification or clearing of that pathogen or toxin,) the Homeopathy Center of Houston immediately recognized sequential homeopathy as the perfect causation-based starting point for autism. The sequence of homeopathic "clearings" peels away each individual layer comprising the client's personal history of drug, chemical, physical, vaccine, or emotional insults and exposures, all arranged event by event in reverse chronological order according to the client's history, or timeline. Each individual trauma is "cleared" encompassing all the effects of its impact—this means, for instance, that clearing any single event includes the use of multiple remedies derived from carefully chosen homeopathic remedies, as well as iso-pathic remedies made from pathogens and toxic chemicals included in the insult, to facilitate the immune system as it rebalances or clears itself in order to heal.

Sequential homeopathy is uniquely able to spur the release of cell memories, toxins, viruses, and bacteria trapped in cells, allowing a reduction of the burdens and demands on the immune system over time. Autism is largely viewed as a collision between genetic predisposition and environmental and vaccine insults. Sequential homeopathy can reduce the body burden, while supporting the natural healing processes to undo the damage left behind through this clearing process, in a natural systematic manner.

As a holistic approach, sequential homeopaths consider the emotional state as well as the physical state. In autism, when a child has limited or no speech, rem-edies that address processing and release trapped emotions can become a major contributor to recovery. If a child processes pent up feelings through dreams or artwork or behavior, the result will always lead to further improvement. Phys-ical healing frequently follows emotional release and healing. Whether recent or farther back historically, as they apply to the event being addressed, emotional healing plays a key role in the child's current level of comfort as well as long-term recovery. Of all ASD therapies, only sequential homeopathy can offer emotional support without the use of drugs.

At the heart of the Houston Homeopathy Method's infrastructure lie vac-cine injury and its reversal. While controversial among the medical discussion of autism, parents of children with autism very frequently report that their child regressed significantly after the administration of one or more vaccines. During the process of clearing each individual child's vaccine record, it is not unusual to see a child briefly regress significantly when their regressive vaccine is cleared, followed by a fairly immediate and often dramatic improvement overall. This would tend to support the parent's assertions that the particular vaccine truly con-tributed largely if not wholly to the child's autism. This phenomenon has been observed repeatedly in hundreds of children who have worked with the Houston Center.

The Homeopathy Center of Houston homeopaths have necessarily gone beyond Hahnemann, Hering and Elmiger in their work with autistic children. Homeopathic analysis of a case typically relies upon a reporting by the client of the most subtle intricacies of their complaints. Because autistic children have limited or no verbal abilities, the Houston homeopaths turned to biomedical research in autism in order to determine what stereotypical behaviors may indicate. Children with autism do not have the benefit of a normally functioning gastrointestinal tract, and because over 70 percent of the immune system resides in the gut, the immune system is also dysfunctional. This means that more supportive remedies must be employed with these children on a daily basis.

Searching for homeopathic solutions to 21st century problems, the approach embraced oligotherapy, gemmotherapy, homotoxicology, cellular reprogramming therapy and German biological medicine. Many of these forms of homeopathic remedies are fast-acting in the area of pain reduction, but with a long-term effect of supporting and improving the efficiency of the entire detoxification and healing process. Most of these children have a history of gut pain, whether expressed or not. Head banging, sudden tantrums, strange posturing and picky eating are all indications of gut discomfort. Proprietary, autism-specific homeopathic combinations developed at the Homeopathy Center of Houston have reduced and relieved gut pain quickly and permanently in many of the children while working through their timelines to the causational issues. After many years of research and study in the biomedical world of autism, a successful case-taking method has been developed to interpret the presenting symptoms as observed by the parents and reported during the monthly consultations. The uniqueness of the Houston Method is its focus on the vaccine injury, biomedical, gut-brain model of autism, and its application of multiple homeopathic approaches to reverse the problems of autism. The method is systematically designed for that model, yet highly individualized by the practitioners to address each child's needs. This has created a program with a more consistent positive response from autistic children than with classical or sequential homeopathy alone and is accomplished without the use of pharmaceuticals, chelation agents, or large amounts of supplements.

Within the first year, with optimum compliance, approximately 75 percent of the parents report significant improvements in their autism and a small number even report recovery. Most of the recovered children required two to three years of work with the center. Some very difficult and intractable cases have shown encouraging and ongoing improvements.

While many therapies involve an inherent risk of permanent regressions, homeopathy in any form cannot bring on a new pathology. It can only bring to the surface healing processes or detoxification of offending agents and the underlying symptoms those agents caused. The most concerning issues faced at the center involve short-term regressions during the detoxification and clearing period. These are usually symptoms brought on during the mobilization and elimination of toxins, or are temporary healing responses—the body's natural means of rebalancing itself. Typically short-lived, and followed by improvements soon after, some of these regressions may happen intermittently for several months, or even last for a week or more. These can include rashes, fevers, or behavioral regressions. However, these resolve, or wax and wane through the process. A worst-case scenario involves one client who repeatedly broke out in a measles-like rash which at one point covered his body for almost ten days. He also developed an intermittent lack of appetite and other regressive behaviors. While the rash was unpleasant to see, after each event, the rash disappeared, the regressions abated, his speech and focus improved and his diet expanded.

Just one of the many recovered cases involves a seven-year-old boy whose parents had tried many biomedical therapies prior to coming to Homeopathy Center of Houston, some of which caused significant worsening, and others caused significant emotional trauma, such as being strapped to a papoose board during lengthy testing procedures or IV chelation. Once he began the Houston Method, each month he experienced a brief, mild worsening of one or two behaviors for a few days at the "peak of the clear," or an occasional mild rash. Each of these mild regressions or physical symptoms was then followed within a few days by marked improvements in speech, eye contact, interaction, or cognitive and academic function. At almost exactly one year after starting the program, he was functioning with no help in school, had caught up to grade level academically, fully recovered his speech and was indistinguishable from any other normal eight-year-old boy in his class—except for his amazing intellectual curiosity!

Development of the general Houston Homeopathy Method was begun by Cindy Griffin, DSH-P, DIHom., BCIM, DCNT through her general practice, where she expanded on Elmiger's original sequential therapy. Her current area of special interest is the effects of glutamate and strep on OCD and aggression. The Houston Homeopathy Method for Autism and ASDs was introduced and has been constantly updated and greatly expanded from Cindy's earlier work by Lindyl Lanham, DSH-P, BS Sp.Ed., BCIM, DCNT when the practice began to see autistic children in 2002. Lindyl's background included work with blind, deaf and autistic children as early as the 1970s at the Texas School for the Blind's Deaf-Blind Annex, followed by ten years as a special education teacher. Later she homeschooled her two sons, the younger being diagnosed with Tourette's syndrome at the age of eight. He has since 90 percent recovered from the tic disorder through homeopathy, has received his baccalaureate degree and is currently in graduate school. The practice was later joined by Julianne Adams, DSH-P, BCIM,

BA Psych, who brought to the method a tireless desire to research strep, nutritional and homeopathic products, and to improve on the method from a holistic viewpoint. Jenice Stebel, DSH-P, DIHom, BCIM has contributed research on the treatment of parasites and strep, as well as being well versed in several special diets for autism. Lynn Rose Demartini, RN, DSH-P, LMT, BCIM, DCN has brought a great deal of medical insight from her years in practice in public health, emergency medicine, massage therapy and as a life-long student of several other holistic therapies. While all homeopaths follow the same basic approach, The Houston Homeopathy Method of sequential homeopathy continues to grow and improve through regular case conferences, and a devotion by all its practitioners to continuing education and research. All practitioners are Board Certified in Integrative Medicine by the American Association of Integrative Medicine (AAIM). Cindy Griffin and Lindyl Lanham are Diplomates of the AAIM College of Natural Therapies, and Lynn Demartini is a Diplomate of the AAIM College of Nursing.

57

THE SMILE CENTER: THE SENSORY MOTOR INTEGRATION AND LANGUAGE ENRICHMENT CENTER

BY MARKUS JARROW

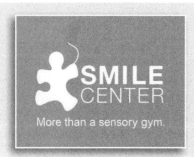

Markus Jarrow, OTR/L, C/NDT

Clinical Director
The SMILE Center
171 Madison Avenue, 5th Floor
New York, NY 10016
(212) 400-0383
markus@smileny.org
www.smileny.org

Huck Ho, OTR/L, C/NDT

Program Director
huckho@smileny.org

The SMILE Center is a brand-new, state-of-the-art, 8,200-square-foot pediatric treatment facility in New York City. It was created in order to provide families with an alternative to a traditional sensory gym. The SMILE Center strives to provide the highest quality of pediatric treatment with a strong emphasis on Sensory Integration, Neuro-Developmental Treatment, and DIR/Floortime. They utilize a unique, intensive, and hands-on treatment approach that addresses the whole child by treating the sensory and postural needs, as well as supporting social-emotional and communication development. They see each child for their unique set of strengths and challenges, and provide them with the opportunities to achieve their potential as individuals and as members of a family and a community.

History

The SMILE Center | The Sensory Motor Integration + Language Enrichment Center was founded by two pediatric occupational therapists, Huck Ho, OTR/L, C/NDT, and Markus Jarrow, OTR/L, C/NDT. Prior to the opening of The SMILE Center, Huck served as Program Director at a large center-based

Early Intervention (zero to three years of age) program in Brooklyn, New York primarily serving children with autism spectrum disorders. Formerly an ABA program, under Huck's leadership the center became the first Early Intervention Program in New York City to implement the DIR/Floortime methodology. Markus previously held a position as clinical coordinator of a large preschool program where he supervised thirty clinicians and oversaw the treatment of more than 125 children with ASD. In 2009, Huck and Markus combined their twenty-five years of experience in pediatric treatment, supervision and administration, and opened The SMILE Center.

The SMILE Center was created in order to provide families with an alternative to a traditional sensory gym. They utilize a unique, intensive, and hands-on treatment approach that addresses the whole child. With strong roots in Early Intervention, The SMILE Center also specializes in the early treatment of babies and young children. They offer children and their families several supplemental treatment options, and have also established a substantial center-based continuing education program that hosts leading clinicians and instructors for monthly conferences. This provides a variety of opportunities for the staff and children/families alike.

Their eclectic approach was developed in response to observing changes in the population of children they had been evaluating and treating for more than a decade. They began to take careful notice of the muscle tone abnormalities and postural control impairments in many of the children diagnosed with sensory impairments and ASD. They noted increasing similarities in alignment and movement patterns to some children diagnosed with neuromuscular or movement disorders. At the same time, they became increasingly aware of sensory-related issues in children being treating for movement and muscle tone abnormalities, particularly in babies and young children. Since both sensory processing and postural control are essential in supporting function, communication and learning, they felt both areas needed equal attention.

While core strength and postural control were considered through traditional Sensory Integration, the approach did not specifically address concerns regarding a child's kinesiology, alignment, and quality of movement. Many children with ASD and sensory integration dysfunction present with low muscle tone and a tendency to rely on end ranges of their joints for stability. This can be illustrated by a child who toe-walks with his back arched, chest out, and his shoulders back. Another example of this is a child that "W"-sits with a rounded back, shoulders forward, and head and neck tilted up. These postures can prevent components of typical movement from occurring that interfere with a child's ability to interact with their world. Both postures prevent side-to-side weight shifting and, in turn, rotation of the trunk. Without rotation, a child's ability to integrate visual, auditory, movement, and spatial information may be significantly impacted.

The primary treatment approaches utilized by pediatric therapists for sensory integration dysfunction and neuromotor impairments typically focus on one or the other. With extensive training in sensory integration and certification in pediatric neuro-developmental treatment (NDT—a hands-on approach to addressing the postural control and movement patterns of children with neuromotor disorders such as cerebral palsy), Huck and Markus began combining these treatment approaches. Collectively, the two approaches provided a framework that addressed both the sensory and motor issues in the wide variety of children they were working with. Having migrated from the ABA methodology, their approach adopted DIR/Floortime principles with an increased focus on increasing meaningful interactions and social-emotional development through child-directed activity.

Mission

The SMILE Center strives to provide the highest quality of pediatric occupational, physical, and speech therapy services with a strong emphasis on sensory integration, neuro-developmental treatment, and DIR/Floortime. With solid foundations in these treatment models, the therapists treat the whole child, by addressing the systemic sensory and postural needs, as well as supporting social-emotional, communicative, and affective development. The goal is to facilitate optimal functional outcomes and autonomy in all of the children that they serve. They see each child for their unique set of strengths and challenges, while providing them the opportunity to develop the skills necessary to achieve their potential as individuals and members of a family and a community. The staff of the SMILE Center takes great pride in their dedication to ongoing training and education in order to maintain solid fundamental pediatric treatment skills and expertise in the latest techniques and specialty therapies.

The interdisciplinary approach utilizes a fundamental framework of treatment that bridges occupational therapy, physical therapy, and speech-language pathology. Each of their therapists receives the training to address both the sensory and motor components of the child in order to more rapidly achieve the functional goals specific to their discipline.

The SMILE Center strongly believes in family training for optimal carryover into the child's natural environment. They provide home programming and home modification consultations in order to create sensory-friendly and enriching learning environments. The SMILE Center's unique sibling groups help brothers and sisters develop more playful, engaging, and rewarding relationships with their siblings on the spectrum through DIR/Floortime supported sessions. This helps to empower the brothers and sisters, as they become active members in the treatment at home, and get trained to assist in carrying out sensory diet activities when possible. Social groups facilitate improved social-emotional, communication, and play skills in order to support more sustained and richer peer interactions with appropriately grouped children.

The SMILE Center provides alternative treatment formats and services to supplement the treatment some families are already receiving. They offer various treatment intensives during the breaks when children are typically out of school. These intensives generally provide four to five hours of daily intensive therapy and DIR/Floortime social groups. They are offered in different formats to meet the needs of different children. The SMILE Center also provides consultations for Therapeutic Listening and Astronaut Training to supplement the treatment that children may be receiving elsewhere.

They work closely with nationally renowned clinicians of all disciplines, with specific expertise in the areas of Sensory Integration, Neuro-Development Treatment, and DIR/Floortime. The SMILE Center hosts leading clinicians for monthly conferences, as well as specific trainings, intensive treatment programs, and ongoing consultations. This further supports their mission to provide the highest quality of care, as their staff continually receives training and mentorship from leading instructors of each discipline.

These educational programs also provide unique opportunities for the families and children of The SMILE Center to participate in conferences and enroll in treatment intensives and consultations with experts in the field. The SMILE Center's one-of-a-kind continuing education program helps to improve the quality of care being provided to children with special needs throughout the community, and also strengthens the networking and relationships amongst therapists in the New York City / Tri-State area.

It is the ultimate goal of The SMILE Center to reach outside of their walls, and provide comprehensive programming and support for children with special needs, their family members, and other community professionals dedicated to child development.

Philosophy

The SMILE Center believes that it takes more than practice to make perfect. Therapists treat the underlying issues of each child as opposed to practicing isolated skills. The dynamic, hands-on approach improves a child's fundamental strengths and therefore enables functional skills to emerge more spontaneously in treatment and in daily life situations. This promotes a more typical developmental sequence as well as mastery and generalization of skills. With supportive training, family members can then provide additional opportunities to further this progress across a variety of natural settings.

Services

- Evaluations and Screenings
- Occupational Therapy
- Physical Therapy
- Speech & Language Therapy
- DIR/Floortime
- Social Groups
- Sibling Groups
- SOS Feeding Groups
- Treatment Intensives
- Therapeutic Listening Consultations
- Astronaut Training Consultations
- Resource Center for Therapeutic Listening Materials
- Manhattan Resource Center for Proloquo2go
- Home Modifications

Specialties

- Sensory Integration
- Neuro-Developmental Treatment
- DIR/Floortime
- Early Intervention
- Therapeutic Listening
- Astronaut Training
- Interactive Metronome
- PROMPT
- Feeding and Swallowing Therapy
- Oral Motor Therapy
- Stabilizing Pressure Input Orthosis (SPIO) Suits
- Augmentative and Alternative Communication

58

SON-RISE PROGRAM

by Raun Kaufman

Raun K. Kaufman

Autism Treatment Center of America
2080 South Undermountain Road
Sheffield, MA 01257 USA
(800) 714-2779
International: 001-413-229-2100
correspondence@autismtreatment.org
www.autismtreatment.org

Raun K. Kaufman is the Director of Global Education and former CEO of the Autism Treatment Center of America. In his work as an international speaker, writer and teacher to families, children, and professionals around the world, Mr. Kaufman brings a distinctive qualification to the realm of Autism treatment—his own personal history. As a young boy, Raun was diagnosed as severely and incurably autistic. His parents developed a unique methodology now known as The Son-Rise Program, which enabled Raun to recover completely from his autism. He holds a degree in Biomedical Ethics from the Ivy League's Brown University and continues to lecture at conferences and symposia worldwide.

Dear parent,
You love your child more than anything in the world. In the early days of your child's life, long before any diagnosis was made, there may have been a hundred different hopes, dreams, and plans you had for your child. And yet, if you are like most parents, you may have been told to discard many of those hopes and dreams and be "realistic" in the face of your child's diagnosis. It can feel extraordinarily challenging when you are told all of the things your child will never accomplish—as if it's been decided ahead of time.

In The Son-Rise Program, the most important place to begin is to know that you don't have to accept the limits that may have been placed upon your child. Your child has the capacity for learning, communicating, experiencing real joy and happiness and developing warm, loving and satisfying relationships.

343

Children on the autism spectrum are capable of great change and even, in some cases, complete recovery.

Who am I to tell you this? My name is Raun K. Kaufman, and, as a young boy, I was diagnosed as severely autistic, with no language and a tested I.Q. of less than 30. Completely mute and withdrawn from human contact, I would spend my days endlessly engaged in repetitive "stimming" behaviors such as spinning plates, rocking back and forth, and flapping my hands in front of my face.

Like many parents today, my parents were told that I would never speak or communicate in any meaningful way and that my autism was a "lifelong condition." The professionals recommended eventual institutionalization.

In an effort to reach me, my parents, authors/teachers Barry Neil Kaufman and Samahria Lyte Kaufman, developed an innovative child-centered program they called The Son-Rise Program. After they worked with me for over three years, I recovered completely from my autism without any trace of my former condition. (After my recovery, my father wrote a best-selling book recounting our story entitled *Son-Rise: The Miracle Continues*—later the subject of an award-winning NBC television movie.) I went on to graduate from the Ivy League's Brown University with a degree in Biomedical Ethics.

Now, I am the former CEO of the Autism Treatment Center of America, and I remain a senior teacher there, as well as lecturing worldwide. As a part of the ATCA, a division of the non-profit organization that my parents founded and at which they still teach, I am so grateful to have the opportunity, with our dedicated staff of almost eighty, to enable parents to help their children in the same way that my parents helped me.

Moreover, I am no fluke. For over a quarter of a century, parents from across the globe have been attending our weeklong training programs, putting in their time, energy, and love, and achieving results with their children that often far outstrip prognoses.

The foundation of The Son-Rise Program rests upon this idea: The children show us the way in, and then we show them the way out. This means that, rather than forcing these children to conform to a world they do not understand, we begin by joining them in their world first. In this way, we establish a mutual connection and relationship, which is the platform for all education and growth. Since autism is fundamentally a social relational disorder, creating interpersonal relationships and social interaction remains our primary focus.

This is the basis of The Son-Rise Program, taught exclusively by the Autism Treatment Center of America. (The Son-Rise Program Start-Up, a 5-day introductory training course for parents and professionals, is offered several times a year on our campus and once a year in London, England.)

The crucial starting point for The Son-Rise Program and one of the first principles taught to parents in the Start-Up course is called *joining*. Instead of stopping a child's repetitive "stimming" behaviors, we join in with these behaviors. The idea is that these children are performing their behaviors for reasons that are important to them (and, as an increasing body of research shows, these behaviors often serve a physiological purpose, as well). When we show interest in what these children are doing, we establish a powerful bond around this common interest. This is so important, because, in response, these children begin to display a genuine interest in us.

Once we have a child's willing engagement, the door is open to help that child to learn and grow. One of our key teaching principles is to *capitalize on each child's own motivation*. With children on the autism spectrum, traditional learning modalities will rarely be motivating. Therefore, we customize the presentation of any curriculum to match each child's highest areas of interest.

Instead of pushing a child to repeat a task (and receive rewards) over and over again as a way to facilitate mastery, we build games and activities around the interests the child already has (such as Thomas the Tank engine, dinosaurs, or physical play). This way, we work *with* each child instead of trying to teach "against the grain." Thus, learning is exponentially increased, with a unique and startling benefit: We have the child's willing and excited cooperation. And when a child has learned something—not memorized it, but learned it—it becomes a generalized skill that he/she can use spontaneously (rather than in a more robotic manner).

In another departure from traditional methods, we use The Son-Rise Program Social Developmental Model to enable parents and professionals to teach *social goals* (communication, eye contact, interactive attention spans, and flexibility) before academic goals. Academic goals, while important, will do nothing to help our children overcome their central challenge of connecting with others socially. As first priority, do we want our children do have more math or more friends? Do we want our children to compensate for their socialization challenges or overcome them?

The single most overlooked area when it comes to autism treatment is *attitude*. Having a non-judgmental, welcoming, and optimistic attitude toward our child determines whether he/she feels safe and relaxed enough to interact with us and learn. We see time and again that children with autism tend to move away from people they perceive as uncomfortable or judging and towards people they see as comfortable, easy, fun and nonjudgmental. Thus, our attitude can provide the impetus for a challenged child to reach out to us, or it can unwittingly act to drive that child away. We spend time in our Start-Up and other programs helping parents with their emotional and attitudinal challenges because it really matters.

So no matter what you are told, please know that there is hope for your child. You are the parent. You have a love, a lifelong commitment, and a day-in, day-out experience with your child that no one else can match. You may sometimes feel pushed aside, but never forget that you aren't *in* the way, you *are* the way.

You have every right to believe in your child. You have every capability to see the possibilities for your child, even when no one else does. And while we cannot know or promise in advance what a given child will accomplish, we will never decide in advance what your child will *not* achieve.

The only reason I can write this letter to you today is because my parents believed in me when no one else on earth did. And that is a special role that you, as a parent, can have with your child. And no one can ever take that from you.

You're not about to give up on your child. Neither are we.

With the deepest respect,
Raun K. Kaufman

59

SOUND-BASED THERAPIES: THE DAVIS MODEL OF SOUND INTERVENTION

BY DORINNE DAVIS

Dorinne S. Davis, MA, CCC-A, FAAA, RCTC, BARA

The Davis Center 19 State Route 10 East, Suite 25
Succasunna, NJ 07876.
(862) 251-4637
info@thedaviscenter.com
www.thedaviscenter.com
www.dorinnedavis.com

Ms. Davis is President/Founder of The Davis Center, the world's premier sound therapy center in Succasunna, NJ. She is the author of four books, including the primer on sound-based therapy, *Sound Bodies through Sound Therapy* and *Every Day A Miracle: Success Stories through Sound Therapy.* She established The Davis Addendum to the Tomatis Effect and designed The Tree of Sound Enhancement Therapy and The Diagnostic Evaluation for Therapy Protocol. She has a radio show on AutismOne.org radio once a month. She is recognized as THE expert on sound-based therapies.

S ound-based therapies use the vibrational energy of sound to make change with learning, development, and wellness challenges with special equipment, specific programs, modified music, and/or specific tones/beats, the need for which is identified with testing. Many sound-based therapies have been demonstrated as helpful to autistic individuals.

While there are many different sound-based therapies which have made change, identifying which methods can be most appropriately used is the foundation of *The Davis Model of Sound Intervention*. This model utilizes the analogy of a tree, *The Tree of Sound Enhancement Therapy,* for discussing how the many therapies make change for each person. *Root System* Therapies address one's sense of hearing. *Seed* Therapies address one's body rhythms. *Trunk* Therapies address the ability to process all basic sound stimulation. *Leaves and Branches* Therapies address auditory processing issues. The *Head* surrounding the Tree portion addresses general wellness. All of the therapies use the vibrational energy of sound to make change for the specified processes.

The pieces of the Tree come together by understanding three key points: 1) There is a connection between the voice, the ear, and the brain supported by five laws known as The Tomatis Effect and The Davis Addendum to The Tomatis Effect; 2) Every cell in your body resonates sound; and 3) Your ear helps stimulate all of your senses by sound vibration, not just hearing.

The *Diagnostic Evaluation for Therapy Protocol (DETP)* evaluates each person's responses for the various levels of the Tree analogy and determines if, when, how long, and in what order any or all of the many different sound-based therapies should be appropriately applied. This battery of tests is key for determining how to best use any sound-based therapy. Assuming that each person starts with *The Root System* therapy is incorrect. Not everyone needs every therapy. The test battery takes the guesswork out of determining if a sound-based therapy is appropriate and provides the order for the correct administration of a sequence of therapies. Currently the assessment can only be obtained at www.thedaviscenter.com.

By using *The Tree of Sound Enhancement Therapy*, some of the various therapies are as follows:

1. The *Root System* therapies are called "Auditory Integration Training," The originator of this type of therapy is Dr. Guy Berard, a French physician, who wanted to establish a program that would create a kind of physical therapy for the ear, which has been demonstrated with this author's research on the acoustic reflex muscle of the middle ear. His method is now known as Berard Auditory Integration Training. The equipment used in his method is either an Audiokinetron or an Earducator. His method can only be applied in a practitioner's office. There are other applications within the generalized term "Auditory Integration Training" that can be used at home. The equipment applicable for home programs are FST, DAA, and BGC and all do a similar yet different type of physical retraining of the acoustic reflex muscle. Each of these programs is modeled after Dr. Berard's work. All "Auditory Integration Training" programs address the person's "sense of hearing." The programs last for ten days and the person listens for ½ hour in the morning and afternoon to specially chosen music played through the appropriate device. While listening, little or no sensory stimulation should occur because it is possible to negate the positive effects of retraining the acoustic reflex muscle.

Symptoms helped: one type of hearing hypersensitivity, lack of sound awareness, inability to discriminate sound differences, sense of self, body movement/rhythm, eye contact, awareness of the world around them, motor skills and more.

Testimonials from parents of autistic children:

    a.   My child no longer covers his ears in uncomfortable listening situations.

    b.   My child no longer reacts to fluorescent lighting.

    c.   My child responds immediately when his name is called.

www.berardaitwebsite.com and www.AITinstitute.org

2.   The *Seed* therapies all make a change with body rhythmical patterns. Our body has many rhythms and patterns such as our heart rate and breath stream. Currently two therapies exist at this level: REI and Cymatherapy.

    a.   REI was developed by Jeff Strong and uses rhythmical drum patterns to stimulate and repair the nervous system. A pair of custom made CDs are created and used for a ten-week period.

        Symptoms helped: inability to "fit in" with the rhythms of those around them, significant sensory processing issues, self-stimulatory behaviors, attention span, sleep, aggression, and more.

        Testimonials from parents of autistic children:

        1. My child fell asleep faster and more calmly.

        2. My child became less aggressive.

        3. My child became less impulsive.

    www.reiinstitute.com

    b.   Cymatherapy represents the work of Dr. Guy Peter Manners, who explored sound as a healing modality. This approach uses sound frequency stimulation on different parts of the body working to balance the body's energy patterns. The current device is called the Cyma1000.

        Symptoms helped: issues with attention, behavior, social connections, cognition, and much more.

        Testimonials from parents of autistic children:

        1. My child waited and listened for instructions.

        2. My child waited his turn better.

        3. My child wanted to be around his family more.

    www.cymatechnologies.com

3.   The *Trunk* therapies are called "Listening Training Programs" and are mod-
     eled after the work of Dr. Alfred Tomatis, the founder of all sound-based
     therapies. The therapies at this level are "core" therapies because they incor-
     porate one of the main points behind The Davis Model of Sound Interven-
     tion—the connection between the voice, the ear and the brain. Dr. Tomatis
     was the first to discover that the voice produces what the ear hears and when
     the distorted frequencies are reintroduced to the ear, the voice regains coher-
     ence or stability. This became known as The Tomatis Effect and he incor-
     porated this process into The Tomatis Method. He differentiated between
     hearing and listening. Hearing is the passive reception of sound and we hear
     without thinking about it. But listening involves mentally thinking about
     what is heard. We must tune into what is heard. By doing so, we cortically
     "recharge" the brain. When recharging the brain, the body's full response to
     sound must be stimulated. Every cell of the body must be stimulated. Every
     sense will be stimulated. Every way that the body responds to sound must
     be stimulated. Listening Training Programs must include air conduction
     vibration of sound, bone conduction vibration of sound, filtered and gated
     music, specific sound delays, and actively incorporating one's speaking and/
     or singing voice in the programming.

     The programs are brain intensive, meaning that the program lasts for
     many days in order to make sufficient change at the cortical level. Practi-
     tioners should incorporate activities that address the person's whole body
     response to sound, not just one type of skill such as academics or sensory
     integration as the full ability to balance the person's skills will not be met.
     Basic programs last for sixty hours, often applied with a break after thirty
     hours. Listening occurs for two hours per day for fifteen days, then a three-
     to six-week break, followed by another fifteen days of two hours per day.
     Some centers administer the second set in eight and seven days with another
     break in between. For people with autism, this basic program is typically
     not enough stimulation to establish sufficient skills for communication, so
     additional sessions are encouraged depending upon each person's needs.
     Follow up sessions should be determined by a proprietary Listening Test
     which shows the levels of progress. Each person's voice should begin to show
     a change in its tonal quality as progress occurs.

     a.   The Tomatis Method was established by Dr. Alfred Tomatis. He felt that
          a good listener was a good learner and by training a person to listen well
          provided them to opportunity to reach their full potential. He identified

the benefit of a dominant right ear, supporting the most direct pathway to the language center in the brain. His method supports learning how to filter out irrelevant information and supports capturing the energizing frequencies of the speech sound spectrum. He uses all of the connections between the voice, the ear and the brain by stimulating the weaker body processes in order to advance overall skill levels resulting in improved listening and enhancement of body sensory needs and communication needs. When using this method at *The Trunk* level make sure it is a full individualized program and not a generic newer program.

Symptoms helped: some hypersensitivities to sound, hyposensitivity to sound, sensory processing issues, oral motor issues, social/emotional connectedness, expressive/receptive language skills, sense of self, inappropriate behaviors, fluency of speech, vestibular imbalances, movement and rhythm, fine/gross motor skills, posture, and more.

Testimonials from parents of autistic children:

1. Within two years following The Tomatis Method, my child was declassified.
2. My child began eating different foods and trying different textures of food.
3. My child's high pitched voice disappeared.
4. My child's reading skills jumped three years growth in six months time.
5. My child began using full sentences to express his thoughts.
6. My child's anxiety to large groups practically disappeared.

www.tomatis.com and www.tomatis-group.com

b. EnListen was developed by Drs. Billie and Kirk Thompson and modeled from the concepts established by Dr. Tomatis. Their proprietary software program provides stimulation with air conduction, bone conduction, sound delays and filters, and active voice work for developing targeted learning skills. This process stimulates growth of new and underutilized neural pathways.

Symptoms helped: weak receptive/expressive language skills, weak motor skills, poor communication skills, sense of self, poor social skills, disorganization, poor reading skills, singing abilities, phonics skills, and more.

Testimonials from parents of autistic children:

1. My child began trying to connect socially with other children around him.
2. My child began combining three or four words in utterances.
3. My child no longer craved spinning.
4. My child began tasting new and different foods.
5. I was able to leave my child playing independently for up to ½ hour at a time.
6. My child's stammer disappeared.

www.enlisten.com

3. Some sound-based therapies are modeled after the work of Dr. Tomatis but do not include ALL of the requirements for a Listening Training Program at The *Trunk* level of *The Tree*. However, they can be inserted at the Upper Trunk/Lower Leaves and Branches of The Tree analogy because they offer more higher functioning changes. Some of these programs are:

a. The Listening Program was developed by Advanced Brain Technologies as a music-based sound stimulation program designed to enhance listening skills and remediate auditory perceptual skills. The basic program included eight CDs that incorporated music and nature sounds to create a balance of exercises for the middle ear muscles. A filtration system and a gating technique is also utilized supporting a full spectrum of sound frequencies. These CDs are listened to for a half hour per day, five days per week for eight weeks typically. Extended sessions are sometimes needed and the program has different levels now. A bone conduction segment has been added with practitioner supervision. The concept is for the brain to receive, process, store and retrieve the information from a person's surrounding sound environment.

Symptoms helped: learning challenges, attention/focus weaknesses, reading challenges, sense of self, communication weaknesses, sensory processing issues, self-regulation, and more.

Testimonials from parents of autistic children:

1. My child began to have an interest in socially interacting with his peers.
2. My child began drawing clearly and writing legibly.
3. My child began to verbally label his drawings.

www.advancedbrain.com

b. The Samonas Method was developed by Ingo Steinbach. Samonas stands for "spectrally activated music of optimum natural structure." By using his Sonas System, he was able to create a system for recording music where the therapeutic value of the music and the effectiveness of the musical recording could be maintained. This new system could only be produced on compact discs. He created CDs that emphasized high frequency listening, presented the sensation of being in the location of the music, created a calming effect on the body, while monitoring the overtone effects of most musical selections. The concept is to experience the energizing effects of sound through the expression of the overtones within the music. The Samonas CD's are generic in nature and no specific "therapy" regimen is currently established for any one type of challenge.

Symptoms helped: vitality, stress, limited concentration, vestibular imbalances, lack of creativity, and more.

Testimonials from parents of autistic children:

1. My child immediately began to notice everything going on around him.
2. My child could focus on an activity for a longer period of time.
3. My child decreased his need to spin constantly.

www.samonas.com

4. The *Leaves and Branches* of *The Tree of Sound Enhancement Therapy* reflects auditory processing skills like memory, discrimination and sequencing skills. These skills are higher functioning skills than basic sound awareness and utilization. These are skills inherent for our understanding of the communication process, including reading. However, these skills need the support of the more foundational skills established in *The Root System, The Seed,* and *The Trunk* of *The Tree* analogy in order for the reception, expression and interpretation of these skills to be well embedded for each person. Without the foundational skills well established, these skills simply become "splinter skills" and testing can show that these skills have improved; but skill testing doesn't show how the body is fully integrating the skills. The Davis Model of Sound Intervention encourages the full integration of all skills to maximize learning and developmental changes. A few of these therapies are:

a. Fast ForWord is a series of programs that use an interactive computer training system to retrain language, reading and learning skills. The initial program targeted receptive language skills and retrained the skill of temporal sequencing—a skill necessary for auditory discrimination, auditory figure ground, and auditory sequential memory. By retraining how the brain comprehends and uses speech information, the person is better able to distinguish the many different components of speech sounds. The basic program still retrains temporal sequencing although the Fast ForWord series of programs now heavily emphasizes skills for reading. The basic program averages between six to eight weeks for approximately 1½ to 2 hours per day.

Symptoms helped: two listening comprehension, phonological awareness, specific language structures, oral language skills, and more.

Testimonials from parents of autistic children:

1. My child wants to listen on the telephone now to his grandparents.
2. My child is able to go shopping with me at the mall now without covering his ears.
3. My child is understanding more of what is being said to him.

www.scilearn.com

b.   Interactive Metronome was developed by James Cassily who thought that learning, cognition and social skills were influenced by the ability to plan and sequence motoric actions. These actions are processed through the sensation of vibration through the ear and are therefore at this level of *The Tree* analogy. Mr. Cassily's theory was that man's intelligence is connected with the ability to process rapid movements and developed a computer-based interactive version of the musical metronome. The purpose of the program is to develop precise control over basic mental functions through the use of body movements. The average program is composed of fifteen one-hour sessions over a period of three to five weeks.

Symptoms helped: attention, motor control, reading, language processing, regulation of behavior, and more.

Testimonials from parents of autistic children:

1. My child began to talk more and became more engaged with those she was communicating with.
2. My child's sleeping patterns improved.

3. My child became less tactilely defensive.
www.interactivemetronome.com

5. The *Head* surrounding *The Tree of Sound Enhancement Therapy* brings the connection between the voice, the ear and the brain full circle and demonstrates the laws within *The Davis Addendum to the Tomatis Effect* as making an important contribution to the full effect of how sound-based therapies make change in learning, development and wellness. Whereas The Tomatis Effect suggests that the voice produces what the ear hears, The Davis Addendum to the Tomatis Effect suggests that the ear also emits (yes, the ear gives out a sound) the same stressed frequencies as the voice and once the imbalanced frequencies are returned to the ear, the voice regains stability or coherence. *The Head* then represents the wellness piece of how sound impacts the entire body. Currently, the science of BioAcoustics is used to help identify how well the body is able to support the changes possible with the other portions of *The Tree* analogy.

Human BioAcoustics was developed Sharry Edwards and after many years of research, the idea of vocal profiling has supported the idea that the body is a mathematical matrix of predictable frequency relationships. Every cell is the body vibrates and emits its own sound frequency. These cellular frequencies must stay "in tune" in order for the body to maintain its wellness. For the autistic person, this piece is often the key for determining if the other many different sound-based therapies will make a change and more importantly maintain any changes.

Symptoms helped: anything related to the body and wellness

Testimonials from parents of autistic children:

1. My child's sound sensitivities decreased dramatically.
2. My child can maintain his focus so much better.
3. My doctor likes supporting my child's detoxing with BioAcoustics.
www.soundhealthinc.com

Overview

The Davis Model of Sound Intervention incorporates all of the many different sound-based therapies only after appropriately using The Diagnostic Evaluation for Therapy Protocol to determine if the therapies are needed, and if so, in the correct order. There are many stories of people using one or another of the therapies with limited or no success, or losing the effects after a period of time. Some people do need more than one therapy and some may need "tuneups" periodically if their body doesn't maintain the support well enough.

Any sound-based therapy can produce change but for some, the change may take place over an extended period of time as the body integrates the changes so that higher ordered skills can develop. To date, most research on these methods have measured skill changes but the responses of sound go further into the body at the cellular and brain level, and researchers are beginning to recognize this fact.

Can there be side effects to this approach? Sound-based therapies can produce skill changes, but the main change goes more deeply to core body needs. Picture the peeling of an onion—each layer represents a layer of development. For some children, many layers need to be removed to get to the heart of their issues and these main issues need to be repatterned so that movement forward can occur. Some people consider this as regression but in reality this repatterning is movement forward—a positive change. It is important not to get "stuck" at this lower functioning level, though, so for many, movement up *The Tree* is necessary to help the person move toward higher progressive levels.

The Davis Model of Sound Intervention offers an alternative approach for addressing the learning, developmental, and wellness challenges associated with autism from a holistic paradigm.

SPEECH-LANGUAGE THERAPY

BY LAVINIA PEREIRA AND MICHELLE SOLOMON

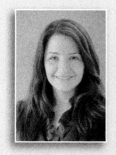

Lavinia Pereira, MA, CCC-SLP

lavinia@firstsoundseries.com

Lavinia Pereira, MA, CCC-SLP is a speech-language pathologist in private practice on Manhattan's Upper East Side. She specializes in the evaluation and treatment of children diagnosed with moderate to severe developmental disorders, including autism spectrum disorders and childhood apraxia of speech.

Lavinia's experience in the field of speech language pathology is multifaceted; she has supervised graduate students at New York University and has guest lectured on the topics of therapeutic planning and treatment techniques at both New York University and Columbia University. She is trained in ABA, Floortime, Oral Motor Therapy, and is a PROMPT trained clinician.

Lavinia earned her Master's degree in Speech-Language Pathology from New York University and holds the Certificate of Clinical Competence from ASHA. She is a licensed speech-language pathologist in New York State.

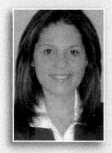

Michelle Solomon, MA, CCC-SLP, PC

michelle@firstsoundseries.com

Michelle Solomon, MA, CCC-SLP, PC graduated from New York University with a Master's degree in Speech-Language Pathology. She holds the Certificate of Clinical Competence from ASHA, has New York licensure in Speech-Language Pathology and earned her degree as a Teacher of the Speech and Hearing Handicapped.

Michelle is currently in private practice in New York City. She specializes in the assessment and treatment of children diagnosed with autism spectrum disorders, childhood apraxia of speech, dysarthria, and other motor speech disorders. In addition, she works with children diagnosed with central auditory processing disorder and language delays/disorders.

Michelle is trained in a variety of techniques including ABA, Floortime, Oral Motor Therapy, Beckman Oral Motor, and is a PROMPT Certified Clinician and PROMPT Instructor.

Together, Lavinia and Michelle develop and present workshops in speech and language development as part of their commitment to educating parents. In addition, they founded *First Sound Series,* a series of interactive, repetitive books developed for children with speech and language delays and motor planning disorders.
www.firstsoundseries.com

It can be an overwhelming process to find a Speech-Language Pathologist (SLP) and once you have, what can you expect during the assessment process? How will he or she teach your child to communicate? Will he or she be trained in the most "cutting-edge" techniques and have enough knowledge about the dynamic disorder of autism? Will the communication skills your child learns in session generalize to your home, school and community? What role will the therapist play outside of the therapy sessions and will this therapy be helpful in teaching your child to communicate effectively?

What is a Speech-Language Pathologist?

A Certified Speech-Language pathologist may also be referred to as an *SLP* or *speech therapist*. This title infers that the individual has completed a master's, doctoral, or other recognized post-baccalaureate degree. In addition, the individual has passed a national examination and successfully completed a supervised, clinical fellowship post graduation. The SLP will then be recognized by ASHA (American Speech-Language-Hearing Association) and earn their Certificate of Clinical Competence (CCC).

An SLP is a "professional who engages in clinical services, prevention, advocacy, education, administration, and research in the areas of communication and swallowing across the life span from infancy through geriatrics" (www.asha.org). SLP's work in a variety of settings including public and private schools, in a client's home, hospitals, rehabilitation clinics, universities, and nursing homes. SLP's work on remediation of feeding and swallowing (Dysphasia) disorders as well as a variety of communication disorders.

SLP's can provide remediation for the following communication disorders:

- **Language disorder:** impairment of receptive (comprehension), expressive (use of spoken), written, and/or other symbol systems;
- **Speech disorder:** impairment of the articulation of speech sounds, fluency or voice;
- **Pragmatic disorder:** impairment of the ability to use and understand social language (verbal and nonverbal);

- **Hearing disorder:** impairment of the auditory system;
- **Central auditory processing disorder:** impairment of the ability to process, retrieve, and/or organize information through the peripheral and central nervous systems;
- **Prosody disorder:** impairment of the suprasegmentals of speech (intonation, stress).

Where can you find an SLP?

Children ages zero to three and school-age children may be eligible for speech and language services through the state in which they reside. Government agencies within your state will be able to provide contact information to begin the assessment process, which will determine eligibility for services. School age children may be evaluated to determine the need for speech-language therapy within the school setting. In addition, licensed therapists in your area can be located by visiting the ASHA website (www.asha.org), asking your child's doctor, or by contacting local support groups and agencies.

What can you expect from the assessment process?

An SLP may be performing the assessment individually or as part of a comprehensive assessment. The following information may be asked of you at the time of your child's assessment (Hegde, 1999):

Case History:

- Prenatal and birth history (complications, C- section)
- Medical (surgeries, illnesses, ear infections)
- Family makeup (siblings, ages)
- Home environment (parent's occupations, single parent household)
- Developmental Milestones (crawling, walking, first words)
- Allergies/ Medications (food, environmental/name, dose)
- Diet Restrictions (gluten free, casein free, picky eater)
- Languages spoken in the home (primary language, additional languages)
- Schooling (name, days/hours per week, contact information)
- Previous and current therapies received (types, length of time, contact information)
- Current ability to communicate (expressive, gestures, signing)
- Receptive language skills (follow directions, understand labels and actions)
- Play Skills (interests, peer interaction, participation in games)

- Behaviors (stereotypical, aggressive, injurious)
- Family history of communication disorders or other relevant disorders/ delays
- Copies of additional reports (neurological, psychological)

Informal Observation:

The clinician will spend time with your child and assess a variety of areas through play, observation, and interactions that elicit the skills in question. The following is a condensed list of several of the areas assessed in an informal observation:

- Expressive and receptive language (gestures, pointing, following directions, comprehension of a variety of concepts, length of utterance, vocabulary, use of questions words, echolalia)
- Play skills (child-directed, symbolic play, narrative play, expanding on ideas)
- Pragmatic language (eye contact, joint attention, turn taking, body in space awareness, reading of facial cues, topic maintenance, conversational exchanges)
- Intelligibility of speech sounds in isolation, words, phrases
- Orofacial assessment (range of motion of articulators—jaw, lips, tongue, dentition)
- Muscle tone (body and face, control of oral secretions, posture, grip)
- Sensitivity to touch (hyper- or hyposensitive)
- Rate and volume of speech appropriate for age
- Feeding skills (manipulation of a variety of textures, tastes, temperatures)
- Behavior (compliance, attention, willingness to try new materials)
- Stereotypical body movements
- Pre-academic/ academic skills (literacy)

Formal Assessment:

The clinician may want to administer standardized tests to further assess speech and language development. Standardized tests yield several different scores (standard score, percentile rank, age equivalency, etc.) and may compare your child's development to that of a typically developing child of the same age. There are a variety of standardized tests that may be appropriate for your child. The SLP will choose tests based on your child's age, development, language abilities and capability of sitting through formal testing procedures.

Once your SLP has completed the assessment he or she will likely write a detailed report of the findings which will be carefully reviewed. Based on the findings, an SLP may recommend further assessments be conducted by other disciplines (Occupational Therapist, Neurologist, Audiologist, Developmental Pediatrician, etc.), may provide an additional diagnosis (Childhood Apraxia of Speech, Dysarthria), or include short and long term goals that are appropriate for your child. It is important that the assessment results and goals are shared with other therapists and teachers working with your child to ensure collaboration and carry-over. The assessment itself can be very overwhelming however, with this information comes the knowledge and power to seek the most appropriate treatment.

What are some of the "cutting edge" treatments being used today?

There are several techniques that are in current use with individuals diagnosed on the Autism Spectrum. Each technique is unique and may or may not be right for your child. The experienced SLP will not only be trained in a variety of techniques, but will know which techniques will be most beneficial and at what point in your child's development each will yield the best results. Below is a list of several highly recognized techniques and a brief description. Additional information can be obtained by visiting their respective websites.

- **PROMPT**: "Prompts for Restructuring Oral Muscular Phonetic Targets," was developed in the 1970s by Deborah Hayden. It has continued to evolve and today is taught and used worldwide by licensed SLP's. PROMPT incorporates the use of organized and systematic tactile (touch) input to the oral musculature to facilitate and/or improve speech production. Seven stages or subsystems (tone, phonatory control, mandibular (jaw) control, labial-facial (lip) control, lingual (tongue) control, sequenced movements (co-articulation), prosody (suprasegmentals) are assessed to determine the child's weaknesses and strengths within a stage and develop core vocabulary that is functional across settings. PROMPT is a dynamic and holistic approach that emphasizes the importance of assessing and targeting the development of the whole client (cognitive-linguistic, social-emotional, physical-sensory) through the use of functional activities and meaningful interactions for communication. Minimally, a licensed SLP must participate in two three-day courses (Introduction to PROMPT and Bridging PROMPT Technique to Intervention), a PROMPT Technique Practicum and complete a four-month self-study in order to become PROMPT Certified. Visit www.promptinstitute.com to learn more about PROMPT, read research articles, or find an experienced PROMPT therapist in your area.

- **Oral Motor (TalkTools Therapy)**: Sara Rosenfeld-Johnson, the founder of Innovative Therapists Int'l, Inc. and TalkTools Therapy tm, is known worldwide for providing educational courses and developing tools designed to assist in implementing oral-motor therapy. Oral motor therapy focuses on assessment and remediation of oral motor deficits (jaw instability, poor lip rounding, poor tongue control, etc.) through the use of specific tools (e.g., horns, bubbles, straws, chewy tubes). In addition, techniques and tools for feeding therapy are utilized to improve strength and coordination. *The Homework Book* is available for clinicians to select exercises for the caregiver to carryover at home. A licensed SLP may participate in a two-day workshop for either treatment planning for oral motor therapy or feeding therapy to become trained in the respective area. Visit www.talktools.net to learn more about oral motor therapy, read articles, find a local therapist who is experienced with oral motor techniques or join a parent group.

- **The Hanen Approach**: The Hanen Approach encourages SLP's to work closely with parents and family members to develop a child's language skills and ultimately increase communication. It is a child-centered approach that can be utilized in a variety of settings and promotes intervention in a naturalistic setting. The program stresses the importance of the family's involvement in a child's success and strives to empower parents to help their child learn to communicate. There are a number of programs available specifically designed for children on the autism spectrum (*More Than Words, Talk-Ability*). Workshops are three days in length. Visit www.Hanen.org to learn more about the programs available, purchase materials, find a trained *Hanen* therapist in your area, and read helpful parenting tips.

- **Beckman Oral Motor:** Developed in 1975 by Debra Beckman for individuals with poor oral motor skills who may not have the cognitive ability to follow directives such as "stick out your tongue." The technique focuses on "increas[ing] functional response to pressure and movement, range, strength, variety and control of movement for the lips, cheeks, jaw and tongue." Beckman recommends multidisciplinary involvement in improving an individual's oral motor skills with the speech-language pathologist assessing and planning the treatment protocol. There are two courses available; Beckman Oral Motor Assessment and Intervention and Beckman Oral Motor Oro-Facial Deep Tissue Release. Visit www.beckmanoralmotor.com to locate a therapist in your area, find information on workshops and or learn how to become involved in research.

Augmentative and Alternative Communication (AAC): is defined as any form of communication (other than oral speech) that is used to express thoughts, needs, wants, and ideas (www.asha.org). AAC is a broad term that encompasses both unaided and aided systems. Unaided communication is the use of signs and gestures without supportive equipment. Aided systems include external devices such as pictures, letters, words, communication books such as PECS (Picture Exchange Communication System), and VOCAs (Voice Output Communication Aids). Children on the autism spectrum are often good candidates for AAC devices as a way to either expand their verbal output or as an alternative to verbal communication. Choosing which type of AAC is most appropriate will be based on your child's communication and motor strengths and weaknesses as well as what is best for your family and the educational setting. Although there is controversy as to which method is most effective with those on the Autism Spectrum, many will use and benefit from a combination of aided and unaided systems (PECS and signing). One commonly used aided system with individuals on the spectrum is PECS.

- **PECS:** Picture Exchange Communication System is an augmentative alternative communication system developed in 1985, by Andrew S. Bondy, Ph.D. and Lori Frost, MS,CCC/SLP. It was specifically developed for children and adults with Autism and related developmental disabilities. The primary goal is functional spontaneous communication via the exchange of pictures. It is considered a visual method and recommended for those with motor impairments due to the ease of retrieving and exchanging a picture with a communication partner. The PECS system consists of six phases: how to communicate; distance and persistence; picture discrimination; sentence structure; answering questions; and commenting. Although certification in the method is not required, it is recommended that any professional or parent using the method consider attending a training session as it is essential to follow the correct protocol. Visit www.pecs.com to learn more about the PECS system, how to become trained or certified, to join PECS user groups, and to purchase products.

How will understanding Autism shape your child's speech-language sessions?

SLP's play a critical role in facilitating the social communication skills of individuals on the autism spectrum (Schwartz & Drager, 2008). Social communication, also known as pragmatics, requires social as well as linguistic skills, which are areas of weakness for this population (Siegel, 1996). Pragmatic skills include eye contact, turn taking, joint attention, topic initiation, maintenance and elaboration. These skills are compromised by the difficulty those with ASD have in imitating others, maintaining attention, generating new ideas, and finding social experiences inherently rewarding. An experienced SLP will treat your child holistically and dynamically, frequently re-assessing and treating all areas of development (cognitive, linguistic, social, physical, sensory, behavior) while maintaining focus on the development of social language skills. For example, your SLP may engage your child in games that encourage turn taking while reinforcing the development of related expressive and receptive language skills and appropriate behaviors.

In addition to significant social language delays, individuals on the autism spectrum often present with challenges (e.g., behaviors, sensory regulation difficulties) that can interfere with learning. Furthermore, different learning styles, limitations, and needs will result in the development of treatment plans that are specifically designed for each individual. One of the biggest challenges your SLP will face will be determining what additional modifications and support strategies should be implemented to facilitate learning. It is the SLP's observations and interactions with your child that will assist in deciding what environmental modifications, behavioral management plans, supporting materials and activities will promote an optimal and motivating setting to learn and support communication.

Environmental modifications: When working with a child on the autism spectrum it is vital that the surroundings are modified to lessen distractions and provide support for additional needs such as sensory and attention deficits.

- Decrease visual distractions (little or no decorations)
- Supportive seating
- Facing away from the window
- Good lighting
- Established work area and sensory or "break" area
- Awareness of noises that might be distracting to the child (buzzing of light, air conditioner/heat)
- Toys and materials out of reach and in enclosed cabinets

Behavior management/regulation: Children with ASD may have behavioral difficulties resulting from frustration, sensory regulation difficulties, self stimulatory behaviors, and/or an inability to communicate their needs and wants effectively. Your SLP will evaluate what behavior management strategies need to be utilized to facilitate a successful session and to develop and maintain a trusting relationship with your child. Just as Autism is a dynamic disorder, a behavioral plan will be a work in progress and continuously altered to meet your child's needs. There are many behavioral modification techniques that can be implemented.

- Use of preferred activities
- Choice boards
- Consistency and following through
- Establishing clear and realistic expectations
- Use of reinforcers (tangible, social, auditory, visual)
- Token system
- Verbal praise
- Replacing negative behaviors with more appropriate behaviors
- Prevention of negative behaviors
- Use of timers to indicate the initiation/completion of a task or transition
- Structured and predictable sessions
- Sensory breaks (physioball, vibration, massage, wheel-barrel walking)

Supporting materials: To maximize learning and your child's ability to communicate the SLP will often use additional supporting materials. These materials enhance nonverbal and verbal communication and provide the structure that children on the autism spectrum often benefit from. In addition, many of these activities foster the development of early sight reading and literacy.

- Use of pictures/words to create a daily schedule
- Use of pictures/words to create an activity schedule for one session to assist in transitioning from one activity to the next
- Written words on objects around room
- Choice board with pictures/words
- Use start-to-finish activities that have a clear beginning and end facilitate
- **Supporting activities**: Children on the autism spectrum often require the use of unique activities to learn various language skills; particularly social language skills. These activities support and encourage communication and interaction.
- Use of routines (daily living activities - dressing, snack time, bedtime routine)
- Use of scripts to learn and practice social scenarios (inviting a peer to play)

- Social stories (address problematic situations by reading stories)
- Repetition of material to foster learning (books, songs, carrier phrases such as "I want___")
- Use of cloze sentences ("Birds fly in the (sky)") and fill-ins ("Ready set (go)")
- "Sabotaging" of materials and environment (desired toy out of reach, piece of a toy missing)
- Group therapy (sessions with typical peers to provide modeling of appropriate social behavior)
- Sessions in a natural setting to promote carryover
- Use of technology (computers, hand held game systems) to encourage independent learning and visual feedback
- Establishing a routine to the sessions
- Keep pace of sessions relative to attention span

How will your SLP facilitate carryover and generalization?

Individuals on the autism spectrum often have difficulty generalizing skills learned in a therapy setting to the "real world." Therefore, working in a naturalistic setting is strongly recommended. A naturalistic setting promotes inclusion in "normal" everyday situations, teaches the individual how to interact with others, and allows for more "teachable" moments. Furthermore, when therapy is provided in a natural setting activities are more purposeful and meaningful which will increase your child's motivation and desire to participate. For example, an SLP would make learning the labels of food more salient if it is taught and experienced in a kitchen with real food items and engaging activities (cooking, cutting, tasting) versus through the use of pictures and pretend play food in an office or bedroom setting.

Speech-language pathologists who work with children on the autism spectrum realize the importance and necessity of carryover and generalization of skills to a variety of settings and across different people. Your SLP will collaborate with other team members (multi-disciplinary approach) to share current goals, strategies, and concerns. For example, your SLP may ask others on the team to encourage a verbal request for a desired toy during their respective sessions. Your SLP in turn may incorporate other team member's goals into their sessions (gripping a writing utensil appropriately, providing scheduled sensory breaks). Communication between the service providers (Occupational therapist, Physical therapists, home-based therapists, Psychologist, Play therapist, etc.) educational providers (teachers, special education itinerant teachers, small class instructors, etc.) and family members/caregivers is essential to your child's ability to transfer what is learned in a speech- language session to other environments and people in their life. Your SLP can promote carryover and generalization in a variety of settings.

Educational settings (outside of the home):

- Your SLP may:
- Observe the classroom and make suggestions
- Spend time with your child in school to demonstrate strategies used in sessions to foster communication
- Train teachers to use PECS, signs, or other aided/unaided AAC
- Collaborate with school therapists
- Keep a shared notebook to communicate successes, goals, concerns on a session to session basis

Home environment:

- Your SLP may:
- Work with parents, extended family members, babysitters
- Provide homework for parents to do each week
- Facilitate sibling interactions
- Suggest appropriate toys, games, and other materials
- Collaborate with home-based therapists
- Participate in team meetings

In the community:

- Your SLP may:
- Teach about the community
- Visit local stores
- Prepare your child for difficult outings/activities (getting a haircut, going to the dentist)
- Teach appropriate behavior and social language for various settings/events in the community

What other roles may the SLP play in your life?

Your SLP will not only work with your child but will also be someone you, the parent, can turn to for suggestions, advice, and to gain knowledge on the constantly changing world of Autism. For example, your SLP may act as an advocate for your child by attending school meetings or writing letters to recommend an increase in services. He or she will share their knowledge on various treatments, local school programs, support groups and therapies available. In addition, your SLP can provide you with resources such as recent books and articles published as well as connect you with other families who are going through similar experience.

Is speech and language therapy helpful for your child?

Yes! "Clinical evidence indicates that children and adults with ASD benefit from assessment and intervention services provided by speech-language pathologists." (Perlock, www.asha.org) Speech-language Pathologists have significantly more training and experience working with children on the autism spectrum than ever before. As the prevalence of Autism continues to rise, SLP's are seeing an increase in the number of children with ASD on their caseload (Schwartz & Drager, 2008). As a result, Speech-language Pathologists now receive training, certification or become familiar with techniques such as applied behavioral analysis (ABA) and relationship development intervention (RDI). Your speech-language pathologist plays a crucial role in your child's development and will aid in the maintenance and generalization of life changing communication skills.

Although speech-language pathologists today have more experience with those individuals on the Autism Spectrum, not every professional will be a "good fit" for your child. There is no exact recipe to working with a child on the spectrum and therefore what works for one child may or may not work for another. An experienced SLP will have training in multiple techniques and find what works for your child. If you are not seeing progress or have doubts about the services your child is receiving please seek out additional resources and recommendations.

As speech-language pathologists who have many years of experience with children on the autism spectrum, we are familiar with the questions and concerns parents may have. The purpose of this chapter was to give you an overview of speech-language pathology and what to expect when your child has been diagnosed with ASD. Our goal was to provide you with the knowledge you need to be an informed parent; which is an empowered parent. You are your child's biggest advocate and the more information you have, the more your child will benefit from speech-language services.

61

STEM CELL THERAPY

by Dr. Frank Morales

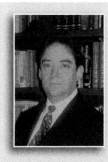

Frank Morales

2805 Hackberry Lane,
Brownsville, TX 78521
(956) 592-5586
Fax: (956) 546-4439
drfrank59@aol.com

Avenida Frida Kahlo 180 Suite #307
Valle Oriente, Sam Pedro, Garza Garcia
Nuevo Leon, Mexico. CP-66260
011-52-868-123-9466
drfrank59@gmail.com

Dr. Morales has dedicated the last nine years of his professional career to stem cell research, establishing some of the first therapeutic protocols primarily in the area of neurology and establishing himself as one of the first physicians to treat autism with adult stem cells. He is a DAN!-certified practitioner and consults with many physicians who treat autism on the use of stem cells for their patients. Dr. Morales currently sits on several scientific committees for stem cell research in Mexico, U.S.A., and China. Dr. Morales is also on the board of directors of the American College for Advancements in Medicine (ACAM). He is also board certified in chelation therapy and heavy metal toxicology, and in nutrition. Dr. Morales is on the Mexican Medical Board of Specialties for Hyperbaric Medicine, and is an active associate professor at several Mexican government training facilities throughout Mexico. Dr. Morales is an associate professor at the Hyperbaric Oxygen Research Facility at the University Politecnico Nacional, based in Mexico City. He is president of the Latin American Hyperbaric Medical Society (Asociacion Latino Americana de Medicina Hiperbarica). Dr. Morales is certified by the American Board of Oxidative Medicine. In addition, he is past president of the International Oxidative Medicine Association, and is medical director of the Rio Valley Medical Clinics and the International World Center for Nutrition, Toxicology and Stem Cell research at the world-renowned AVE medical facility in Monterrey, Mexico. Dr. Morales recently organized a team of physicians and researchers, who together have established a state-of-the-art facility, which is opening the door to a new frontier of regenerative medicine. In addition, Dr. Morales is medical director of Investigaciones Immunologicas de Mexico SA de CV.

Dr. Morales participates as medical director for several research foundations, researching ultraviolet light therapy and photodynamic therapy. He has led several research projects in different parts of the world, i.e. Tanzania and Uganda in Africa. Dr. Morales is on the teaching faculty at the Dental Institute of Mexico (Instituto Odontologico de Matamoros, Mexico), where he participates in the Biological Dentistry & Stem Cell Departments of Research and Clinical Practice.

It is only appropriate that we start with a basic description of stem cells, as there is a wide misconception when it comes to the different types of stem cells. In short, there are three types of adult stem cells. The first, embryonic stem cells, are the most controversial. They are divided into two types: the fertilized ovum, which creates the blastocyte stem cell, and the fetal tissue, which is primarily tissue aborted at six to twelve weeks. The embryonic ovum stem cells—although considered most powerful, or in scientific nomenclature, totipotent—are encoded with information to create a placenta and finally a human being. Animal studies have demonstrated that embryonic blastocyte stem cells involve an increased risk of tumor growth. There is still much research that needs to be performed in this field if we are ever to use them as a therapeutic modality in humans.

The second category of stem cells is the adult stem cells, which consist of two types: First are the adult autologous stem cells, which are one's own stem cells harvested primarily from bone marrow, stimulated peripheral blood, and adipose, or fat, tissue. Second are allogeneic stem cells, from another source than one's own body. These include primarily umbilical cord blood stem cells (UCBSc), Wharton's jelly from the placental cord, amniotic fluid, and the placenta matrix.

The third category of stem cell is from a recently discovered technique developed to manipulate an adult cell back to its embryonic state, called an induced pluripotent stem cell (IPS). The IPS stem cells show promising preliminary results, but are yet to be proven as safe and efficacious as the other types. The two basic types of stem cells found in these different categories are the hematopoietic or progenitor stem cells labeled as CD 34 and mesenchymal stem cells (MSC). The CD 34 stem cells are considered pluripotent and multipotent, with the capacity to replenish and regenerate dying and damaged cells and tissues. MSC stem cells have the capacity to reproduce into all tissue types and have recently been found to be anti-inflammatory and immunomodulating. Children with ASD suffer from hypoperfusion and immune dysregulation, the two major conditions that are quite evident.

Hypoperfusion is decreased blood flow to the brain, meaning that the brain does not receive enough oxygen and cannot function normally. Anytime there is not enough blood flowing to the brain, the brain cells become inflamed and make more nitric oxide. This creates very porous cell membranes, and they receive too much calcium, which damages the mitochondria, which are the energy producers for the cells. As a result, the brain cells die from lack of food.

Immune deregulation is sometimes found in children with autism spectrum disorders (ASD). These children have immune systems that do not respond normally to stimulation and fail to control signals that are very important for regulating immune destruction of bad cells or infected tissue. When the body signals the immune system for help in healing or regulating a certain cell or certain tissue, it unfortunately fails, and subsequent healing does not occur in children with ASD—hence the chronic states of illness in these children.

Children with ASD most often have continually suppressed immune systems and chronic inflammation, and suffer from autoimmune responses. Most if not all autoimmune diseases are the response of our own immune system being malinformed, due to the immune system being stimulated secondary to a chronic inflammatory state, caused by gluten and dairy intolerance, to name a few. This immune deregulation causes autoimmune disorders, which have the immune system constantly attacking many of the body's own good cells.

Autoimmune disorders include Crohn's disease, multiple sclerosis, rheumatoid arthritis, and lupus erythematosus, to name a few. Certainly ASD is included as well. Immune deregulation is very apparent in the gastrointestinal health of children with ASD. The majority of ASD patients suffer from symptoms of bloating, diarrhea, gas, and gastrointestinal lesions, as well as constant and chronic inflammation of their gastrointestinal systems.

We have discovered that the combination of CD34 and mesenchymal stem cells (MSC) has the potential to treat the most common characteristic symptoms of ASD, namely hypoperfusion and immune dysregulation.

The use of adult stem cells for ASD is a new concept based on the capabilities of immune modulation by correcting immune abnormalities and neural hypoperfusion, which appear to be broadly consistent in children with autism, where a correlation of altered inflammatory response and hypoperfusion with symptomatology is apparent in most cases reported.

The ability of adult stem cells to help in the healing process in many diseases, chronic and acute, is now very apparent, due not only to our experience of having treated over a thousand patients for a variety of diseases to date, but the added number of patients treated worldwide. Adult stem cells have more than proven their safety and efficacious use in many areas of medicine. We are currently living in a very exciting time in medicine, with advances made in the area of cell therapies and the compilation of information that has been established by the intensive and dedicated work on the human genome, which have created a great arsenal for the medical practitioner of the future. This will give well-prepared physicians a great advantage in how they will approach the prevention and treatment of disease. As stem cells are currently being used to treat thousands of patients throughout the world to date for repair, regeneration, and immunomodulation, we are slowly starting to incorporate the knowledge acquired from the human genome to help our patients prevent most, if not all, disease.

The credit for development of the therapeutic use of intravenous (IV) and intrathecal (injecting into the spinal fluid for direct access to the brain) adult stem cells for ASD goes to several of us who have been courageous enough to take the first steps to bring forth the use of adult allogeneic stem cells. In 2007, several colleagues and I authored a paper, which, to my knowledge, was the first to report the use in combination of CD34 progenitor and mesenchymal (MSC) stem cells via intrathecal (spinal injection) and intravenously (IV) for the treatment protocol of ASD.

In the historical archives, one can find references to oral and intravenous use of bone marrow, the primary site of adult stem cells. The actual story of hematopoietic cell transplantation really starts after the Second World War, with the first and only use of the atom bomb, or nuclear weapons, on Japan. The radiation and the effects it had on humans and their failure of bone marrow attracted the attention of scientists, who became interested in learning more about the direct and predictably fatal effects that radiation had on bone marrow and its failure to continue to produce cells. Several researchers were able to demonstrate that transfusions from healthy marrow and spleen could reverse the otherwise lethal effects that radiation had on the production of cells from the bone marrow.

Our success rate is a superior 75 to 80 percent, with all cases showing a positive documented response. The changes have ranged from a minimal to a full-remission response.

We strongly believe our superior success rate is contingent on the approach taken by our internationally renowned team of experts, who cover all aspects of ASD.

LP is a three-year-old female who had an uneventful delivery with normal development until after her vaccines at age two. LP developed fever and flulike symptoms, with a constant runny nose immediately after the vaccines. Several months later, the flulike symptoms decreased. For the next six months, she experienced a steady deterioration, with loss of social interaction and lack of spontaneous speech, followed by development of gastrointestinal complications with classical overgrowth of fungal and bacterial infection. By age three, she had developed a total picture of ASD, with diffuse hypotonia, floppy child syndrome, and avoidance of direct eye contact. LP was evaluated and put through our extensive ASD protocol, setting up a favorable terrain for stem cell therapy. Four months after the ASD protocol and the infusion of stem cells, LP immediately had positive changes, with improvements in sleeping patterns allowing her to sleep through the night without disruption, bowel movements becoming normal, connectedness, and eye contact, followed by regaining of spontaneous speech. She has shown continued improvement, with steady developmental gains over the next four months. LP has returned for a second stem cell infusion. Now, at age five, she is a completely normal developing child, currently exhibiting excellent and undeniable gains in mathematical and social skills.

The low level of risk is quite evident after more than several thousand documented infusions of adult stem cells having established their safety and efficacy, with no documented cases of any negative side effects.

The worst documented cases have been with patients who do not prepare accordingly.

The expense and time put into therapy with stem cells, without getting any evident results, can be quite disappointing and give a false impression of the efficacy of adult stem cells. The proper evaluation and specific protocols for the preparation of the infusion of stem cells are key factors for the success of adult stem cell therapy.

The future of cellular therapy is extremely promising as we head into the new era of medicine. The understanding of the human genome, along with our recent development and understanding of gene therapy, will allow us to drastically change the way we approach disease. We will not only cure, but have the ability to prevent disease. Although adult stem cells hold a very promising possibility of cure, we must maintain a multifaceted approach in treating these children. Stem cells are not a standalone miracle cure, but work in synchronization and get best results when patients are prepared and are followed accordingly.

62

SUPPLEMENT THERAPY: RESCUE, REPAIR, AND RECONNECT

BY MICHAEL PAYNE

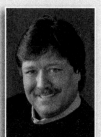

Michael Payne, MS, CRC, CNS

Living Well Today
8002 Discovery Dr. Ste. 102
Richmond, VA 23229
(804) 523-7801
info@startlivingwelltoday.com
www.startlivingwelltoday.com

Living Well Today was founded in 2002 by Michael Payne, MS, CRC, CNS. Over the past five years, Michael has focused on nutritional solutions to neurological and autoimmune disorders serving over 2,000 families with Autism. He believes that each child has a different story, "when you have seen one child with autism, you have seen one child with autism." After working with so many children, Michael has found that rarely does one strict protocol solve something as complex as autism. Being well versed in many protocols, Michael is able to help navigate through the complexities of biomedical treatment. He is a founding member of the board of advisors for Xymogen, a nutriceutical company based in Orlando, Florida and is on the international speaker forum for GUNA, Inc., a biotherapeutic company based in Milan, Italy. Michael is a sought-after lecturer in the autism community.

From the time Bernie Rimland gave B6 and magnesium to his son, it became clear that cellular nutrition is essential for our kids. At the same time, somewhere in the Midwest, Carl Pfieffer noted that use of B6, zinc and targeted amino acids improved detoxification for individuals with mood disorders. Their contributions became the incubator for aware parents and innovative practitioners to explore the use of nutritional supplementation as biomedical treatment for children with autism.

Cutting-edge supplement treatments remain in the purview of parent driven organizations and scientists searching for answers to this complex dance between genetics, environment and neuro-immune conditions. For years we have focused on methylation defects, gut immaturity, immune dysregulation, and toxicity as the primary cause of spectrum disorders. Scientifically researched nutritional supplementation offers a solution to many of these difficult issues.

THE RESCUE PHASE:

Most spectrum kids are what I call "on without the off switch." Mom and Dad need relief from sleepless nights and constant motion due a confluence of issues that imbalance gamma-aminobutyric acid (GABA)/glutamate in the central nervous system. Our starting point is at least two of the following

GABA, inositol, theanine and MAGNESIUM

GABA is the most important and widespread inhibitory neurotransmitter in the brain. GABA controls rhythmic theta waves regulating "cooling" neurotransmitters such as noradrenaline, dopamine, and serotonin. Constant excitation can lead to irritability, restlessness and even seizures. A starting dose of 250 mg twice a day can shift the worried and tense child away from anxiety to a sense of well being. Titrated doses over a month can reach 1000 mg three times a day for the most extreme cases. As with any supplement, the most important regulator of dose is "mommy" radar. One in ten kids cannot handle any GABA dose due to absence of a feedback loop that converts GABA to glutamate and actually increases the behaviors that we are trying to stop.

My research indicates adding theanine in doses of 100 mg to 200 mg often adds to the calming process. While more aligned with glutamate, theanine crosses the blood-brain barrier producing a psychoactive effect by increasing GABA and dopamine in NMDA receptors. I have not observed any side effects.

If your child suffers from obsessive thoughts or repetitive behavior inositol offers relief. Studied since the 1970s, this wonder molecule regulates the cingulate gryus reducing repetitive behaviors. Large doses of up to three grams twice a day have been used safely. This is one of the hidden jewels in the supplement toolbox.

After following the rescue phase for a few days symptoms will begin ameliorate and we can began the next step.

THE REPAIR PHASE:

Our first line of defense against the world is the digestive system. The intestine is a complex matrix of specialized cells that help us determine what is for us and what is against us. It is not unusual for a group of mommy warriors to spend the day talking about what they found in the diaper as the content, tone and texture are highly correlated with the health of our kids. Gut immaturity compromises the immune system, alters nutritional absorption, and affects cognitive processes. A weakened intestinal tract allows opportunistic microbes to populate turning the biofilm into a murky biosludge. And so the spiral begins. Here are cutting-edge formulas I developed after years of trial and error: The rule of thumb, Fighters in the morning Helpers at night!

Fighters

PROTEOLYTIC ENZYMES, OLIVE LEAF, WILD BEAR'S GARLIC, CHORELLA, CILANTRO, MODIFIED CITRUS PECTIN and MODIFILIN

Gentle Biofilm starts with the use of proteolytic enzymes upon rising to remove the protective protein cover of the microbial or bacterial infection. Then twenty minutes later, a mixture of olive leaf, Wild Bear's Garlic, chorella and cilantro, a food based group of antiviral and detoxification agents, are administer to deal with the newly exposed infection and toxic metals. Additional binders such as modified citrus pectin from grapefruit or modifilin, a brown seaweed that grabs onto toxic metals while protecting thyroid metabolism and GI health, are added twenty minutes later to "mopup" unleashed toxic substances. Once a day is enough but some kids can repeat this program after school.

Helpers

LACTOBACILLUS RHAMNOSUS, SEACURE, IGG2000, MULTI IMMUNE, TRANSFER FACTOR and PROBIOTICS

Why would you want helpers at night? From a chronobiological point of view, we know that digestion and immunity are very active during the night giving the helper treatments more coverage.

Many individuals concerned about digestive health know the virtue of good bacteria known as probiotics. Yet little discussion is given to the fact that the right bacteria produces sIGA and creates a barrier keeping harmful bacteria from entering the body through the bowel wall. Lactobacillus Rhamnosus GG, Biffido Bacterium Lactis Hn019, Lactobacillus Aciddophilus La-14, Lactobacillus Plantarium Lp115 and Biffidobacterium Bl-05 are scientifically studied human strain probiotics that support immunity and bowel function. When added to IGG

2000, a serum derived immunoglobulin that reduces the inflammation and binds pathogens, there is an exponential healing effect. Additional supplementation such as Seacure or Butter Oil, which are fermented foods that promote the rapid healing of leaky gut syndrome and Multi-Immune Transfer Factor that educates the intestinal immune system to recognize self vs not self provides a powerful stimulus for long term health of the gastro intestinal tract. Many strains of probiotics, prebiotics and homeostatic soil organisms exist but as usual "mommy radar" and not science will determine use.

Cellular Nutrition

Cellular nutrition is essential for all systems of the body. As far back as sixth grade science class we extoled the virtues of mitochondria as the energy powerhouse of life. Without these important engines immunity, detoxification and endocrine functions are impaired. Here are the essential elements needed for cutting-edge support of cellular nutrition:

Magnesium plays a role in energy metabolism, nerve function regulation of blood sugar and protein synthesis. Symptoms of magnesium deficiency include loss of appetite, fatigue, brain fog, and muscle weakness. I use 100 mg to 300 mg per day. Nighttime use can relax the body and assist sleep when given after dinner.

Selenium is an important trace mineral that serves as an antioxidant preventing cellular damage caused by free radicals. It helps support immune function, rids the body of heavy metals, and plays a major role in thyroid regulation. A modest amount of 200 mcg is important but high dose my result in selenosis. More is not always better.

Vitamin C is widely to known to support immune system; many people take it at the first sign of cold. However vitamin C is essential for preserving intracellular glutathione. Studies indicate that our kids have low glutathione which is important for detoxification of pesticides, lead and other heavy metals. Doses start at 500 mg and may range as high as 3000 mgs in complex cases.

Vitamin B complex is another nutrient essential to mitochondrial function. *Thiamine, riboflavin,* and *niacin* promote the completion of the Krebs cycle in formation of NADH. Doses for each vary depending on your child but in general 10 mg to 25 mg of each is useful.

Zinc is an essential mineral important in immune activating T-lymphocytes, which fight infections. It is required for multiple enzyme actions. Used in various treatments for mood modulation to krytopyrrole I use between 20 mg to 40 mg per day.

Coenzyme Q10 is a fat-soluble substance called ubiquinone that acts as an antioxidant to protect against neurological disease. At the cellular level it acts as a guardian for the mitochondria. New reduced forms of CoQ10 are reported to be more active. Typically I use 50 to 300 mg per day.

No cellular nutrition discussion would be complete without *essential fatty acids* (EFA). A broad range of theories exist but without EFA the lipid bilayer and receptor sites of cells are impaired. Typically, I have chosen a blend of omega 3-6-9 as a starting point. Mixtures that overweigh DHA to support cognitive function are important for many of kids. The addition of *acetyl-l-carnitine*, *phosphocholine* and *serine* increase nutrient transport and communication. Many supplements combine these nutrients for a synergistic blend.

Methylation and Detoxification

One datapoint on which we all agree is that all of our kids have problems with methylation. Where we disagree is how to treat the issue. Some give high dose, some give low dose. Some take supplements, some take drug analogs or give injection. A symphony of genetics, clinical observation and of course, mommy radar, will determine which strategy is best for your child.

Correcting methylation spurs detoxification. Many factors such as transsulfuration, ammonia, lead and mercury toxicity can determine outcome. Any of the aforementioned stressors can truncate the cycle causing toxicity or redistribution of toxins increasing autistic behaviors. Following the step program that I have outlined will mitigate many of the issues. Here are the cutting edge supplements for methylation. Start with B-12 in methyl and hydroxy forms, I then add methyltetrahydrofolate and increase zinc. After that settles we add trimethylgylcine phosphatidylcholine, Methionine and SAMe as needed. In select cases, I often use OSR and molybdenum to preserve intracellular glutathione. Start low and go slow, the methylation symphony will play in tune.

> NOTE: If ammonia is an issue, use charcoal flush twice a week with horsetail, magnesium malate, and tetrahydrobiopterin (BH4). Ammonia protocol alone has positive effect on speech and behavior.

THE RECONNECT PHASE:

For years we have focused on the gut-brain connection, methylation and chelation as the primary treatment for spectrum disorders. While useful, this process is only part of the puzzle. In a recent study we noted that the brain is the "super observer" of the immune system regulating detoxification through the intercellular matrix. What if we missed it? Just maybe it is the brain and brain-gut connection that needs to be addressed first and not relegated to an afterthought. I have observed that a systematic approach to brain connectivity and cell signaling enhancement could be a key for many of our complex cases and would improve clinical outcomes for the non responder and responder alike.

When you have seen one child with autism, you have seen one child with autism! Over the past ten years we have seen many treatments come and go, but the systematic approach of Rescue, Repair, and Reconnect has helped many in the community. The journey continues as many well-meaning individuals are searching for next treatment. However, I offer one caveat when pursuing bio-medical treatments—between supplement schedules, doctor's visits, and therapy sessions, remember to remember the gift that is your child.

A culmination of ten years of work, The Solamar Intensive by Living Well Today is a brain centered program that reduces inflammation and supports communication between the endocrine, immune and neurological systems producing outstanding results for our kids.

63

TRADITIONAL AND INDIGENOUS HEALING

BY DR. LEWIS MEHL-MADRONA

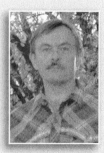

Lewis Mehl-Madrona, MD, Ph.D., MPhil

Education and Training Director
Coyote Institute for Studies of Change and Transformation
Burlington, VT and Honolulu, HI

Department of Family Medicine
University of Hawaii School of Medicine, Honolulu, HI

PO Box 9309, South Burlington, VT 05407.
mehlmadrona@gmail.com
(808) 772-1099

Dr. Lewis Mehl-Madrona graduated from Stanford University School of Medicine and completed his family medicine and his psychiatry training at the University of Vermont College of Medicine. He earned a Ph.D. in clinical psychology at the Psychological Studies Institute in Palo Alto and also became a licensed psychologist in California. He took a Master's in Philosophy degree from Massey University in New Zealand in Narrative Studies in Psychology. He is American Board certified in family medicine, geriatric medicine, and psychiatry. He is the author of *Coyote Medicine*, *Coyote Healing*, *Coyote Wisdom*, *Narrative Medicine*, and most recently, *Healing the Mind through the Power of Story: The Promise of Narrative Psychiatry*. He is the Education and Training Director for Coyote Institute for Studies of Change and Transformation, based in Burlington, Vermont and in Honolulu, Hawaii, and is Clinical Assistant Professor of Family Medicine at the University of Hawaii in Honolulu.

Recently, traditional cultural healings have become more widely discussed in the area of autism thanks to Rupert Isaacson's recent book and film about taking his son to African and then to Mongolian healers. Significant improvement occurred through this journey/interaction, though not cure. Parents are ever vigilant for new sources of miracles, and, thanks to the book, several parents of my patients are making the journey to Mongolia this next summer.

Isaacson noticed immediate improvement in his son's language skills when he started riding horses. He had previously trained horses for a living, but had never seen a horse and a child bond so spontaneously. Rowan's tantrums were nearly driving Isaacson and his wife, Kristin Neff, to divorce. All the while, his son was withdrawing more and more. Isaacson began riding Betsy, a neighbor's horse, with his son.

According to preliminary analysis of an ongoing study by Dismuke-Blakely, hippotherapy has been shown to increase verbal communication skills in some autistic children in as little as eighteen to twenty-five minutes of riding once a week for eight weeks. "We see their arousal and affect change. They become more responsive to cues. If they are at a point where they are using verbal cues, you get more words," Dismuke-Blakely said. "It's almost like it opens them up. It gives us access."

After about three weeks, Isaacson says, Rowan's improved behavior was translating into the home and outside world as well. But not consistently. In late 2004, Isaacson brought a delegation of African Bushmen from Botswana to the United Nations. The traditional healers of the group offered to work with Rowan. "For the four days while they were with him, he started to lose some of his symptoms. He started to point, which was a milestone he hadn't achieved," Isaacson said. When the tribal healers left, Rowan regressed.

Isaacson decided to visit healers in Mongolia, the oldest horseback culture on Earth. Just trekking across the Mongolian prairie on horseback changed his son's behavior dramatically.

> "Rowan came back without three key dysfunctions that he had. He went out to Mongolia incontinent and still suffering from these neurological firestorms—so tantruming all the time and cut off from his peers, unable to make friends—and he came back with those three dysfunctions having gone. He's . . . becoming a very functional autistic person," Isaacson said (Bonifield, 2009).

Traditional healers abound here in North America, though the journey to reach them is less far, and probably less exotic. Traditional healing in North America includes elements of ceremony, manual medicine, energy medicine, storytelling, hypnosis, and psychotherapy. Indeed, traditional medicine could be the standard from which we evaluate more modern forms of psychotherapy, medicine, or healing. Traditional healers have been assisting children and adults diagnosed with autism for as long as this label has existed. Traditional healers use their gifts to assist the individual and the family to transform to the extent that the spirits who assist the healers can facilitate. Traditional healers do their work throughout the world, as evidenced by a brief mention of them in a South African medical article about autism (Mubaiwa, 2008).

Elsewhere (Mainguy & Mehl-Madrona, 2009), we have written about how traditional healers in North America go about doing this, and have compared the methods of traditional healers to those of contemporary creative arts therapists in terms of their use of art, music, and drama. For example, the Bonny Method of Guided Imagery and Music therapy integrates visual and auditory experience into a unified journey, similar to what traditional healers do

While considering traditional healers, we must not underestimate the use of the horse as a means to improve balance, strength, and motor coordination. As responsive, moving, and exciting living beings, horses can motivate and stimulate the child with autism in unique ways. Being on a horse may provide strong sensory stimulation to muscles and joints, impact the balance and movement sense detected by sensory receptors in the inner ear, and provide varied tactile experiences as the rider hugs or pats the horse. The therapist addresses communication goals by asking the rider to follow simple or multistep directions, such as "turn to face backwards and give me high five." The rider is encouraged to communicate directions to the horse to "go" or "whoa," by using words, sign language, or pointing to pictures. In addition, pulling on the reins indicates stop, and a kick tells the horse to get going. Clients are taught to relate appropriately to the horse with gentle pats. The consequences of inappropriate behaviors are easy to implement. The horse stops. Good behavior is rewarded with short trots.

Within the indigenous worldview, all healing is fundamentally "spiritual healing." Spirits are the source of all inspiration for healing. Spirits are everywhere. Spirits guide the treatment. Healers are adept at narratives without words. The sacred songs of ceremonies convey rich cultural messages through music. Elders teach people diagnosed with autism to participate in their specific sociocultural context, through whole body communication. Rather than teaching a set of behaviors, the elders encourage increased self-awareness/self-other awareness, leading to more overt social interactions.

Music therapy principles can link to what elders do with children diagnosed with autism, and can play an important role for parents of children with autism by fostering relationships and developing positive interactions. Most approaches to music therapy rely on spontaneous musical improvisation just as elders do.

Drumming has its impact in both traditional healing and musical therapy. Dance movement therapy and drama therapy are used with autistic children, just as traditional healers incorporate people diagnosed with autism into ongoing dance ceremonies. Body-centered therapies can bring important comfort to individuals struggling with autism, and parallel the spontaneous cultural therapies into which elders introduce autistic individuals.

Bernard Williams (1993) has proposed that all cultures share a "belief-desire-intent" psychology. Boyd (2009:257) notes that animals other than humans understand the concepts of desire and intention. Human children understand intention in their first year and desire by their second year. Belief-desire-intention represents a fundamental cross cultural psychology (Saxe, 2004; Premack & Premack, 2003). Autistic individuals lack the capacity to understand others' beliefs, desires, and intentions. Through stories and ceremony, traditional healers attempt to provide them with a better sense of others' beliefs, desires, and intentions.

Indigenous healers conceptualize illness very differently from conventional medicine.[2] Contemporary medicine bases its diagnoses on structural changes in tissues, while indigenous cultures are more concerned with disharmony and imbalances in social relationships (Mehl-Madrona, 2003). Medicine is noun based, while indigenous thought is verb based. While biomedicine traces the sources of structural tissue changes, indigenous healers contemplate the source for disturbances in the harmony of individuals within their communities and in all their relationships. When the harmony within relationships is disturbed, imbalances result that lead to illness and therefore to suffering. The two views are not necessarily contradictory. They can be linked, though not within the restricted perspective of contemporary biomedicine. The linkage occurs from our observation that sufficient degrees of disharmony and imbalance lead to tissue damage. It is associated with suffering. For example, different cytokines (messenger molecules of inflammation) are out of balance for a variety of disease (arthritis, asthma, diabetes). Different imbalances are seen for each disease; what is consistent is the presence of imbalance.

Most people spontaneously experience mental images while listening to music (Goldberg,1995). The musicality of traditional healers may be an important aspect of their ability to provide assistance to people with a diagnosis of autism.

The "natural history of disease" concept of biomedicine compares and contrasts to one of disharmony and imbalance, in which larger levels of disharmony are associated with greater strength for those forces that oppose health. To accept this, we must accept the idea that how we live and the stories we enact relate to the health of our bodies, and that our psychological resilience parallels, in some manner, our physical resilience. Biomedicine has difficulty traveling here, though the concept is becoming more commonly discussed in narrative medicine circles (Mehl-Madrona, 2007).

Storytelling seems to evoke a response from children with autism. They lack the usual intense interest in monitoring other people, and lack a well-developed theory of mind. They are relatively unable to tell a good story. Through the telling of stories in an inherent musicality, the elders help children to develop an interest in others, especially since so many of the characters in the stories are animals.

Ceremony

Here is a ceremony I watched an elder do with a person diagnosed with autism: The mother brought the son to the elder's home and we sat in the living room. We chatted while normal household activity transpired and then the elder took us into a small bedroom that he reserved for his healing activities. He took an iron pot and put sage into it. He lit that sage, and waved the smoke all around the child. He sang a song that I recognized as a spirit calling song. Then he talked to Hank, the child, about new beginnings, about letting everyone go and starting over. Then he drummed and sang with the child and prayed more. He waved his eagle feather over Hank and blessed him. He sang another prayer song and began a long chant with Hank. When it was over, Hank told him about six white geese feathers he found. He talked about and orange and gold sunset with geese and some buffalo horns he found.

Elsewhere, we (Mainguy & Mehl-Madrona, 2009) published three case stories of children who worked with elders:

Case 1. Regina was a twenty-four-year-old adult who had been diagnosed with moderately severe autism. She had lived most of her life in Pittsburgh, but had recently been brought back to her home reserve in upstate New York because her mother feared for her own health and wanted Regina to develop relationships with other relatives to sustain her, in the event that her mother became too ill to care for her or died.

When Regina first arrived, she showed minimal interest in any social relationships. Her interest instead was in cemeteries, which she visited for hours, as well as standing in what appeared to be strange postures for hours, or massaging herself. She also talked incessantly about the internal organs of the abdomen. When the traditional healer met her, the healer sat in the cemetery with her, speculated about which internal organ might be trying to speak, and gifted her with a new toy pickup truck. The healer also brought a drum. While they were doing other activities, the healer began to drum . . . and drum . . . and drum. Eventually Regina was engrossed in the drumming, nodding her head in rhythm. Finally the healer handed Regina the drum and invited her to play. Almost magically, another drum appeared and they banged away together.

I know that Regina's mother had given the healer tobacco in request for his help with Regina, but could afford little else. She had barely enough money to stay stocked with cigarettes. The healer clearly cared about Regina, as did others in the community. He kept coming to visit her. Slowly but surely they developed a relationship focused upon the drums. Subtly, the elder began to add singing and chanting to the drumming. Regina began humming along. Over time she began to learn the words. The elder sat with her periodically. The elder also gave Regina a can of paint and let her paint anything she wished on the elder's house. Michael spent hours on this project in which the elder, joined him occasionally, painting along with him or chatting away.

Eventually Regina began attending ceremonies. She appeared proud to be within the sweat lodge ceremony *(inipi)*, drumming. The elder gave her a special sweat drum to bring to ceremony. Regina was beginning to form social awareness. Over the course of the next two years, Regina became progressively more oriented into the healer's *hocokah*, or circle of people who relied upon him. Then her mother died. Regina cried, but virtually the entire community came out for him. The funeral lasted four days, as was customary. Regina was seamlessly integrated into the community. She danced at powwows. Over four years, she had developed a social self.

Case 2. Brad was a three-year-old child diagnosed with autism. Consistent with contemporary health care, Brad had waited eighteen months from recognition to diagnosis. No services were available to him once diagnosed. Donald lived on a reserve about two hours from any major urban area. Friends of Brad's mother encouraged her to connect with me. My first response, despite whatever else could be done, was to introduce Brad and his mother to one of the local healers. I encouraged Mary Jane, Brad's mother, to start coming to ceremony and bringing Brad, who was initially relatively new to human contact. This example convinced me that community could overcome great obstacles. We watched Brad make great strides to catch up with his age-mates. More than just the drumming and singing and dancing, Brad became a most adorable powwow dancer, even when he was clueless about how to dance. His mom learned to make elaborate costumes, which made up for his missed steps and puzzled expressions on his face.

More than the support for Brad, was the support for his single mother. People often underestimate the support that a community can provide, despite poverty and adverse conditions. Faye had previously run in a hard group—drugs, heavy drinking, and gangsters. The shock of Brad's diagnosis opened a door in her heart to embrace the traditional stories of her Cree origins. She sat for long talks with elders. She began learning traditional ways. Three years later, Brad was dramatically improved.

Case 3. Ralph was eight years old, and insisted on dressing like a rabbit. He wouldn't go outside without his bunny ears. He liked wearing bunny shoes as well. Ralph liked to watch fire. He lit matches whenever possible and stared at the flame until the fire burned his fingers. His parents lived in fear that he would burn down the house. He communicated very little, except through lighting fires.

Ralph couldn't sit unless he was wearing his bunny ears and his bunny shoes. Otherwise, he would pace incessantly. If enough time elapsed without his bunny slippers, he would begin to bang his head against the wall.

When Ralph's family moved back to the reserve (because a house opened in which they could live), Ralph was slowly adopted by the community. At first people were scared of him. With time, he grew on everyone. The elder began to invite him to light the fire to heat the stones for the sweat lodge ceremony. Others let him burn their garbage. Others protected him when he ventured into dangerous places on the reserve, and kept him from hurting himself. Eventually Ralph had free run of the entire reserve, because everyone took care of him.

Over time, Ralph became interested in the pipe. I suppose it was because it kept being lit on fire. Here is a story the elder told this autistic boy about his sacred pipe:

Ralph seemed to listen to the elder's stories indirectly. He slowed his play, attending longer to a particular object, and returned to his former speed and easy distractibility only after the story ended. Over time, Ralph began to act as if he were more aware of the elder. He slowly developed a sense of social relatedness, though it took four years for him to have a conversation with the elder. By eight years, Ralph was interacting almost normally. He seemed to respond to the containment by the community, to the persistent efforts of the elder to engage him, to the music, the rhythm, the consistency of humans in his life, and to the presence of his family.

Explanation

In each of my stories, the elders relied heavily upon drumming and singing to integrate the diagnosed with autism individuals into their circles of concern. In keeping with their general approach, they were completely permissive and non-judgmental, refusing to accept the autism diagnosis. Rather, as one elder said, "That's just how Michael is. He's okay. When he wants to be different, he will be. Until then, let him be." Within this permissive and accepting approach, Michael was encouraged to attend all ceremonies and powwows. The protection of the elder assured a minimum of teasing. Michael was encouraged to dance, regardless of how clumsy he looked. "We dance," the elder said, "because that is our nature."

Drama therapy is also used with autistic children, and relates directly to what elders do. Drama includes physical exercises that emphasize embodiment, discovery of the way we present ourselves in roles, and encourages a gently paced exploration of the self in the context of others (Landy, 1996). Drama therapy uses mirroring, a technique that encourages two people to mirror the movements of each other without words, which promotes understanding. Adding vocalization and then emotions can happen through mimicking correspondent facial and body tension. Therapists use a "back to back" game, which can be used to work with physical contact without eye contact. This gives the patient some indication of the impact of his strength on another body. Emotions, as different social attitudes can be sculpted on the other body, varying from a low to a high amount of physical contact, and playing on the repertoire of different social attitudes.

Thus, a traditional healing approach to autism uses elements of what conventional medicine calls spiritual healing, energy medicine, drama therapy, music therapy, and relationship to call forth a healing response. I suspect these approaches have evolved over thousands of years of trial and error with the affected person and have a stronger degree of success (based upon their sustainability) than we have yet appreciated.

TRANSCRANIAL MAGNETIC STIMULATION

BY JOSHUA BARATH, DR. ESTATE SOKHADZE,
DR. AYMAN EL-BAZ, DR. GRACE MATHAI, DR. LONNIE
SEARS, DR. MANUEL F. CASANOVA

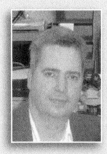

TRANSCRANIAL MAGNETIC STIMULATION

BY JOSHUA BARATH, DR. ESTATE SOKHADZE,
DR. AYMAN EL-BAZ, DR. GRACE MATHAI, DR. LONNIE
SEARS, DR. MANUEL F. CASANOVA

minicolumns and provided an overview of the field in recent reviews of the literature appearing in *Brain* and in *Brain, Behavior and Evolution*. Dr. Casanova serves as an editor to four journals and recently retired as the chairperson of the Developmental Brain Disorders Branch Study Section (NIH). He was a member of the Scientific Advisory Board for the National Alliance for Autism Research (NAAR) and a founding member of the Tissue Advisory Board for the Autism Tissue Program (ATP). He currently serves with the Advisory Board of Families for Effective Autism Treatment (FEAT).

Transcranial magnetic stimulation (TMS) allows scientists to stimulate the brain non-invasively in alert, awake patients. The first TMS device that could stimulate focal regions of the brain was developed in Sheffield, England by A.T. Barker and colleagues in 1985 (Barker et al., 1985). TMS operates based on Faraday's law of electromagnetic induction (1831), which describes the process by which electrical energy is converted into magnetic fields and vice versa. The TMS apparatus achieves the induction of a magnetic field by using a power supply to charge capacitors, which are then discharged through the TMS coil and this creates a magnetic field pulse. The principle of electromagnetic induction proposes that a changing magnetic field induces the flow of electric current in a nearby conductor—in this case the neurons below the stimulation site. Typically TMS coils are designed to produce magnetic fields in the range of 1 tesla (T), which is powerful enough to cause neuronal depolarization. The focal point of stimulation is about 1 cm² in area, and maximal induction is proposed at 90 degrees to the magnetic field (see George & Belmaker, 2007).

TMS can be administered in a single-pulse manner where single or paired pulses are delivered non-rhythmically and not more than once every few seconds or repetitively (rTMS) where pulses are delivered at specific frequencies in trains with precise inter-train intervals (ITI). Generally, single-pulse TMS is used for physiological research or diagnostic purposes while rTMS is used to alter the excitability and function of targeted areas of cortex. rTMS can be divided into low-frequency rTMS (≤1Hz) and high-frequency rTMS (>1 Hz), which categorically affect cortical excitability in different ways. Studies have shown that low-frequency or "slow" rTMS (≤1 Hz) increases inhibition of stimulated cortex (e.g., Boroojerdi et al., 2000), whereas high-frequency rTMS (>1 Hz) increases excitability of stimulated cortex (e.g., Pascual-Leone et al., 1994). It has been proposed that the effect of "slow" rTMS arises from increases in the activation of inhibitory circuits (Pascual-Leone et al., 2000). Additionally long-term potentiation and long-term depotentiation of synaptic currents may respectively be models for understanding the mechanisms of high- and low-frequency rTMS (see Hoffman & Cavus, 2002 for review).

rTMS is a simple outpatient procedure lasting approximately 20 minutes. Patients are seated in comfortable, reclining chair and are fitted with a swim cap to outline the TMS coil position and aid in its placement for each session. Before the procedure begins the "motor threshold" is determined in each patient. "Motor threshold" is the intensity of the pulse delivered over the motor cortex that produces a noticeable motor response. Sensors are applied to the hand muscle (i.e., the first dorsal interosseous) opposite the site of stimulation and motor responses are monitored with physiological monitoring tools on a PC computer. The output of the machine is gradually increased by 5% until a 50μV deflection on the monitor (i.e., electromyograph) or a visible twitch of the muscle is observed. Once the patient's "motor threshold" is determined the coil is moved to the site of stimulation (e.g., the prefrontal cortex) and the pulse intensity is adjusted relative to the patient's "motor threshold." Common dosing schedules include one to two visits per week, and typically patients are welcome to read a book or magazine during the procedure (Fig. 1)

TMS is generally regarded as safe without lasting side effects. Reported side effects include a mild, transient tension-type headache on the day of stimulation and mild discomfort due to the sound of the pulses; earplugs are recommended especially at higher frequencies of stimulation. Given the modulatory effect of rTMS on cortical excitability, there is a very small risk of inducing a seizure with rTMS (see Wasserman et al., 1996). Given this risk, participants with epilepsy or a family history of epilepsy are generally excluded of rTMS studies, and as a safety precaution, most rTMS studies adjust the stimulation intensity below the participant's "motor threshold" (e.g., 90 percent of motor threshold). rTMS is generally considered safe for use in pediatric populations, as no significant adverse effects or seizures have been reported (see Quintana, 2005 for review).

rTMS has been applied to a wide variety of psychiatric (e.g., ADHD, depression) and neurological disorders (e.g., Parkinson's disease). A number of studies report an improvement in mood after repeated frontal lobe stimulation in depression (e.g. George et al., 1995), and it has been found that rTMS may improve certain symptoms associated with anxiety disorders, like post-traumatic stress disorder (PTSD) and obsessive-compulsive disorder (OCD) (see George & Belmaker, 2007). In attention deficit hyperactivity disorder (ADHD), TMS has proven to be a useful tool for investigating neurophysiological mechanisms underlying ADHD symptomatology. In Parkinson's disease (PD) most studies to date have shown beneficial effects of rTMS on clinical symptoms (Wu et al., 2008).

Within the context of autism spectrum disorders (ASDs), rTMS has unique applications as a treatment modality. ASD is associated with disturbances in social interaction and communication, restricted and stereotyped behavioral patterns, and frequently abnormal reactions to the sensory environment (American Psychiatric Association, 2000; Charman, 2008). It has been suggested that a wide range of deficits in autism might be understood by disrupted information integration in the brain, and more specifically, high local connectivity at the expense of deficiencies in long-range connectivity (Rippon et al., 2007) and an increase

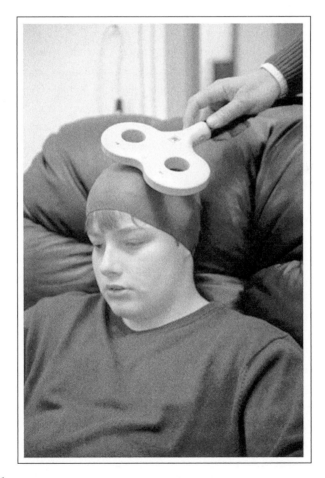

Figure 1.

in the ratio of cortical excitation to cortical inhibition (Rubenstein & Merzenich, 2003). Locally overconnected neural networks may explain the superior ability of autistic children in isolated tasks (e.g., visual discrimination), while, at the same time, deficiencies in long-range connectivity may explain other features of the disorder (e.g., lack of social reciprocity). Higher-than-normal cortical noise and an increase in the ratio of cortical excitation to inhibition may explain the strong aversive reactions to auditory, tactile, and visual stimuli frequently recorded in autistic individuals as well as a higher incidence of epilepsy (Gillberg & Billstedt, 2000).

One possible explanation for higher-than-normal cortical noise and abnormal neural connectivity in ASD is the recent finding of minicolumnar abnormalities. Minicolumns are considered the basic anatomical and physiological unit of the cerebral cortex (Mountcastle, 2003), and contain pyramidal cells that extend the cortical width surrounded by a neuropil space consisting of several species of GABAergic, inhibitory interneurons (i.e., double-bouquet, basket, and chandelier cells) (Casanova, 2007). Double-bouquet cells in the peripheral neuropil space of minicolumns provide a "vertical stream of negative inhibition" (Mountcastle, 2003) surrounding the minicolumnar core. Our preliminary studies indicate that minicolumns are reduced in size and increased in number in the autistic brain, especially the prefrontal cortex (Casanova et al., 2002ab, 2006ab). More specifically, minicolumns in the brains of autistic patients are narrower and contain less peripheral, neuropil space (Casanova, 2006ab). The lack of a "buffer zone" normally afforded by lateral inhibition and appropriate neuropil space may adversely affect the functional distinctiveness of minicolumnar activation and could result in isolated islands of coordinated excitatory activity (i.e., possible seizure foci); this autonomous cortical activity may hinder the binding of associated cortical areas, arguably promoting focus on particulars as opposed to general features. In addition the effect of loss of surround inhibition may result in an increase in the ratio of cortical excitation to inhibition and signal/sensory amplification, which may impair functioning, raise physiological stress, and adversely affect social interaction in patients with ASD.

We hypothesize that contrary to other inhibitory cells (i.e., basket and chandelier), whose projections keep no constant relation to the surface of the cortex, the geometrically exact orientation of double-bouquet cells and their location at the periphery of the minicolumn (inhibitory surround) makes them the appropriate candidate for induction by a magnetic field applied parallel to cortex (Fig. 2). Over a course of treatment "slow" rTMS may restore the balance

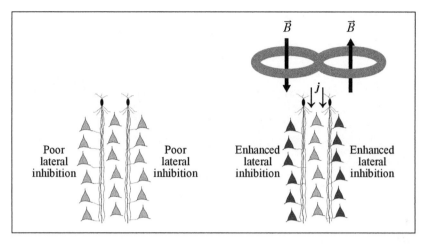

Figure 2.

between cortical excitation and cortical inhibition and lead to improved long-range cortical connectivity.

Thus far our laboratory has focused on clinical, behavioral, and neuroimaging outcome measures, in order to access the effectiveness of rTMS in ASD. One neuroimaging modality that has unique applications to ASD research is electroencephalography (EEG). EEG is the noninvasive measurement of the summation of postsynaptic currents via scalp electrodes; the oscillatory frequency ranges of the postsynaptic currents can be divided into delta (0–4 Hz), theta (4–8Hz), alpha (8–12Hz), beta (12–30Hz), and gamma (30–80Hz) frequencies. It is well known that the generation of normal gamma oscillations directly depends on the integrity of networks of inhibitory interneurons within cortical minicolumns (Whittington et al., 2000). Additionally, the synchronization of cortical activity over wide-ranging cortical regions in the gamma range has been linked to the connectivity or "coherence" of assemblies of neurons working on the same object (percept, idea, cognition) (Brown et al., 2005).

In one of our recent papers (Sokhadze et al., 2009b), we measured the EEG gamma band in twelve children with ASD and twelve controls during a visual attention task and then measured the EEG gamma band in the ASD group after six sessions of "slow" rTMS to the prefrontal cortex. We hypothesized that the ASD group would have excess gamma band activity due a lack of cortical inhibition, and treatment with "slow" rTMS would help restore inhibitory tone (i.e., reduce excess gamma band activity). We also analyzed clinical and behavioral

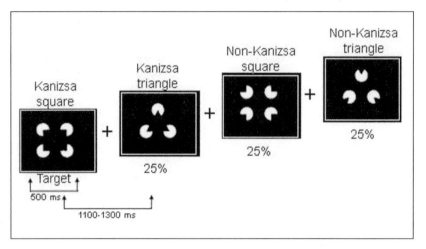

Figure 3.

questionnaires assessing changes in symptoms associated with ASD after rTMS treatment. The visual attention task employed Kanizsa, illusory figures which have been shown to readily produce gamma oscillations during visual tasks (Fig. 3). Subjects are instructed to press a button when they see the target Kanizsa square and ignore all other stimuli: Kanizsa stimuli consist of inducer disks of a shape feature and either constitute an illusory figure (square, triangle) or not (colinearity feature); in non-impaired individuals gamma activity has been found to increase during the presentation of target visual stimuli compared to nontarget stimuli.

We found that the power of gamma oscillations was higher in the ASD group and had an earlier onset compared to controls—especially in response to nontarget illusory figures over the prefrontal cortex (Fig. 4); additionally there was less of a difference in gamma power between target and nontarget stimuli in the ASD group particularly over lateral frontal and parietal recording sites. After six sessions of "slow" rTMS in the ASD group the power of gamma oscillations to nontarget Kanizsa figures dramatically decreased at frontal and parietal sites on the same side as the stimulation site, and there was more of a difference between gamma responses to target and nontarget stimuli. According to clinical and behavioral evaluations the ASD group showed a significant improvement on the repetitive behavior scale (RBS) which assesses repetitive and restricted behavior patterns associated with ASD (e.g., stereotyped, self-injurious, compulsive, and restricted range) (Bodfish et al., 1999). More recently, our laboratory has

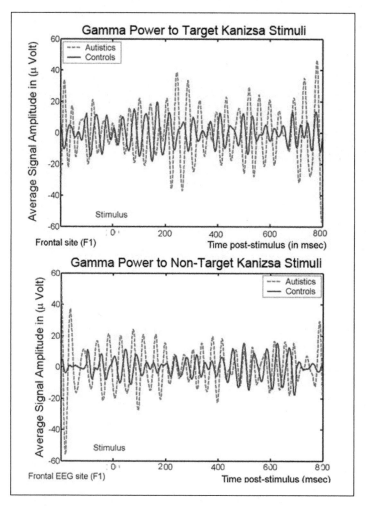

Figure 4.

analyzed gamma coherence before and after twelve sessions of "slow" rTMS in fourteen subjects with ASD. Analysis at four sites of EEG over frontal and parietal sites revealed significantly lower coherence in the ASD group before rTMS, while after rTMS there was a significant improvement pointing to an increase in global cortical connectivity.

We have also been interested in investigating event-related potential (ERP) abnormalities in ASD: ERPs provide a neurobiological measure of perceptual and cognitive processing and represent scalp-recorded, transient changes in the

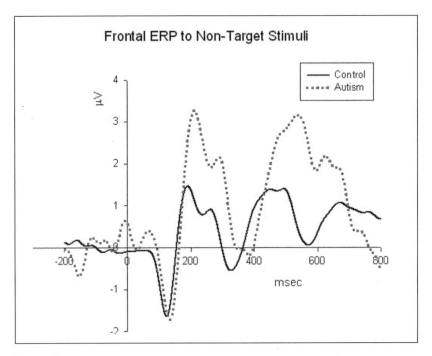

Figure 5.

electrical activity of the brain in relation to the onset of a stimulus. In a previous paper (Sokhadze, et al. 2009a), we investigated ERPs in a three-stimuli, visual task of selective attention in eleven high-functioning children and young adults with autism spectrum disorder and eleven age-matched, typically developing control subjects. Patients with ASD showed significantly higher and longer cortical responses to irrelevant, visual stimuli compared to controls (Fig. 5). In a follow-up paper (Sokhadze, et al. 2009c), we investigated the effects of six sessions of "slow" rTMS stimulation to the frontal cortex on performance in this three-stimuli, visual task of selective attention, as well as clinical and behavioral questionnaires in thirteen individuals with ASD. Low-frequency rTMS minimized early cortical responses to irrelevant stimuli in this task and increased responses to relevant stimuli, indicating improved selectivity and better stimulus differentiation. Additionally, in agreement with our previous results (Sokhadze et al., 2009b), we found a significant reduction in repetitive behavior according to the RBS.

Our findings of excessive gamma oscillations and ERP responses in visual tasks are in agreement with other studies noting that neural systems in the brains of autistic patients are often inappropriately activated (e.g., Belmonte & Yurgelin-

Todd, 2003); this may be due to a disruption in the ratio between cortical excitation and inhibition (Casanova et al., 2002ab; Casanova, 2006ab; Rubenstein and Merzenich, 2003). In autism, increased cortical activity made evident by gamma and ERP responses indicate that activity induced by perceptual processes starts earlier and continues longer, because the neural networks subserving cognitive processes involved in combining information processing are not functioning normally. A reduction in the ability to decrease these cortical responses may reflect inhibitory deficits, and may result in the brains of autistic patients being over-activated. Abnormally large cortical responses to sensory stimuli (i.e., signal/sensory amplification) may play an important role in the manifestation of symptoms of ASD (e.g., sensory hypersensitivity, impaired social interaction). Enhanced and weakly differentiated responses to both target and nontarget stimuli in sensory specific cortical areas (e.g., visual cortex at occipital EEG sites) and low functional connectivity support the hypothesis of abnormal regional activation patterns (local over-processing vs. global underprocessing).

Overall, our preliminary results show promising results for TMS as a treatment modality targeting core symptoms of ASD. Treatment with "slow" rTMS decreased excess gamma activity and amplified ERP responses in ASD patients during visual tasks and improved the signal differentiation between processing relevant and irrelevant stimuli (Sokhadze et al., 2009bc). Additionally, "slow" rTMS dramatically improved the coordinated activity or coherence between different regions of the brain and significantly improved repetitive and restricted behavior patterns associated with ASD. Our results suggest that low-frequency rTMS may improve the inhibitory tone and decrease the ratio of cortical excitation to inhibition in ASD, and this may lead to improved long-range connectivity. TMS has the potential to become an important therapeutic tool in ASD treatment and may play an important role in improving the quality of life of many with the disorder.

VIRUSES AND AUTISM

BY DR. MARY MEGSON

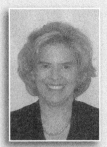

Mary Megson, MD

Office Information:
Pediatric & Adolescent Ability Center
7229 Forest Avenue
Suite 211
Richmond, VA 23226

(804) 673-9128
Fax: (804) 673-9195

info@megson.com
www.megson.com

Dr. Megson is a developmental pediatrician who has worked in the field of pediatrics for more than twenty years. As a developmental specialist in pediatrics, she devotes her career to children with developmental issues, which include ADHD, ADD, autism spectrum disorder, Asperger's syndrome, and developmental delays. She is board certified by the American Board of Pediatrics, a Fellow of the American Academy of Pediatrics and a Member of the Society of Developmental Pediatrics. Dr. Megson travels all over the world speaking at international conferences.

Viruses are a known cause of autism, including cytomegalovirus (CMV), rubella, herpes and measles.[1] The immune reaction to these viruses causes inflammation, an autoimmune response and subsequent changes in brain function.[2] Live attenuated viruses in vaccines set up a low-grade presence in the body creating immunity, but antibodies to these viruses may cross-react with human tissue, causing autoimmune reactions all over the body.

Children may acquire these viral infections at birth, in the perinatal period and beyond. Signs of viral infections in children with autism, due to increased Th2 response and immune suppression, are often not the usual signs of acute infection: nasal congestion, fever, cough and/or nausea and vomiting. Chronic viral infections cause other symptoms: low endurance, rashes that come and go, and prolonged or intermittent low-grade fever. The children tire easily, have chronic congestion after allergy elimination, and are irritable.

Labs are nonspecific. Increased IgM antibodies suggest recent infection. Increased IgG antibodies suggest past infection. Extremely high antibody titers far after exposure may suggest ongoing exposure. White blood counts are very high or low, most often with increased lymphocytes and monocytes. Often natural killer cells are low.

Treatment includes nutritional support, such as extra vitamin A, C, and zinc. Cod liver oil contains 14-hydroxy-retro-retinol needed to turn on T cells to fight viruses.[3] Monolaurin is a natural antiviral known to be effective against mumps and rubella. Unfortunately, there is no lab test that proves chronic viral infections are present. Some clinicians use antiviral therapies such as vancyclovir empirically for a limited period of time and continue based on clinical response.

With autism, it is important to recognize that the effects of a particular virus may be far from the area of infection. For example, the antibody to measles cross-reacts with intermediate filaments.

These function to form the tight junction barrier between cells that line the gut wall and the blood-brain barrier. Many children after MMR develop "leaky gut syndrome," probably as a result of making cross-reactive antibodies to measles. Indeed, many of the antineuronal antibodies found in autistic children are anti-intermediate filaments in the nervous system.[4]

Other treatments such as transfer factor, bovine colostrum and intravenous immunoglobulin (IVIG) are sometimes used. Dr. Jaquelyn McCandless has had some success using low-dose naltrexone, an opiate antagonist to prevent depression of the antiviral component of the immune system. Formal studies are ongoing using this approach.[5] Always, the benefit to the patient should far outweigh the risk of exposure to the intervention. Natural antivirals include garlic, olive leaf extract, probiotics, and others.

Another important defense against viral infections includes eating a healthy diet, getting adequate sleep and exercise, and avoiding stress in the child's life.

VISION THERAPY

BY DR. JEFFREY BECKER

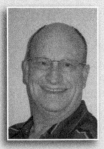

Jeffrey Becker OD

NeuroSensory Center of Eastern Pennsylvania
250 Pierce Street, Suite 317
Kingston, Pennsylvania 18704
(570) 763-0054
Jbecker@Keystonensc.com
www. Keystonensc.com

Dr. Becker is a neurodevelopmental/behavioral optometrist with board certification and specialty training in neurosensory disorders. Dr. Becker is a Defeat Autism Now! (DAN!)-certified clinician. He is the director of Vision Rehabilitation Services for the Neurosensory Center of Eastern Pennsylvania. He has participated in multiple research projects involving neurologically impaired individuals. He has spoken about vision and learning at national and international autism conferences. He most recently published an article in *The Autism File* is titled "Vision Therapy Can Help Children with Spectrum Disorders." Dr. Becker is also an adjunct faculty member of Misercordia University, Dallas, Pennsylvania, where he teaches vision rehabilitation courses to master's-level occupational and physical therapy students. In more than twenty-seven years of clinical and research experience, Dr. Becker has examined and treated over 3,000 patients who are neurologically impaired with neurosensory disorders.

"Vision" refers to how the visual system coordinates function between the two eyes and the brain (Cohen, et al., 1988). We ask questions like: Do both eyes perceive the same image at the same time? Do both eyes move in unison? Do both eyes have equal focusing power? Do both eyes do all these visual requirements easily, fluidly, and for an extended length of time? If the answer to any of these questions is "No," then vision therapy may be indicated. Vision therapy is done in a sequential manner that mirrors normal developmental processes. This allows the child to most readily relearn the visual skills that were lost, or to learn those that were never developed. It is therefore necessary to start with very easy tasks and work toward more difficult tasks. The Piagetian approach to development indicates that this is the best way to remediate vision-related problems.

The therapy has been used by optometrists for years in the general population in those who have visual functioning disorders and now it can be adapted to autism spectrum disorder (ASD) individuals by developmental/behavioral optometrists (Trachman et al. 2008). It is important that these clinicians have specific training with these disorders through DAN! and other agencies such as Autism Research Institute (ARI).

Fifty-three percent of children who are poor readers have some form of visual functioning disorder, and it has been estimated that up to 80 percent of children with special needs have significant visual functioning disorders that affect the learning and developmental process (Cohen, et al., 1988).

Success is based on visual, subjective, and functional findings. Success rates vary depending on the initial functional loss. Studies indicate that success rates range from 63 percent to as high as 89 percent. This depends on the frequency and number of sessions completed (Cohen, et al. 1988).

DG, an eight-year-old boy, sat in my examination chair after his mother had completed all the appropriate intake forms as recommended by the Defeat Autism Now! protocol. She tried to control her son as he attempted to touch the bright instruments in my examination room. The paperwork indicated that DG had been diagnosed with ASD at two years of age. He was in and out of different programs and, at one time, was labeled as dyslexic. The interview proceeded typically, but his mother was not quite sure why she was here with her son, even though an observant occupational therapist had suggested she make an appointment with me. She said, "I've had my son's eyes checked before every school year, and he has always had 20/20 vision." My comprehensive neurosensory examination, along with the functional and developmental vision examination, indicated that the other eye care specialists were correct. DG did have 20/20 visual acuity in both eyes. But they had apparently not assessed another aspect of vision, which is very important (Holmes, et al., 2008). DG had significant eye tracking and eye focusing problems, reduced convergence difficulty with depth perception, and vestibular inaccuracies.

At this point, I explained to DG's mother the difference between sight (acuity) and vision. Sight is the ability to see a certain size object at a certain distance. The standard means to assess acuity was conceived by Herman Snellen in 1862, and since that time we have referred to normal sight as 20/20. The top number indicates the distance of the observer from the acuity chart, and the bottom number is the size of the letter being viewed. All this really means is that a person can see a certain size letter at a certain distance. This terminology is, of course, important for many aspects of our lives. However, even more important to our children with ASD, like DG, is functional/behavioral vision. Deficits with their visual systems can be very disabling.

Children with ASD, like DG, appear more likely to have visual functioning disorders than the general population (Taub, 2007). When doing the intake form for DG, it was noted that he disliked doing any near point tasks. He preferred to run randomly around the room, picking up items along the way. He would briefly look at them and then put them down quickly when he saw another item to view, examining the new item for a very short period of time. This behavior was repeated consistently. His mother noted that she felt DG was very smart because he could easily memorize songs and verses. (My experience has been that ASD children are very smart but are unable to utilize their intelligence in the positive and productive manner that we all expect.) He would not engage in eye contact and would attend to objects out of the corner of his eyes. Instead of moving his eyes, he turned his head to see objects.

DG's evaluation, which took over two hours, indicated visual functional deficits that needed to be remediated in order for DG to be able to function visually in the world. This two-hour evaluation included tests with the Sensory View diagnostic system (NeuroSensory Centers of America, 2009). This system assists in the evaluation of myelin health, eye movements, balance, proprioception, and dynamic visual acuity. After these tests are done, an additional evaluation is done to assess depth perception, visual suppressions, visual focusing, ocular health, and the ability of the eyes to work together. These tests, which are done by an eye care specialist trained in these procedures, need to be done without the use of the phoroptor, an instrument normally utilized in routine eye examinations.

Vision therapy can be done in an office by a trained therapist, in an outpatient rehabilitation center, or at home. Vision rehabilitation to correct most oculomotor, eye focusing, and eye deviation deficits typically continues for six to eight months when done two or three times per week. Treatment also requires home participation for thirty to forty-five minutes per day for five days per week on an outpatient basis. This does not mean that the rehabilitation cannot be concluded earlier (or later) than this prescribed time. Program length is dependent on the child's participation level and attendance.

Due to DG's particular needs, I began his therapy program in my office. The eye movement exercises I prescribed consisted of computer-based therapy, as well as handheld therapy techniques. Both techniques have the same end result, but I have found that the computer techniques seem to work more quickly, and the results are more consistent in nature than those using the handheld therapies. The disadvantage of the computer therapies is that many children with ASD have difficulties sitting at the computer for any length of time, thus making the sessions more frustrating for them. Therefore, we incorporated both therapy techniques into DG's treatment program.

The computer programs we have had success with come from a company in Gold Canyon, Arizona (HTS, 2009). The programs can be tailored for each child and his or her skill level. We can incorporate therapies for all visual deficits, including gross motor, fine motor, vestibular, and focusing issues, into this program. The computer programs allow easy progression for each child and can be modified when a child has difficulty with certain tasks. I review progress at least two times per month but usually more frequently, making sure that the child is meeting the proper goals.

Case Example

DG's mother was completely amazed at her son's progress. His eye contact improved, his visual stimming significantly decreased, and his school performance accelerated. His teachers wanted to know what his mother had done to get him this far. He was a more pleasant child, according to what others told DG's mother. Most importantly, DG now knows that he can do these tasks and has improved self-esteem.

Once the in-office rehabilitation program is completed, a reduction in rehabilitation time is given to the child, and a phase-out program is begun for several months. This is done to monitor and maintain all visual skills that are learned and to make sure the child has adapted adequately to the new visual functioning environment.

As a final step, DG was given a home maintenance program to follow and is checked every three months in the office to confirm that he has not regressed. The home maintenance program can be a computer-based program (HTS) or the procedures that are outlined in the next section. It is very important to do this program with the understanding that these visual skills have been learned and can easily be unlearned, if not reinforced on a routine basis at home (Becker et al., 2009).

RISKS: none, except for the time commitment

Checklist for possible developmental visual deficits related to asd. If you can answer yes to two or more of these signs, your child should engage in a complete neurosensory and developmental vision evaluation:

1. Child likes to look out of the corners if his/her eyes when doing either near point or distance viewing.
2. Child only does near tasks for short periods of time, then goes back to task after a few short minutes.
3. Child turns head to the left or right to view distant or near objects.
4. Child bends head to either shoulder when viewing distant or near objects.
5. Child covers or closes an eye when looking at near point tasks.
6. Child likes to visually stim with his hands in front of one eye or another.
7. Child moves closer and closer to near point tasks over a short period of time.
8. Child rubs eyes frequently.
9. Child's eyes tend to water when doing near point tasks.
10. Child likes to turn head up or down and moves head in strange positions to do near point tasks.

How to Find a Qualified Eye Care Specialist

To locate a neurodevelopmental optometrist in your area, log onto www.nora.cc (Neuro-Optometric Rehabilitation Association). When making an appointment, ask the following questions:

1. How frequently does the doctor examine children with autism spectrum disorders?
2. Does the doctor do functional vision testing, not just acuity testing?
3. Does the doctor prescribe vision therapy, and who carries out the therapy?
4. How long is the examination process with the doctor? (It should last at least sixty to ninety minutes to get a good understanding of the child's deficits.)
5. Will the doctor write and correspond with the school and/or other professionals?

THERAPIES OF THE FUTURE

ANTI-ALLERGIC, ANTI-INFLAMMATORY, AND OTHER FUTURE TREATMENTS

BY DR. THEO THEOHARIDES

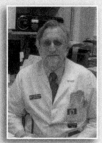

Theoharis C. Theoharides, MS, Ph.D., MD

Department of Pharmacology and Experimental Therapeutics
Tufts University School of Medicine
136 Harrison Avenue
Boston, MA 02111, USA
(617) 636-6866
Fax: 617-636-2456
www.mastcellmaster.com

Professor of Pharmacology, Internal Medicine and Biochemistry
Director, Molecular Immunopharmacology and Drug Discovery Laboratory,
Tufts University School of Medicine, Boston, MA, USA.
(www.mastcellmaster.com)
Clinical Pharmacologist, Massachusetts Drug Formulary Commission (1986–2010)

Scientific Director, Algonot, LLC, Sarasota, FL
www.algonot.com

Dr. Theoharis Theoharides is the Director of the Molecular Immunopharmacology and Drug Discovery Laboratory, as well as a Professor of Pharmacology, Biochemistry and Internal Medicine at Tufts University, Boston, MA. He received all his degrees from Yale University, is a member of seventeen scientific societies and has published over 270 research papers and two textbooks. Dr. Theoharides is much more than just an eminent physician and pharmacologist; he goes a step further in posing new theories and defining the cutting edge of mast cell research. He was the first to show that mast cells can be stimulated by non-allergic triggers, such as stress hormones, to secrete inflammatory mediators selectively without histamine. Based on his discoveries, Dr. Theoharides proposed the novel concept that mast cells play a critical role in brain inflammation and autism. Dr. Theoharides extends his expertise beyond theory into practical options and offers hope for patients with diseases such as autism which, to date, have defied treatment.

O ver the last few years, much useful evidence has been produced on autism, especially with respect to the identification of autism susceptibility genes. However, no single or even cluster of genes can explain the dramatic rise in autism prevalence over the last twenty years. Additionally, more efforts should be directed at understanding what contributes to the pathogenesis of autism, rather than focusing primarily on the neurologic sequelae. Now it is time to move from informational to translational research, where one can identify old or new potential targets in order to develop novel and effective treatments.

Mast cells, which are a type of immune cell, and the stress hormone corticotropin-releasing hormone (CRH) in conjunction with the neuropeptide neurotensin, can disrupt the protective gut-blood-brain barriers and lead to brain inflammation. Enteroviruses, neuropeptides, stress hormones, and toxins could all contribute to brain inflammation and autism through mast cell activation, especially in age and genetically vulnerable patient subpopulations. (Refer to Chapter 45 on NeuroProtek.)

For instance, many autism patients have evidence of "allergic symptomatology," but there has been minimal attempt to help autism patients and their parents understand that "allergic symptoms" may fall under different diagnoses, such as:

Allergy

Angioneurotic edema

Atopy

Atopic dermatitis

Autoinflammatory diseases (involving interleukin-1 release)

Eczema

Food allergy

Food intolerance

Idiopathic urticaria

Idiopathic mast activation disorder

Mastocytosis

Nonclonal mast cell activation syndrome

Non-IgE food allergy

Urticaria pigmentosa

Note: It is important for patients and their caregivers to understand that many of these subcategories *do not* test positive on skin prick and RAST test to the known antigens. As no specific antigen is implicated, these patients *cannot* be treated with immunotherapy.

The American Academy of Allergy, Asthma and Immunology (of which I am also a fellow) last year produced a DVD with The Mastocytosis Society, Inc. (TMS) entitled *Mast Cell Activation Symptomatology* given free (www.tmsfora-cure.org) to all physicians, and for $1 to anyone else. The DVD provides an illustrative insight to the fact that allergies are only one aspect of mast cell activation.

There are no truly anti-allergic drugs available. Cortisone, a steroid, is the only drug that would come close to it by suppressing the immune system response, including mast cell function. However, cortisone cannot be given for long periods of time, especially to children, because of its numerous side effects, including increased risk for infections, inhibition of long bone growth plates, fragile bones, and depression. Despite the limitations described above, some available treatments can be very useful in reducing allergic-type symptoms/inflammation and may, therefore, benefit at least some autistic patients.

Available Formulations

NeuroProtek: See chapter 43.

Cyproheptadine (Periactin) is a combined histamine-1 and serotonin receptor antagonist, and produced significant improvement (as 4 mg orally per day) over that of the antipsychotic haloperidol in a double-blind trial of 40 children with autism, randomized to either haloperidol and cyproheptadine vs. haloperidol and placebo. The apparent benefit of cyproheptadine may be related to the higher platelet serotonin levels reported in over 40 percent of patients with autism. Although high platelet serotonin may not reflect availability in the brain, it could affect the neuroenteric plexus that utilizes serotonin.

Disodium cromoglycate (cromolyn, Gastrocrom) is a potent inhibitor of *rodent* mast cell histamine secretion, but weak inhibitor of human mast cells. Nevertheless, it is often used (100 mg orally two or three times/day) to treat GI symptoms in mastocytosis patients.

Ketotifen (Zaditen), is a histamine-1 receptor antagonist not available in the U.S.A., and has been reported to also partially inhibit mast cell activation and is often used (2–4 mg orally once per day) for treating symptoms associated with mastocytosis, but also for eosinophilic esophagitis and gastroenteritis.

Hydroxyzine (Atarax) is a potent histamine-1 receptor antagonist, which also partially inhibits mast cell activation and has mild anti-anxiety actions. It is often used (5–25 mg orally once per day usually at night—it also exists as an elixir of 5 mg/teaspoon) for treating symptoms associated with allergies and mastocytosis, but also ADHD.

Rupatadine (Rupafin) is a newer histamine-1 receptor antagonist, available in Europe and Latin America, but not yet in the U.S.A. Rupatadine also inhibits mast cell release of inflammatory mediators and can also be used (10–20 mg orally per day) for eosinophilic esophagitis and gastroenteritis. These drugs may be more appropriate for the subgroup of autistic patients with allergic symptoms.

New Future Treatments

CRH-receptor antagonists

Many autistic patients are anxious and cannot handle stress. Research has shown that the stress hormone corticotropin-releasing hormone can stimulate mast cells to release proinflammatory molecules. CRH receptor antagonists could have a double benefit by reducing stress and reducing CRH-induced mast cell activation.

UCP2 Inducers

Recent research has shown that the mitochondrial uncoupling protein 2 (UCP2) has an inverse relationship with mast cell activation. UCP2 regulates the production of reactive oxygen species and buffers intracellular calcium, both of which are increased in autistic patients. Given this base knowledge, UCP2 expression in peripheral lymphocytes from patients with autism should be investigated, and UCP2 inducers should be identified for therapy.

In summary, there are several autism treatments on the horizon, but additional research with a focus on practical use of data with real-life applications is critical in order to implement the autism treatments of the future. It is important to investigate mast cell-associated triggers and mediators in patients with autism, especially at the time the diagnosis is suspected or made. Such efforts could help clarify the pathogenesis of autism and identify potential biomarkers, as well as define new therapeutic targets. Moreover, by aggressively addressing "allergic symptomatology" in patients with autism, behavioral exacerbations may be reduced or prevented.

68

RESEARCH AT THE UNIVERSITY OF LOUISVILLE AUTISM CENTER

BY DR. MANUEL CASANOVA, DR. ESTATE SOKHADZE, DR. AYMAN EL-BAZ, JOSHUA BARUTH, DR. GRACE MATHAI, DR. LONNIE SEARS

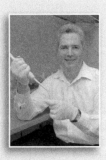

Manuel F. Casanova, MD (1,2)
Estate Sokhadze, Ph.D. (1)
Ayman El-Baz, Ph.D. (3)
Joshua Baruth, MS (2)
Grace Mathai, Ph.D. (4)
Dr. Lonnie Sears, Ph.D. (4)

1. Department of Psychiatry and Behavioral Sciences
2. Department of Anatomical Sciences and Neurobiology
3. Department of Bioengineering
4. Department of Pediatrics

University of Louisville Health Sciences Center
500 South Preston Street, Building 55A, Room 217
Louisville, KY 40202

From a traditional neurological perspective, the clinical syndrome of autism is characterized by abnormalities in higher-order cognitive abilities, complex behavior, and the presence of seizures in a significant number of patients. In autism, these symptoms occur in the absence of long tract signs, blindness, or deafness. This constellation of symptoms is associated in neurology with dysfunction of the outer gray matter of the brain or neocortex. Research studies support the suggested localization, as studies of eye tracking movements have documented generalized abnormalities in the integrative circuitry of neocortex. Functional

410

MRI studies have similarly revealed abnormalities in neocortical activation to different tasks (e.g., theory of mind, face recognition, executive functions, and language) suggesting underdevelopment of higher-order integrating connections of the neocortex in autism. The reported increase in volumes of gray and white matter confirms the presence of neocortical abnormalities and in its connections through the white matter.

The above characteristics of cognition in autism suggest problems with information processing that are expressed in different ways in different tasks. Across characteristics, it appears that as tasks get more demanding or require reliance on global versus local information, performance fails; emergent skills normally present are absent, thus making it impossible to assume the processing load as demands increase. The question many researchers would like to answer is: What is the underlying mechanistic framework for these cognitive abnormalities or is there a unifying framework at all? One possibility is that disturbance of global precedence and possibly even hypersensitivity to complexity may arise from the use of sharply tuned, narrowly focused receptive fields in cortical connections. This may result from an abnormality in the internal structure of neocortical minicolumns, which may be amenable to therapeutic interventions.

A comprehensive program of basic, applied, and outcomes research has been created at the University of Louisville with the goal of increasing our understanding of autism. The Autism Center aims to study how the brain analyzes information, what the underlying deficits might be, and to explore possible clinical interventions and determine the efficacy and quality of those interventions. The research director of the University of Louisville Autism Center is Dr. Manuel Casanova, Associate Chair for Research and the Gottfried and Gisela Kolb Chair in Psychiatry.

Research at the Autism Center of the University of Louisville presently focuses on how the brain processes signals. Information processing is viewed as a common characteristic of the behavioral and cognitive abnormalities in autism, and thus an organizational framework for hypothesis testing. Initial research has looked at the anatomy of the cell minicolumn, the smallest cortical unit capable of information processing. Previous studies have found this anatomical and functional unit of the brain to be altered in patients with autism. More specifically, minicolumns in the brains of autistic patients were described as being narrower and more numerous per linear length of tissue section examined as compared to controls. Since the minicolumn reiterates itself millions of times throughout the brain, variations in the total number and width of minicolumns can result in macroscopic changes of the brain's surface area and/or gyrification. In this regard, our Autism Center is currently trying to establish a correlation between autopsy and neuroimaging (postmortem MRIs) findings in autism. The intent is to develop markers of the condition that can be detected while the patient is alive. Another innovative aspect of the research is an attempt to validate current diagnostic screening techniques against autopsy findings.

Basic research within the Autism Center includes the study of functional circuitry associated with the impact of stimulus saliency, novelty, and typicality on information processing from the visual perceptual or local level processing to the conceptual level processing. Topographical studies of the cell minicolumn indicate a gradient of severity spanning idiotypic (least affected) brain regions to heteromodal regions (most affected). Our results thus suggest that lower levels of visual processing performed by idiotypic (e.g., calcarine) cortex will be spared or even enhanced. How this normal function translates into higher-level processing deficits (e.g., working memory, executive functions, complex figure recognition tasks) and abnormalities typical of autism is a major aim of our Autism Center.

At the Autism Center, diffusion tensor imaging (DTI) is being used to investigate microstructural abnormalities in white matter pathways between brain structures related to the signs and symptoms of autism, and the molecular mechanisms involved in cell-cell interaction in the cortex of autistic patients and controls. Computer programs and algorithms are being created that help define morphometric measures of cortical circuitry. Findings from these minicolumnar studies are being modeled as simulations of cell migration during brain development to define a time window of vulnerability for the condition.

Applied research focuses on investigating the human side of the disorder through studies of lifespan, treatment, and social and vocational activities. Case definition strategies are being explored by measuring variables on cases and controls and interview data on spouses and other relatives to allow the investigation of the impact of autism on the family. Future studies will include an attempt to define autism as a spectrum based on how far from the mean persons score on the Social Responsiveness Scale, and clinical trials to study the impact of possible therapeutic interventions on automatic information processes.

Outcomes research seeks to understand the end results of medical, psychosocial, behavioral, and educational interventions. For individuals with chronic conditions, end results include those personal experiences that influence quality of life, morbidity, and mortality. Outcome research also helps in predicting the impact of various influences. As part of the diagnostic endeavors, the clinical core of the Autism Center explores case definition and risk factors for autism. As an immediate benefit, these studies provide patients and their relatives evidence about benefits, risks, and results of treatments so they can make more informed decisions.

Clinical colleagues in the Systematic Treatment of Autism and Related Disorders program (STAR) at the University of Louisville pursue applied and outcomes research initiatives, which also include translational research on the effectiveness of clinic-based and community-based interventions for autism. Particular attention to outcomes of teacher training in autism, effectiveness of social skills interventions, parent training and outcomes, and services research are highlighted.

The Autism Center at the University of Louisville is exploring ways to translate some of our initial neuropathological findings on minicolumns into a clinical intervention. The value of each minicolumn's output is insulated to a greater or lesser degree from the activity of its neighbors by inhibition in its peripheral neuropil space. This allows for gradations in amplitude of excitatory activity across a minicolumnar field. It has been posited that reductions in inhibitory activity may explain some symptomatology of autism, including increased incidence of seizures and auditory-tactile hypersensitivity. Our Autism Center is using the specificity of repetitive transcranial magnetic stimulation (rTMS) to induce electricity in conductors at right angles to an expanding or collapsing magnetic field (law of electromagnetic induction). This effect may be of benefit when selectively attempting to activate the inhibitory cells and fibers surrounding the minicolumn. These anatomical elements have as a geometric preference being perpendicular to the cortical surface. The basic idea is for slow rTMS to increase the activity of inhibitory cells in minicolumn which will then enhance spatial contrast needed to enhance functional discrimination in patients with autism. Results of a preliminary study seem to indicate that this is the case (Sokhadze and others 2009).

RESEARCH BEING CONDUCTED AT THE SEAVER AUTISM CENTER

BY DR. DAVID GRODBERG, DR. ALEXANDER KOLEVZON, AND DR. JOSEPH BUXBAUM

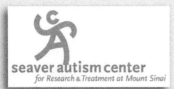

David Grodberg, M.D.

Assistant Professor of Psychiatry
Seaver Autism Center
Mount Sinai School of Medicine
New York, NY

Alex Kolevzon, M.D.
Assistant Professor of Psychiatry and Pediatrics
Clinical Director, Seaver Autism Center
Mount Sinai School of Medicine
New York, NY 10029

Joseph Buxbaum, Ph.D.
G. Harold and Leila Y. Mathers Professor of Psychiatry, Neuroscience, Genetics and Genomic Sciences
Director, Seaver Autism Center
Mount Sinai School of Medicine
New York, NY 10029

www.seaverautismcenter.org
theseavercenter@mssm.edu
(212) 241-0961

Dr. Grodberg trained at the Yale Child Study Center, where he developed expertise in developmental psychopathology in autism and other developmental disorders. In formulating a child's psychiatric diagnosis, he considers the longstanding effects of neurobiology on development as well as the day-to-day difficulties children experience in their social, communicative and emotional functioning. Dr. Grodberg also serves as the school psychiatrist for the Association for Metroarea Autistic Children. He participates as an investigator on several clinical studies at the Seaver Autism Center and was awarded an NIH National Research Service Award grant. Dr. Grodberg is conduction his own research in imaging in autism as well.

Dr. Kolevzon is the Clinical Director of the Seaver Autism Center at Mount Sinai School of Medicine. An Assistant Professor of Psychiatry and Pediatrics, Dr. Kolevzon has published numerous papers on autism as well as three books designed for medical student and resident education. He has extensive clinical expertise in the psychopharmacology of autism and related conditions, and as an investigator on many clinical trials, his research is focused on developing new pharmacological treatments. He is also extremely committed to medical student and residency training and education, and is the Associate Residency Training Director in Child and Adolescent Psychiatry at Mount Sinai. He is an active teacher, mentor, and clinical supervisor, and has received many teaching awards as well as a grant to support innovative educational endeavors.

Dr. Buxbaum is a world-renowned molecular geneticist and serves as the Director of the Seaver Autism Center. His research has focused on understanding the molecular and genetic basis of autism spectrum conditions to allow for a better understanding of etiology, and lead to the development of novel therapeutics. Dr. Buxbaum is the G. Harold and Leila Y. Mathers Professor of Psychiatry, Neuroscience, Genetics and Genomic Sciences at Mount Sinai and he has received numerous awards for his research, including most recently from the Eden Institute Foundation for his 'commitment and dedication to improving the quality of life in individuals with autism." (2008) Dr. Buxbaum has published over 100 publications in esteemed journals, and his work on autism and related conditions has been published in major journals including *Nature*, *Nature Genetics*, *Proceedings of the National Academy of Sciences*, *Molecular Psychiatry*, and *Biological Psychiatry*.

OVERVIEW

Autism research has proliferated over the past twenty years, due to the combined efforts of families, foundations, academic researchers, and the National Institutes of Health (NIH). Investigators around the world have created partnerships and consortia to advance the understanding and treatment of autism spectrum disorders (ASD). Nationally, the new administration in the White House has invested billions of dollars into research at the NIH, and recently sixty million dollars was earmarked specifically for autism research. Locally, autism consortia are being formed to prioritize critical areas for research, as task forces work to ensure that individuals with ASD receive collaborative cross-agency services statewide with emphasis on early intervention, service coordination, information dissemination, and research.

The rate at which ASD is being diagnosed has increased dramatically in recent years, as has autism awareness in the popular culture. The Centers for Disease Control reports the prevalence of ASD at 1 in 110 children [1] and the American Academy of Pediatrics is now recommending routine early screening for ASD. Screening tools have been validated and behavioral, educational, and pharmacological approaches to working with children and adults with ASD are being systematically studied across the U.S and internationally. Importantly, the Food and Drug Administration (FDA) has recently approved the use of two medications for irritability associated with autism.

During this time, the Seaver Autism Center for Research and Treatment at Mount Sinai School of Medicine in New York City has stood at the forefront of advances in autism research. This Center was founded with a grant from the Beatrice and Samuel A. Seaver Foundation in 1993 and has been generously funded in part by the foundation ever since. Beatrice Seaver passed away in 1992 and left the majority of her estate to the foundation which was instructed to use foundation assets to support medical research in New York City. The Trustees decided to create an Autism Center at Mount Sinai at a time when only a handful of foundations in the U.S. supported work in autism.

Under the direction of Dr. Joseph D. Buxbaum, today the Seaver Autism Center functions as a collaborative effort that combines psychiatry, psychology, neurology, molecular genetics, and neuroimaging into an integrated series of unique research programs. Additionally, the Seaver Autism Clinical Program provides state-of-the-art assessment and treatment in ASD. In recognition of advances in research and an everchanging field, we have also introduced cutting-edge genetic testing to our clinical practice in ASD. The center also strives to translate scientific efforts into state-of-the-art community care and has alliances with numerous support groups and community agencies in New York.

This chapter will summarize the ongoing programs at the Seaver Autism Center in genetics, experimental therapeutics, neuroimaging, as well as the Clinical Program.

GENETICS IN THE SERVICE OF PATIENT CARE

Recently, there have been major changes in the understanding of the etiology of ASD. The Seaver Autism Center has been a lead site of several large genetic consortia, including the Autism Genome Project (AGP, www.autismgenome.org/) and the Autism Case-Control (ACC) study. [2, 3] These initiatives have identified several new causal genetic loci underlying specific cases of ASD. This has led to a profound shift in our thinking, such that ASD can now be conceived of as having multiple independent causes where in many cases the cause can be largely attributed to a specific etiological event. This perspective, called the "multiple rare variant hypothesis,"[4] raises both great challenges and great opportunities. One challenge is that this complexity may necessitate studying and/

or treating different forms of ASD differently. The opportunities are that with these rare causal variants, it becomes possible to give a genetic diagnosis for some cases of ASD, to have more predictive power regarding risk of recurrence in siblings, and to think about novel targeted therapeutic approaches.

To take a concrete example from recent work carried out by Dr. Buxbaum at the Seaver Autism Center, we, together with our international collaborators, identified the cause of ASD in a boy as a novel mutation in the PTEN gene. Once this mutation was identified, it could be concluded that this was the cause of the ASD, which immediately led to genetic counseling opportunities. The mother of the child was pregnant, but after being informed by genetic counselors that the mutation in her affected child occurred spontaneously and would not recur, her concern about her unborn child was allayed. Furthermore, PTEN mutations are associated with tumor syndromes, and as a result of identifying the mutation, a surveillance program could be implemented. [5]

With these causal genetic variants, one can explicitly model them in mouse and other model systems. For example, several groups have mutated the mouse PTEN gene and studied neurobiology and behavior of these mice, which should ultimately lead to therapies based on the insights learned from these animal models. The most dramatic example of such an approach is the recent large-scale clinical trial in Fragile X Syndrome (FXS). [6] FXS accounts for approximately 2 percent of ASD cases. Detailed analysis of mouse and other models of FXS gave rise to a hypothesis that dysregulation of a glutamate receptor in the synapse underlies some of the cognitive deficits in the disorder. As a result of this hypothesis, drugs that targeted this receptor were tried in mice and other model organisms that had mutations that mimic FXS, and these drugs were shown to correct some of the cellular and behavioral deficits observed in the mice. Since January 2008, there are now large-scale clinical trials in FXS with drugs targeting these pathways.

The Laboratory of Molecular Neuropsychiatry has been studying the genetics of ASD, for over ten years. Currently, the laboratory carries out genetic analyses, identifying known and novel genetic causes for ASD in patient samples, and also makes use of mouse model systems to evaluate the mechanisms by which genetic variants can cause ASD, as well as to evaluate potential therapies. The rationale for genetic analyses in ASD is several-fold as already described. First, there is compelling evidence for a large, albeit complex, contribution of genetics to ASD. Second, in some cases, by identifying genetic causes for ASD, there can be immediate benefits to the families, including awareness of recurrence risk, and potential medical conditions to be aware of. In very rare, but growing instances, experimental therapeutics are available to individuals with specific genetic causes of ASD. Third, knowing genetic causes can lead to functional studies in experimental systems, including animal models, which can be used to develop and evaluate therapeutics.

The Laboratory of Molecular Neuropsychiatry has taken advantage of the evolving methods of genetic analyses to look at genes that increase risk for ASD (i.e., susceptibility genes) as well as gene mutations and chromosomal abnormalities that are causal for ASD. We have identified causes of ASD in individuals, including mutations that are causal for ASD (e.g., mutations in the *PTEN* gene), and chromosomal abnormalities that are causal for ASD (e.g., duplications in 15q11-13 and 22q11). [7] We have also identified risk factors for ASD, including single nucleotide polymorphisms that increase risk (e.g., the SLC25A12 genes[8]) and chromosomal changes that increase risk, including duplications in the regions of the X-chromosome. [7] Most recently, the laboratory has joined together with five other sites to conduct the largest extensive sequencing genetic study in ASD to date, involving thousands of families. For more information, please visit the National Institute of Mental Health (NIMH) sequencing network website (www. nimh.nih.gov/health/topics/autism-spectrum-disorders).

With these various causal and susceptibility loci for ASD, we are now able to create mouse model systems that have alterations in these loci and these mice can be studied for their neurodevelopment and behavior. We have implemented a large battery of behavioral and neuoroanatomical tests and the mice we have characterized to date show deficits in social communication, social memory, and learning, as well as other deficits. Ultimately these mice will represent important model systems to evaluate therapeutics. (Parts of this section on genetics were originally written by Dr. Buxbaum, printed in the Fall 2009 issue of *Autism Spectrum News,* and can be viewed for free at www.mhnews-autism.org).

The Family Studies Research Program conducts a wide range of studies investigating the familiality of autism symptom domains and performs extensive clinical evaluations in an attempt to determine how autism-related difficulties with social interactions, communication skills, and/or restricted and repetitive behaviors and interests may run in families. The program works with all available family members to assess behavioral traits that may run in families and attempt to locate genes associated with these characteristics in individuals and with autism and their families.

The Experimental Therapeutics and Clinical Trials Program at the Seaver Autism Center conducts treatment studies for children and adults that target specific symptoms of ASD, including repetitive behaviors, aggression, language delays, motor skills deficits, and social impairment. The center has a long history of conducting key clinical trials in psychopharmacological interventions as part of the NIH Studies to Advance Autism Research and Treatment (STAART) Centers Program. Our mission is to bridge the gap between new discoveries at the basic science level to the design of large clinical trials and exportation to the community. We are extremely committed to investigating best practices in the treatment of autism, and are currently participating in several national, multi-center, clinical trials of medications to treat core and associated symptom domains in autism. We are currently also conducting important studies examining novel therapeutics, including oxytocin, social skills group therapy, Luminenz-AT, and *Trichuris suis* ova.

Oxytocin

Oxytocin is a nine-amino-acid peptide and is well known for its peripheral effects on facilitating uterine contractions during parturition and milk let-down. However, oxytocin also plays an important role in social attachment and affiliative behaviors, including sexual behavior, mother-infant and adult-adult pair-bond formation, and separation distress. Moreover, oxytocin plays a role in repetitive behaviors and stress reactivity. Investigators in our center have found that synthetic oxytocin administered via intravenous infusion to adults with ASD produced significant reductions in repetitive behaviors and facilitated social cognition/memory. [9] We are currently conducting an important study examining the effect of intranasal oxytocin on complex social cognition and empathic accuracy in adults with ASD.

Social Skills Groups

This research program is designed to evaluate changes in behavior and in the brain associated with social skills treatment in children with ASD. The study compares two commonly used approaches to social skills groups—a play-based approach and a cognitive behavioral approach. We use tests of social functioning as well as functional magnetic resonance imaging (fMRI) to examine changes in both social behavior and activity in the brain following treatment.

The Neuroimaging Program is focused on the neural basis of deficits in social communication and executive functioning associated with ASD. We use fMRI to examine brain activity as individuals with ASD perform tasks related to core aspects of social cognition, including imitation, empathy, language comprehension, and emotion processing. This approach allows us to probe for differences in activation and functional organization in the autistic brain, which will ultimately inform intervention research and the development of treatment strategies. We also use fMRI in conjunction with ongoing treatment studies (both behavioral and pharmacological), which enables us to look at how brain function is affected by treatment, and perhaps also whether certain patterns of brain activity predict response to treatment. Other neuroimaging techniques, such as structural MRI, magnetic resonance spectroscopy (MRS), and diffusion tensor imaging (DTI), allow us to examine differences in brain structure, connectivity, and chemistry, respectively. Current neuroimaging studies include: The Neural Basis of Sensory and Perceptual Symptoms in Autism; Informational and Neural Bases of Empathic Accuracy in Autism Spectrum Disorder; and Anterior Cingulate and Fronto-Insular Related Brain Networks in Autism.

The Clinical Program is staffed by a team of professionals across a range of disciplines, all with specialized training in ASDs, and all of whom are actively involved in both clinical and research activities of the Seaver Center. Clinicians are selected based on unique expertise working with children, adolescents, and adults; specific expertise is available for those individuals with ASDs who have complex needs and may be considered difficult to assess and treat. Importantly, this expertise also includes the treatment of underserved populations within the autism spectrum, including very young children and high-functioning adults.

The Clinical Program provides the following outpatient services:

- *Comprehensive Assessment and Evaluation*, including diagnostic testing, genetic testing, neuropsychological testing, academic testing, speech, and psychiatric evaluations.
- *Early Intervention (EI) Evaluations*. EI evaluations are conducted for children under age three suspected of exhibiting symptoms of ASD. These evaluations will yield comprehensive reports, referrals, and recommendations for families.
- *Treatment through Psychosocial and Medication Interventions*. Treatment options will include, but are not limited to medication management, social skills groups, parent training sessions, cognitive behavior therapy, and sibling support.

- *Service Coordination* will entail helping individuals and their families attain early intervention services, facilitating school placements for children, and assisting adolescents and adults with employment and job placement.
- *Community Outreach and Training*, such as lectures and workshops provided to parent groups, agencies, and schools. An annual conference is also held each spring to address current scientific trends and discoveries

In addition, given the host of medical conditions associated with ASD, including gastrointestinal, eating/weight management, allergy, and sleep disturbance, the Seaver Autism Center Clinical Program works closely with physicians from other specialties at Mount Sinai for referrals and follow-up care.

The Seaver Autism Clinical Program is carefully integrated with our robust research portfolio, and provides access to the most recently developed genetic testing and progressive treatments delivered by experts at the leading edge of their field. At the same time, ongoing research efforts at the Seaver Center benefit from the ability to invite patients receiving treatment in the clinical program to participate in future research.

Conclusion

The Seaver Autism Center for Research and Treatment is an interdisciplinary, translational, and collaborative effort between clinicians and scientists at Mount Sinai School of Medicine and institutions across the United States and abroad. We are extremely grateful to all the individuals and families who participate in our research. Our team believes the key to success lies in translating the knowledge gained from research into developing innovative treatments that meaningfully impact individual and community care. It is our vision that using state-of-the-art molecular genetics, neurobiological, and clinical resources, we are now posed to make significant breakthroughs in identifying genetic subtypes of ASD and developing targeted treatments. For more information, please visit our website at: www.seaverautismcenter.org, or call us at (212) 241-0961

FINAL
THOUGHTS

A SOCIAL WORKER'S VIEW FROM THE TRENCHES

BY BONNIE WARING

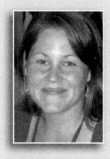

Bonnie Waring LMSW

Community and Resource Coordinator
Rebecca School
40 East 30th Street
New York, NY 10016
(212) 810-4120 ext.309
BWaring@rebeccaschool.org
BFWaring@aol.com

Mrs. Waring is a social worker and currently the community and resource coordinator of the Rebecca School in Manhattan, NY. She is a graduate of Fordham University's Graduate School of Social Service. She helped establish a grant-funded, community-based initiative serving families that have loved ones with autism in Queens, New York, along with running an after-school program for children with special needs.

E very child is unique, whether they are typically developing or have neu-rodevelopmental delays. This idea—the idea of individuality—is finally breaking through and gaining understanding in the world of interventions for autism spectrum disorders (ASDs). As a social worker in the field, I have had the privilege of visiting many treatment centers, schools, recreational facilities, and community centers, and to attend workshops and seminars, all of which related to autism. From my observations, it seems that a new way of thinking has been evolving. This new way of thinking embraces a "whole picture" vision when working with people with ASD.

This "whole picture" idea can be interpreted in many ways when applied to people with ASD. One way emphasizes looking at the body or individual as a whole—that is, acknowledging how all aspects of body functioning can be connected in a system that works together. Some treatment centers and schools are integrating this idea into practice by offering services and therapies that encompass a more dynamic view of the body. Government health agencies and many professionals agree there is no single intervention or treatment for a person with autism. Treatments or interventions have many levels, touching upon all the nuances, characteristics, medical concerns and personality traits of each individual with ASD. This individuality of treatment plans for people with ASD is crucial. Moreover, the need to involve the families with these plans is of utmost importance.

Families raising individuals with ASD play a huge part in the successful implementation of almost all of the treatment and intervention options out there in the world of autism. For example, a doctor tests for allergies in a child with ASD and finds that the child is allergic to the protein gluten. In order to successfully help the child with this medical concern, we must take the family into consideration. What type of support will this family need to successfully remove gluten from their child's diet? How much will it cost the family to purchase gluten-free items? Can they afford it? Will all members of the family need to go on the diet in order for it to be successful, for example, so that gluten-containing items are removed from the home? Will the family be able to help their child implement the gluten-free diet in other settings besides the home? These are just a few of the types of questions that are taken into consideration when professionals and families attempt to carry out an effective plan.

Another example of the importance of the family involves the implementation of school and therapeutic interventions. Although interventions that encompass this "whole picture" thinking have been around for years, the push in acceptance seems to be a more recent phenomenon. As stated above, children are distinctive in every way. Families typically know their child best, their unique likes and dislikes, their passions and their fears. These details are necessary and can have great meaning to the success of interventions, so family members offering input to school staff and therapy team members is crucial. Reciprocally, the generalization of skills learned in school and therapy sessions requires family involvement. In other words, skills learned outside of the home must be supported by the family in the home. Families need to be educated on how to support their child in this generalization process.

This idea of the family being a huge piece to each child's puzzle leads to the concept of self care. I work with many parents raising children with ASD, and I often find myself asking them: "And what about you? How are you feeling?

What are you doing to take care of yourself?" The family is a factor in all aspects of the child's life. Self care for families is essential in looking into this "whole picture" notion. Many schools and other agencies dedicated to helping people with autism offer family support groups and other outlets of self care.

I understand this notion of a push toward a more "whole picture" view of people with ASD has been presented in a general fashion and that many of these ideas of intervention and treatment have existed for years. However, it is my opinion that some of these ideas are only now beginning to be recognized as important. I also understand that differing viewpoints exist. But I see a greater acceptance of the need to build treatment and intervention plans in an individualized way, and I know the value of a team approach in achieving this. I look forward to building the foundation that supports success together.

AFTERWORD

BY TERI ARRANGA

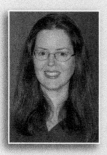

Teri Arranga

(714) 680-0792
tarranga@autismone.org
www.autismone.org
www.autismfile.com

Teri Arranga serves as the director of AutismOne, the editor of
the U.S. and Canada edition of *The Autism File* magazine, and a
program host on the VoiceAmerica Health and Wellness Channel.
She has been involved with a number of media projects, including
consulting for award-winning filmmaker Lina Moreco of Canada. Teri received the
National Autism Association's Believe Award for 2008. She has been an active advocate in
the autism community for many years, including broadcasting events in Washington, D.C.
Teri and Ed Arranga have two boys on the spectrum, Jarad and Ian.

This chapter is a paradox: an afterword, by definition, offers closing remarks
on the topic of a book. But this book is a door, and through this door we
will move forward into the future for children with autism, their siblings, and all
children.

This book illuminates treatment options. Children already affected by autism
can and do recover or significantly improve when a combination of biomedical
and behavioral/educational therapies are employed. Doreen Granpeesheh, PhD,
BCBA-D, whom you met in this book, agrees: "While behavioral/educational
and biomedical practitioners have individually helped provide successful treatment models for autism, working together, these interventions have led to the
best possibilities for successful outcome."

Along the way, we have discovered causes and the physiological conditions
underlying an autism diagnosis, and we have learned ways to support the body
in healing and restore functional skills that regressed or were delayed. And, just
as importantly, we have learned that applying this knowledge to young siblings

of affected children can stave off autism before it sets in. What does this mean for siblings and firstborns?

The door into the future is prediction and prevention. No longer must families fear. They can march confidently into the future, rehabilitating an affected child while preventing autism from developing in additional family members. For first-time parents the same bright star of hope shines.

According to Martha Herbert, MD, PhD, a pediatric neurologist at Massachusetts General Hospital/Harvard Medical School and director of the TRANSCEND Research Program:

> The future of autism will involve a much tighter integration of clinical treatment with research. Both will shift their emphasis from temporary amelioration of downstream symptoms to targeting upstream root causes with treatments that have broad and sustained impact on outcome. Research will respectfully learn from effective treatments and shed insight on their mechanisms of effectiveness. There will be a deeper understanding of how brain and sensorimotor systems interact with whole-system physiological processes, and a greater skill in knowing what to strategically target to get the maximal effect. Treatments will become less drastic, more physiologically sophisticated, more coordinated, safer and more effective. The medical system will recognize precursor signs of autism in infants in medical as well as behavioral domains, and as things to be addressed early and with determination before they get worse and tip over into autism or more severe autism. Preventive measures such as reducing toxic exposures and having healthy low-allergen, nutrient-rich diets and balanced lifestyles will move from marginal concerns to become central to the way we live so that optimal health and safety in the preconception, pregnancy, and infancy periods are supported by equal safety over the whole course of life and throughout society. Community support and care will be restored and all will be valued for their intrinsic worth.

Kenneth Bock, MD, author of *Healing the New Childhood Epidemics: Autism, ADHD, Asthma, and Allergies* (Random House, 2007), adds:

> To me, the future in autism is to, hopefully, be able to provide optimized individualized biomedical and behavioral treatments to each

affected child starting at as young an age as possible. This is predicated on increasing awareness of early subtle signs and symptoms and, thusly, initiating prompt interventions. Furthermore, increasing research and subsequent clinical approaches to the prediction and prevention of autism spectrum disorders is paramount. Recognizing the importance of environmental factors acting in concert with genetic vulnerabilities makes the addition of government and corporate leaders to the present driving force of parents, clinicians, and researchers an essential ingredient for success in this process.

David Humphrey, JD, president of The Autism Forum, speaks to us further about the hope of prediction of regressive autism and prevention with treatment after birth:

Can the debilitating effects of autism be predicted and prevented? Yes, we have all the pieces in front of us. We just need to put them together to see a future of hope honoring the sanctity of life for these children. In years past, treatment appeared to be a wacky notion. Autism was seen then as a hardwired, genetic condition that could not be treated. Today, most professionals have changed their position. Professionals now stress the importance of early intervention and treatment. The history of autism has been a series of erroneous professional beliefs corrected by the parents' determination for treatment, which has resulted in innumerable success stories. Most of these same professionals would be surprised to know that today parents with autism in their family are actively and successfully preventing new siblings from developing regressive autism. Many doctors treating children with autism are preventing most of the younger siblings from developing ASD. Even though this is anecdotal, as an attorney, I call this "direct eyewitness testimony." Direct eyewitness testimony in the law is considered very reliable, especially if numerous stories are the same from unrelated individuals. This observation needs to be part of a study to verify what is happening for the benefit of the scientific community.

Dr. Doreen Granpeesheh sums it up nicely: "Early identification of children who are at risk for autism is now a necessary goal. By identifying early signs of autism in the young siblings of affected children, practitioners will be able to focus on the early treatment of autism and, in time, bring about the prevention of autism as a whole."

———————————————∽⊙⊙∼———————————————

I join in spirit with the staff of Skyhorse Publishing in extending my best wishes for the future to you, your family, and your children. We are a team with our children: Together we will find the answers. Together we will have a voice.

Take joy in your child today.

With love, hope, and great respect,

— **Teri Arranga**

REFERENCES

THERAPIES

Chapter 2. Animal-Assisted Interventions and Persons with Autistim Spectrum Disorders, by Dr. Aubrey Fine

American Pet Products Association. (2009). *Industry Statistics & Trends*. Retrieved August 16, 2009, from: www.americanpetproducts.org/press_industrytrends .asp

Barol, J. (2006). *The Effects of AAT on a child* (unpublished thesis). New Mexico Highland University.

Dayton, L. (2010, January 23). Pets are a natural remedy for owners' health. *The Australian* (Sydney, Australia).

Delta Society. (1996). *Standards of practice in animal-assisted activities and therapy*. Bellevue, WA: Delta Society.

Fine, A. H., & Eisen, C. (2008). *Afternoons with Puppy: Inspirations from a therapist and his therapy animals*. West Lafayette, Indiana: Purdue University Press.

Friedmann, E., Locker, B. Z., & Lockwood, R. (1990). Perception of animals and cardiovascular responses during verbalization with an animal present. *Anthrozoos, 6*(2), 115–134.

Grandin, T., Fine, A., & Bowers, C. (In Press). The use of therapy animals with individuals with autism. In A. Fine (Ed.) *The Handbook on Animal-Assisted Therapy: Theoretical Foundations and Guidelines for Practice* (3rd Ed.). New York: Elsevier Science Press.

Grandin, T., & Johnson, C. (2005). *Animals in translation*. New York: Scribner.

Journal of the American Veterinary Medical Association. (1998). Statement from the committee on the human-animal bond. *Journal of the American veterinary medical association, 212*(11), 1675.

Levinson, B. (1969). *Pet Oriented Child Psychotherapy*. Springfield, IL: Charles C. Thomas Publisher.

Martin, F. & Farnum, J. (2002). Animal assisted therapy for children with pervasive developmental disorders. *Western Journal of Nursing Research, 24*, 657–670.

McNicholas, J. & Collis, G. M. (2000). Dogs as catalysts for social interactions: Robustness of the effect. *British Journal of Psychology, 91*, 61–70.

McNicholas, J., & Collis, G. (2006). Animals as supports. Insights for understanding animal assisted therapy. In A. Fine (Ed.), *Handbook On Animal Assisted Therapy* (2nd Edition, pp. 49–71). San Diego, CA: Academic Press.

Ming Lee Yeh, A. (2008). Canine AAT model for autistic children. At Taiwan International Association of Human-Animal Interaction International Conference, Tokyo Japan, 10/5–8/2008.

Odenthal, J., & Meintjes, R. (2003). Neurophysiological correlates of affiliative behavior between humans and dogs. *Veterinary Journal, 165*, 296–301.

Olmert, M. D. (2009). *Made for Each Other*. Philadelphia: De Capo Press.

Wells, D. L. (2009). The effects of animals on human health and well-being. *Journal of Social Issues, 65*(3), 523–543.

Chapter 3. Anthroposophical Curative Education and Social Therapy, by Dr. Marga Hogenboom and Paula Moraine

Autism: a Holistic Approach Bob Woodward and Dr. Marga Hogenboom; Floris Books, 2001.

Holistic Special Education Camphill Principles and Practice. edited by Robin Jackson; Floris Books, 2006.

Chapter 5. Antifungal Treatment, by Dr. Lewis Mehl-Madrona

Ashwood P, Van de Water J. (2004). Is autism an autoimmune disease? *Autoimmunology Review, 3*(7-8):557–562.

Ashwood, P., Anthony, A., Torrente, F., & Wakefield, A. J. (2004). Spontaneous mucosal lymphocyte cytokine profiles in children with autism and gastrointestinal symptoms: mucosal immune activation and reduced counter regulatory interleukin-10. *Journal of Clinical Immunology, 24*(6):664–673.

Azcarate-Peril, M. A., Bruno-Barcena, J. M., Hassan, H. M., Klaenhammer, T. R. (2006). Transcriptional and functional analysis of oxalyl-coenzyme A (CoA) decarboxylase and formyl-CoA transferase genes from Lactobacillus acidophilus. *Applied Environmental Microbiology, Mar, 72*(3): 1891–1899.

Baggio, B., Gambaro, G., Zambon, S., Marchini, F., Bassi, A., Bordin, L., Clari, G., Manzato, E. (1996). Anomalous phospholipid in n-6 polyunsaturated fatty acid composition in idiopathic calcium nephrolithiasis. *Journal of the American Society of Nephrology, Apr, 7*(4): 613–620.

Chetyrkin, S. V., Kim, D., Belmont, J. M., Scheinman, J. I., Hudson, B. G., Voziyan, P. A. (2005). Pyridoxamine lowers kidney crystals in experimental hyperoxaluria: a potential therapy for primary hyperoxaluria. *Kidney International, 67,* 53–60.

Crook W. (1999). *The Yeast Connection.* Newton, MA: Professional Books.

Edelson (2006).The Autism Yeast Connection. At www.ei-resource.org/articles/autism-articles/the-candida-yeast%11autism-connection/. Last Accessed 09 Feb 2010.

Fomina, M., Hiller, S., Charnock, J. M., Melville, K., Alexander, I. J., Gadd, G. M. (2005). Role of oxalic acid oversecretion in transformations of toxic metal minerals by Beauveria caledonica. *Applied Environmental Microbiology, Jan 71*(1): 371–381.

Ghio, A. J., Roggli, V. L., Kennedy, T. P., Piantadosi, C.A. (2000). Calcium oxalate and iron accumulation in sarcoidosis. *Sarcoidosis Vasc Diffuse Lung Dis, Jun, 17*(2): 140–150.

Great Plains Laboratory. (2008). OXALATES CONTROL IS A MAJOR NEW FACTOR IN AUTISM THERAPY. July 2008 Newsletter.

Hornig, M., Lipkin, W. I. (2001). Infectious and immune factors in the pathogenesis of neurodevelopmental disorders: epidemiology, hypotheses, and animal models. *Ment Retard Dev Disabil Res Rev 7*(3): 200–210.

Jepson, B., Johnson, J. (2007) *Changing the Course of Autism: A Scientific Approach for Parents and Physicians*. New York: Sentient Publications.

Kumar, R., Mukherjee, M., Bhandari, M., Kumar, A., Sidhu, H., Mittal, R. D. (2002). Role of Oxalobacter formigenes in calcium oxalate stone disease: a study from North India. *Eur Urol Mar, 41*(3): 318–322.

Rimland, B. (1988). Candida caused Autism? *Autism Research Review International, 2*(2): 3.

Money, J., Bobrow, N. A., Clarke, F. C. (1971). Autism and autoimmune disease: A family study, *J Autism Child Schizophr, 1*:146.

Pardo, C. A., Eberhart, C. G. (2007). The neurobiology of autism. *Brain Pathology, 17*(4):434–447.

Rosseneu, S. *Aerobic gut flora in children with autism spectrum disorder and gastrointestinal symptoms.* Presented at Defeat Autism Now! Conference. San Diego, CA, October 3, 2003.

Ruijter, G. J. G., van de Vondervoort, P. J. I., Visser, J. (1999). Oxalic acid production by Aspergillus niger: an oxalate non-producing mutant produces citric acid at pH 5 and in the presence of manganese. *Microbiology 145*: 2569–2576.

Kornblum, Lori, *Feast Without Yeast: Four Stages to Better Health*, Madison, WI: Institute of Nutrition.

Shaw, W., Kassen, E., Chaves, E. (1995). Increased urinary excretion of analogs of Krebs cycle metabolites and arabinose in two brothers with autistic features. *Clinical Chemistry 41*, 1094–1104.

Shi, L., Fatemi, S. H., Sidwell, R. W., Shirane, Y., Kurokawa, Y., Miyashita, S,, Komatsu, H., Kagawa, S. (1988). Study of inhibition mechanisms of glycosaminoglycans on calcium oxalate monohydrate crystals by atomic force microscopy. *Urol Res, 27*(6): 426–431.

Stubbs, E. G. (1976). Autistic children exhibit undetectable hemagglutination-inhibition antibody titers despite previous rubella vaccination. *J Autism Child Schizophr., 6*(3):269–274.

Stubbs, E. G., Crawford, M. L. (1977). Depressed lymphocyte responsiveness in autistic children. *Autism Child Schizophr, 7*(1):49–55.

Takeuchi, H., Konishi, T., Tomoyoshi, T. (1987). Observation on fungi within urinary stones. *Hinyokika Kiyo May; 33*(5):658–661.

Vargas, D. L., Nascimbene, C., Krishnan, C., Zimmerman, A. W., Pardo, C. A. (2005). Neuroglial activation and neuroinflammation in the brain of patients with autism. *Ann Neurol, 57*: 67–81.

Vulvar Pain Foundation. Reducing Oxalate. http://vulvarpainfoundation.org/Low_ oxalate?treatment.htm Last accessed 8 February 2010.

Wakefield, A. J., Anthony, A., Murch, S. H., et al. (2000). Enterocolitis in children with developmental disorders. *Am J Gastroenterol, 95*: 2285–2295.

Chapter 6. Applied Behavior Analysis, by Jennifer Clark

Lovaas, O. I. (February 1987). "Behavioral Treatment and Normal Educational and Intellectual Functioning in Young Autistic Children." *Journal of Consulting and Clinical Psychology, 55*(1): 3–9.

Chapter 7. Aquatic Therapy, by Andrea Salzman

1. Salzman, A. (2009). *Aquatic Therapy Boot Camp: Aquatic Therapy University.* Plymouth, MN. For more information: (800) 680-8624. www.aquatic-university.com

2. Salzman, A. New therapy pool especially for children with autism. Aquatic Therapist Blog. Plymouth, MN. July 08, 2008. www.aquatictherapist.com/index/2008/07/new-therapy-pool-especially-for-children-with-autism.html

3. Bloorview Kids Rehab. Programs & Services: Community Programs: Snoezelen. January 19, 2010. www.bloorview.ca/programsandservices/communityprograms/snoezelen.php.

4. Aquatic Therapy University. 2010 Pediatric Certification Track. Aquatic Sensory Integration for the Pediatric Client: Using Water to Modulate Vestibular, Tactile, Proprioceptive, Visual & Auditory Input. Minneapolis,MNcampus.Formoreinformation:(800)680-8624.www.aquatic-university.com

5. Aquatic Resources Network. Aquatic Sensory Integration for the Pediatric Client (Distance learning DVD and manual). Plymouth, MN. For more information: (800) 680-8624. www.aquaticnet.com.

6. AquaticNet Social Network. Autism work group. Aquatic Resources Network. Plymouth, MN. To join discussion group: www.aquatictherapist.ning.com.

7. Vonder Hulls, D. S.; Walker, L. K., Powell, J. M. (2006). Clinicians' perceptions of the benefits of aquatic therapy for young children with autism: a preliminary study. *Phys Occup Ther Pediatr*, 26(1-2):13–22.

8. Huettig, C.; Darden-Melton, B. (2004). Acquisition of aquatic skills by children with autism. *Palaestra, 20*(2):20–46.

9. Bumin, G., Uyanik, M., Yilmaz, I., Kayihan, H., Topcu, M. (2003). Hydrotherapy for Rett syndrome. *J Rehabil Med, 35*(1): 44–45.

10. Yilmaz, I., Yanardag, M., Birkan, B., Bumin, G. (2004). Effects of swimming training on physical fitness and water orientation in autism. *Pediatrics International, 46*(5):624–626.

11. Aetna. Clinical Policy Bulletin: Pool Therapy, Aquatic Therapy or Hydrotherapy (Number: 0174). Revised April 3, 2009. www.aetna.com/cpb/medical/data/100_199/0174.html.

12. Salzman, A. Coding Confusion. Advance for Physical Therapy & Rehab Medicine. Merion Publications. King of Prussia, PA. November 8, 2004. http://physical-therapy.advanceweb.com/Article/Coding-Confusion.aspx.

13. Salzman, A. A Poolside Practicum: Part I. PTs can use aquatic therapy to teach transitions in children with autism. Advance for Physical Therapy & Rehab Medicine. Merion Publications. King of Prussia, PA. October 20, 2008. http://physical-therapy.advanceweb.com/Article/A-Poolside-Practicum-Part-I.aspx.

14. Salzman, A. A Poolside Practicum: Part II: PTs can use aquatic therapy to teach transitions in children with autism. Advance for Physical Therapy & Rehab Medicine. Merion Publications. King of Prussia, PA. November 18, 2009.
http://physical-therapy.advanceweb.com/Article/A-Poolside-Practicum-Part-II.aspx.

15. Salzman, A. A Poolside Practicum: Part III: PTs can use aquatic therapy to enhance body awareness and kinesthesia. Advance for Physical Therapy & Rehab Medicine. Merion Publications. King of Prussia, PA. December 1, 2008. http://physical-therapy.advanceweb.com/Article/A-Poolside-Practicum-Part-III.aspx.

16. Salzman, A. A Poolside Practicum: Part IV: PTs can use aquatic therapy to alter tactile processing.Advance for Physical Therapy & Rehab Medicine. Merion Publications. King of Prussia, PA. December 29, 2008. http://physical-therapy.advanceweb.com/Article/A-Poolside-Practicum-Part-IV.aspx.

17. Salzman, A. A Poolside Practicum: Part V: PTs can use aquatic therapy to enhance vestibular input. Advance for Physical Therapy & Rehab Medicine. Merion Publications. King of Prussia, PA. January 27, 2009. http://physical-therapy.advanceweb.com/Article/A-Poolside-Practicum-Part-V.aspx.

18. Salzman, A. Poolside Practicum: Part VI: PTs can use aquatic therapy to offer visual challenges. Advance for Physical Therapy & Rehab Medicine. Merion Publications. King of Prussia, PA. February 24, 2009. http://physical-therapy.advanceweb.com/Article/A-Poolside-Practicum-Part-VI.aspx.

Chapter 8. Art Therapy Approaches to Treating Autism, by Nicole Martin and Dr. Donna Betts

American Art Therapy Association (2009a). *About art therapy.* Retrieved January 6, 2010 from www.arttherapy.org/aboutart.htm.

American Art Therapy Association (2009b). *How did art therapy begin?* Retrieved January 6, 2010 from www.arttherapy.org/faq.htm#howbegin.

Betts, D. J. (2003). Developing a projective drawing test: Experiences with the Face Stimulus

Assessment (FSA). *Art Therapy: Journal of the American Art Therapy Association, 20*(2), 77–82.

Betts, D. J. (2009). Introduction to the Face Stimulus Assessment (FSA). In E. Horovitz & S.

Eksten (Eds.), *Art Therapy Handbook: Assessment, Diagnosis, and Counseling.* Springfield, IL: Charles C. Thomas.

Evans, K., Dubowski, J. (2001). *Art Therapy with Children on the Autistic Spectrum: Beyond Words.* London: Jessica Kingsley.

Gilroy, A. (2006). *Art therapy: Research and Evidence-Based Practice.* London, UK: Sage Publications. (Reviews research on ASD from pages 144–146.)

Kramer, E. (1979). *Childhood and Art Therapy: Notes on Theory and Application.* New York: Schocken Books.

Martin, N. (2008). Assessing portrait drawings created by children and adolescents with autism spectrum disorder. *Art Therapy: Journal of the American Art Therapy Association, 25*(1), 15–23.

Martin, N. (2009a). *Art as an Early Intervention Tool for Children with Autism.* London: Jessica Kingsley.

Martin, N. (2009b). Art therapy and autism: Overview and recommendations. *Art Therapy: Journal of the American Art Therapy Association, 26*(4), 187–190.

Stack, M. (1998). Humpty Dumpty's shell: Working with autistic defense mechanisms in art Therapy. In M. Rees (Ed.), (1998), *Drawing on Difference: Art Therapy with People Who Have Learning Difficulties.* London: Routledge.

Other Recommending Reading

Betts, D. J. (2001). Cover story: Weekend outings provide creative outlet: Individual expresses himself through art therapy. *The Advocate: Magazine of the Autism Society of America, 34*(3), 20–21.

Betts, D. J. (2001). Special report: The art of art therapy: Drawing individuals out in creative ways. *The Advocate: Magazine of the Autism Society of America, 34*(3), 22–23, 29.

Emery, M. J. (2004). Art therapy as an intervention for autism. *Art Therapy: Journal of the American Art Therapy Association, 21,* 143–147.

Chapter 11. Center for Autism and Related Disorders, Inc. (CARD), by Dr. Doreen Granpeesheh, Dr. Jonathan Tarbox, and Dr. Michele Bishop

Howard, J. S. (2006). Paper presented at the Annual Meeting of the California State University, Fresno, Applied Behavior Analysis Conference.

Stokes, T. F., & Baer, D. M. (1977). An implicit technology of generalization. *Journal of Applied Behavior Analysis, 10,* 349–367.

Chapter 13. Chelation: Removal of Toxic Metals, by Dr. James Adams

J. B. Adams, M. Baral, E. Geis, J. Mitchell, J. Ingram, A. Hensley, I. Zappia, S. Newmark, E. Gehn, R.A. Rubin, K. Mitchell, J. Bradstreet, J.M. El-Dahr, "The Severity of Autism Is Associated with Toxic Metal Body Burden and Red Blood Cell Glutathione Levels," *Journal of Toxicology,* vol. 2009, Article ID 532640, 7 pages, 2009. www.hindawi.com/journals/jt/contents.html

J. B. Adams, M. Baral, E. Geis, J. Mitchell, J. Ingram, A. Hensley, I. Zappia, S. Newmark, E. Gehn, R.A. Rubin, K. Mitchell, J. Bradstreet, J.M. El-Dahr Safety and Efficacy of Oral DMSA Therapy for Children with Autism Spectrum Disorders: Part A - Medical Results BMC Clinical Pharmacology 2009, 9:16 www.biomedcentral.com/1472-6904/9/16

J. B. Adams, M. Baral, E. Geis, J. Mitchell, J. Ingram, A. Hensley, I. Zappia, S. Newmark, E. Gehn, R.A. Rubin, K. Mitchell, J. Bradstreet, J.M. El-Dahr Safety and Efficacy of Oral DMSA Therapy for Children with Autism Spectrum Disorders: Part B - Behavioral Results BMC Clinical Pharmacology 2009, 9:17 www.biomedcentral.com/1472-6904/9/17

Bernard S et al, Autism: a novel form of mercury poisoning. *Med Hypotheses.* 2001 Apr;56(4):462–71.

James et al, Metabolic endophenotype and related genotypes are associated with oxidative stress in children with autism. *Am J Med Genet B Neuropsychiatr Genet.* 2006 Dec 5;141(8):947–56.

Nataf R et al., Porphyrinuria in childhood autistic disorder: implications for environmental toxicity. *Toxicol Appl Pharmacol.* 2006 Jul 15;214(2):99–108

Bradstreet J., Geier DA, Kartzinel JJ, Adams JB, Geier MR, A Case-Control Study of Mercury Burden in Children with Autistic Spectrum Disorders, *J. Am. Phys. Surg* 8(3) 2003 76–79.

Holmes AS, Blaxill MF, Haley BE. Reduced levels of mercury in first baby haircuts of autistic children. *Int J Toxicol.* 2003 Jul-Aug;22(4):277–85.

Windham et al, Autism spectrum disorders in relation to distribution of hazardous air pollutants in the San Francisco bay area. Environ Health Perspect. 2006 Sep;114(9):1438-44.

Palmer RF et al., Environmental mercury release, special education rates, and autism disorder: an ecological study of Texas. Health Place. 2006 Jun;12(2):203–9.

Chapter 15. Craniosacral and Chiropractic Therapy, by Dr. Charles Chapple

Goddard, Sally. (2005). *Reflexes, Learning and Behavior, a Window into the Child's Mind.* Eugene, OR: Fern Ridge Press.

Chapple, Charles W., D.C., F.I.C.P.A. (2007). Making the Connection Between … Primitive Reflexes, Sensory Processing Disorders and Chiropractic Solutions. *SI Focus Magazine Winter 2007,* 8–9.

Chapple, Charles W.D.C., F.I.C.P.A. (2005). A Biomechanical Approach for the Improvement of…Sensory, Motor and Neurological Function with Individuals with Autistic Spectrum Disorder (ASD), Pervasive Developmental Delay (PDD), and Sensory Processing Disorder (SPD). *SI Focus Magazine Autumn 2005,* 6–9.

Dodd, Susan B. A. (2005). *Understanding Autism.* Elsevier Australia.

Koester, Cecilia, M.Ed. (2006). *Movement Based Learning…For Children of All Abilities,* Reno, NV: Movement Based Learning Inc.

Kranowitz, Carol Stock, M.A. (2005). *The Out of Sync Child…Recognizing and coping with Sensory Processing Disorder,* New York: Penguin Group.

Melillo, Robert, DC. (2009). *Disconnected Kids,* New York: Perigee.

Upledger, John E., D.O., F.A.A.O. and Jon D. Vredevoogd, M.F.A. (1983). *Craniosacral Therapy,* Seattle: Eastland Press.

Williams, Stephen D.C., F.C.C. (paed), F.C.C. (2005). *Pregnancy and Paediatrics: A Chiropractic Approach.* Southampton, UK: Stephen P. Williams.

Chapter 16. Dance/Movement Therapy, by Mariah Meyer LeFeber

Adler, J. (2003). From autism to the discipline of authentic movement. *American Journal of Dance Therapy, 25*(1), 5–16.

American Dance Therapy Association. (2008). Retrieved October 28, 2008 from www.adta.org/about/factsheet.cfm.

Berrol, C. (2006). Neuroscience meets dance/movement therapy: Mirror neurons, the therapeutic process and empathy. *The Arts in Psychotherapy, 33,* 302–315.

Canner, N. (1968). *And a Time to Dance.* Boston: Beacon Press.

Erfer, T. (1995). Treating children with autism in a public school system. In F. J. Levy, J. P. Fried, & F. Leventhal (Eds.), *Dance and Other Expressive Arts therapies* (pp. 191–211). New York: Routledge.

Hartshorn, K., Olds, L., Field, T., Delage, J., Cullen, C., & Escalona, A. (2001). Creative movement therapy benefits children with autism. *Early Child Development & Care, 166,* 1–5.

Kestenberg, J. A., Loman, S., Lewis, P., & Sossin, K. M. (1999). *The meaning of movement: Developmental and clinical perspectives of the Kestenberg Movement Profile.* New York: Brunner-Routledge.

Levy, F. (2005). *Dance Movement Therapy: A Healing Art.* Reston, VA: National Dance Association.

Loman, S. (1995). The case of Warren: A KMP approach to autism. In F. J. Levy, J. P. Fried, & F. Leventhal (Eds.), *Dance and Other Expressive Arts Therapies: When Words Are Not Enough* (pp. 213–224). New York: Routledge.

Meekums, B. (2002). *Dance Movement Therapy: A Creative Psychotherapeutic Approach.* London: Sage Publications.

Wolf-Schein, E., Fisch, G., & Cohen, I. (1985). A study of the use of nonverbal systems in the differential diagnosis of autistic, mentally retarded and fragile x individuals. *American Journal of Dance Therapy, 8*(1985), 67–80.

Chapter 18. Dietary Interventions for Autism, by Karyn Seroussi and Lisa Lewis, Ph.D.

1. MacCabe DF, et al. "Neurobiological effects of intraventricular propionic acid in rats: possible role of short chain fatty acids on the pathogenesis and characteristics of autism spectrum disorders." *Behav Brain Res.* 2007 Jan 10;176(1):149–69.

2. Jyonouchi H, Geng L, Ruby A, Zimmerman-Bier B. "Dysregulated innate immune responses in young children with autism spectrum disorders: their relationship to gastrointestinal symptoms and dietary intervention." *Neuropsychobiology.* 2005;51(2):77–85.

3. Jyonouchi H, Geng L, Ruby A, Reddy C, Zimmerman-Bier B. "Evaluation of an association between gastrointestinal symptoms and cytokine production against common dietary proteins in children with autism spectrum disorders." *J Pediatr.* 2005 May;146(5):605–10.

4. Vojdani A, O'Bryan T, Green JA, McCandless J, Woeller KN, Vojdani E, Nourian AA, Cooper EL. "Immune response to dietary proteins, gliadin and cerebellar peptides in children with autism." *Nutr Neurosci.* 2004 Jun;7(3):151–61.

5. Reichelt KL, Knivsberg. "Can the pathophysiology of autism be explained by the nature of the discovered urine peptides?" *AM. Nutr Neurosci.* 2003 Feb;6(1):19–28. Review.

6. Buie T, Winter H, Kushak, R. "Preliminary findings in gastrointestinal investigation of autistic patients." 2002. Harvard University and Mass General Hospital.

7. Millward C, Ferriter M, Calver S, Connell-Jones G. "Gluten- and casein-free diets for autism spectrum disorder." *Cochrane Database Syst Rev.* 2004;(2):CD003498.

8. Garvey J. "Diet in autism and associated disorders." *J Fam Health Care* 2002;12(2):34–8.

9. Knivsberg AM, Reichelt KL, Hoien T, Nodland M. "A randomised, controlled study of dietary intervention in autistic syndromes." *Nutr Neurosci* 2002 Sep;5(4):251–61.

10. Lucarelli S et al. "Food allergy and infantile autism." *Panminerva Med.* 1995 Sep;37(3):137–41.

11. *Summary of Biomedical Treatments for Autism* by James B. Adams, Ph.D., April 2007, published online at http://autism.asu.edu.

12. According to the Food Allergy & Anaphylaxis Network, eight foods account for 90% of all food allergies. These include milk, egg, peanut, tree nuts (walnuts, cashews, etc.), fish, shellfish, soy and wheat.

13. Oski, Frank A., MD1996 *Don't Drink Your Milk.* Teacher Services, Inc.

14. Iacono G, Cavataio F, Montalto G, Soresi M, Notarbartolo A, Carroccio A. Persistent cow's milk protein intolerance in infants: the changing faces of the same disease. *Clin Exp Allergy* 1998 Jul;28(7):817–23.

Chapter 19. Drama Therapy, by Sally Bailey

Attwood, T. (1998). *Asperger's syndrome: A guide for parents and professionals.* London: Jessica Kingsley.

Bailey, S. (2009a). Performance in drama therapy. In D. R. Johnson & R. Emunah (Eds.), *Current Approaches in Drama Therapy,* 2 ed. (pp. 374–392) Springfield, IL: Charles C. Thomas Publisher.

Bailey, S. (2009b). Theoretical reasons and practical applications of drama therapy with clients on the autism spectrum. In S.L. Brooke (Ed.), *The Use of the Creative Therapies with Autism Spectrum Disorders* (pp. 303–318). Springfield, IL: Charles C. Thomas Publisher.

Bailey, S. (2006). Ancient and modern roots of drama therapy. In S. L. Brooke (Ed.), *Creative Arts Therapies Manual: A Guide to the History, Theoretical Approaches, Assessment, and Work with Special Populations of Art, Play, Dance, Music, Drama, and Poetry Therapy* (pp. 214–222). Springfield, IL: Charles C. Thomas Publisher.

Bolding, G. (2007, November 9) Student overcomes autism with acting. *The Kansas State Collegian*, p. 3.

Blair, R. (2008). *The Actor, Image, and Action: Acting and Cognitive Neuroscience.* London: Routledge.

Grandin, T. (2002). Teaching tips for children and adults with autism. [Electronic Version]. *Center for the Study of Autism.* Retrieved on August 2, 2005 from www.autism.org/temple/tips.html.

Iacoboni, M. & Dapretto, M. (2006, December 7). The mirror neuron system and the consequences of its dysfunction. *Nature Reviews: Neuroscience,* 942–951, Retrieved July 27, 2008 from www.csulb.edu/~cwallis/cscenter/mnc/abstracts/nn2024.pdf.

Iacoboni, M., Molnar-Szacks, I., Gallese, V., Buccino, G., Mazziotta, J.C., & Rizzolatti, G. (2005). Grasping the intentions of others with one's own mirror neuron system. *PLoS Biology, 3*(3) 79e. Retrieved January 23, 2006 from www.plosbiology.org.

Jensen, E. with Dabney, M. (2000). *Learning Smarter: The New Science of Teaching.* San Diego: The Brain Store.

McConachie, B. (2008). *Engaging Audiences: A Cognitive Approach to Spectating in the Theatre.* New York: Palgrave Macmillan. North Shore ARC brochure: *The Spotlight Program: Innovative drama-based social pragmatics for students ages 6–22.* Retrieved January 11, 2009 from http://spotlightprogram.com/Documents/Spotlight%20Brochure.pdf.

Posner, M., Rothbart, M. K., Sheese, B. E., & Kieras, J. (2008). How arts training influences cognition. In C. Ashbury & B. Rich (Eds.), *Learning, Arts, and the Brain* (pp. 1–10). New York: Dana Press.

Oberman, L. M. & Ramachandran, V. S. (2007). The simulating social mind: The role of the mirror neuron system and simulation in the social and communicative deficits of autism spectrum disorders. *Psychological Bulletin, 133*(2), 310–327.

Ramachandran, V. S. & Oberman, L. M. (2006, November). Broken mirrors: A theory of autism. *Scientific American,* 63–69.

Regan, T. (Director). (2007). *Autism: The Musical.* [Motion picture]. United States: Bunim-Murray Productions.

Chapter 20. Early Start Denver Model, by Dr. Sally J. Rogers

1. Rogers, S.J., & Dawson, G. (2009). *Play and engagement in early autism: The Early Start Denver Model.* NY: Guilford.

2. Rogers, S. J., Herbison, J., Lewis, H., Pantone, J., & Reis, K. (1986). An approach for enhancing the symbolic, communicative, and interpersonal functioning of young children with autism and severe emotional handicaps. *Journal of the Division of Early Childhood, 10*(2), 135–148.

3. Rogers, S. J., & Lewis, H. (1989). An effective day treatment model for young children with pervasive developmental disorders. *Journal of the American Academy of Child and Adolescent Psychiatry, 28,* 207–214.

4. Stern, D. (1985). *The interpersonal world of the human infant.* New York: Basic Books.

5. Koegel, R.L., O'Dell, M., & Dunlap, G. (1988). Producing speech use in nonverbal autistic children by reinforcing attempts. *Journal of Autism and Developmental Disorders, 18(4)*, 525–538.

6. Schreibman, L., & Pierce, K. (1993). Achieving greater generalization of treatment effects in children with autism: Pivotal response training and self-management. *Clinical Psychologist, 46*, 184–191.

7. Dawson, G., Webb, S. J., Wijsman, E., Schellenberg, G. D., Estes, A., Munson, J. et al. (2005). Neurocognitive and electrophysiological evidence of altered face processing in parents of children with autism: Implications for a model of abnormal development of social brain circuitry in autism. *Development and Psychopathology, 17, 679–697*.

8. Rogers, S. J., & DiLalla, D. L. (1991). A comparative study of the effects of a developmentally based preschool curriculum on young children with autism and young children with other disorders of behavior and development. *Topics in Early Childhood Special Education, 11(2)*, 29–47.

9. Rogers, S. J., Lewis, H. C., & Reis, K. (1987). An effective procedure for training early special education teams to implement a model program. *Journal of the Division of Early Childhood, 11(2)*, 180–188.

10. Rogers, S. J., Hayden, D., Hepburn, S., Charlifue-Smith, R., Hall, T., & Hayes, A. (2006). Teaching young nonverbal children with autism useful speech: A pilot study of the Denver Model and PROMPT interventions. *Journal of Autism and Developmental Disorders, 36(8)*, 1007–1024.

11. Vismara, L.A., Colombi, C., & Rogers, S.J. (2009). Can one hour per week of therapy lead to lasting changes in young children with autism. *Autism, 13(1)*, 93–115.

12. Dawson, G., Rogers, S., Munson, J., Smith, M., Jamie, W., Greenson, J., et al. (2009). Randomized controlled trial of the Early Start Denver Model: A developmental behavioral intervention for toddlers with autism: Effects on IQ, adaptive behavior, and autism diagnosis. *Pediatrics, doi/10.1542/peds.2009–0958*.

13. Koegel, R.L., Koegel, L.K., & Surratt, A. (1992). Language intervention and disruptive behavior in preschool children with autism. *Journal of Autism and Developmental Disorders, 22(2)*, 141–153.

14. Koegel, L.K., Koegel, R.L., Hurley, C., & Frey, W.D. (1992). Improving social skills and disruptive behavior in children with autism through self-management. *Journal of Applied Behavior Analysis, 25(2)*, 341–353.

15. Ratner, N., & Bruner, J. (1978). Games, social exchange, and the acquisition of language. *Journal of Child Language, 5*, 391–402.

Chapter 22. Enzymes, by Dr. Devin Houston

1. Ehren, J., Moron, B., Martin, E., Bethune, M. T., Gray, G. M., Khosla, C. (2009). A food-grade enzyme preparation with modest gluten detoxification properties. *PLos ONE 4*(7): e6313.

2. Scalbert, A., Johnson, I. T., Saltmarsh, M. (2005). Polyphenols: antioxidants and beyond. *Am. J. Clin. Nutr, 81*(S1): 21.

3. Scalbert, A., Williamson. G. (2000). Dietary intake and bioavailability of polyphenols. *J. Nutr. 130*: 2073S.

Chapter 23. Equine Therapy, by Franklin Levinson and Dr. Nicola Start

Brown, Sue-Ellen. 2004. "The Human-animal bond and self psychology: Toward a new understanding." *Society & Animals* 12:1. PP. 67-86

Ewing, C.A., P.M. MacDonald, M. Taylor, and M.J. Bowers. "Equine-Facilitated Learning for Youths with Severe Emotional Disorders: A Quantitative and Qualitative Study." *Child and Youth Care Forum 36, no. 1* (2007)

Karol, J. "Applying a Traditional Individual Psychotherapy Model to Equine-Facilitated Psychotherapy (EFP): Theory and Method." *Clinical Child Psychology and Psychiatry 12, no. 1,* 2007: 77.

Latimer & Burke (2009) [TK]

McCormick A, McCormick M. *Horse Sense and the Human Heart: What Horses Can Teach Us About Trust, Bonding, Creativity and Spirituality.* Deerfield Beach, Florida: Health Communications, Inc. 1997.

McCulloch, Leonard J. "Horse Whispering, Psychotherapy, and Traumatic Brain Injury" Outlook Volume 2, Issue 1.Winter 2001

Melson G.F. *Why the wild things are: Animals in the lives of children.* Cambridge and London University Harvard Press.2001:115.

Nebbe, 2003 [TK]

Wolf, E. S. *Treating the Self: Elements of Clinical Self Psychology.* New York/London: The Guilford Press, 1988

Chapter 25. Food Selectivity and Other Feeding Disorders in Autism, by Dr. Petula Vaz and Dr. Cathleen Piazza

Bachmeyer, M. H., Piazza, C. C., Fredrick, L. D., Reed, G. K., Rivas, K. D., & Kadey, H. J. (2009). Functional analysis and treatment of multiply controlled inappropriate mealtime behavior. *J Appl Behav Anal, 42*(3): 641–658.

Cohen, S. A., Piazza, C. C., & Navathe, A. Feeding and nutrition. In: Crocker ILRAC (Ed.). (2006). *Medical Care for Children and Adults with Developmental Disabilities.* Baltimore: Paul H. Brooks Publishing Co.

Freeman, K. A., Piazza, C. C. (1998). Combining stimulus fading, reinforcement, and extinction to treat food refusal. *J Appl Behav Anal, 31*:691–694.

Gulotta, C. S., Piazza, C. C., Patel, M. R., Layer, S. A. (2005). Using food redistribution to reduce packing in children with severe food refusal. *J Appl Behav Anal, 38*:39–50.

Keen, D. V. (2008). Childhood autism, feeding problems and failure to thrive in early infancy. *Eur Child Adolesc Psychiatry, 17*: 209–216.

Kelley, M. E., Piazza, C.C., Fisher, W. W., Oberdorff, A. J. (2003). Acquisition of cup drinking using previously refused foods as positive and negative reinforcement. *J Appl Behav Anal, 36*: 89–93.

Kerwin, M. E. (1999). Empirically supported treatments in pediatric psychology: severe feeding problems. *J Pediatr Psychol, 24*: 193–214; discussion 215–216.

Kodak, T., Piazza, C. C. (2008). Assessment and behavioral treatment of feeding and sleeping disorders in children with autism spectrum disorders. *Child and Adolescent Psychiatric Clinics of North America, 17*: 887–905.

Laud, R. B., Girolami, P.A. , Boscoe, J. H., Gulotta, C. S. (2009). Treatment outcomes for severe feeding problems in children with autism spectrum disorder. *Behavior Modification, 33*: 520–536.

Mueller, M. M., Piazza, C. C., Moore, J. W., et al. (2003). Training parents to implement pediatric feeding protocols. *J Appl Behav Anal, 36*: 545–562.

Mueller, M. M., Piazza, C. C., Patel, M. R., Kelley, M. E., Pruett, A. (2004). Increasing variety of foods consumed by blending nonpreferred foods into preferred foods. *J Appl Behav Anal, 37*: 159–170.

Munk, D. D., Repp, A.C. (1994). Behavioral assessment of feeding problems of individuals with severe disabilities. *J Appl Behav Anal, 27*: 241–250.

Najdowski, A. C., Wallace, M. D., Doney, J. K., Ghezzi, P. M. (2003). Parental assessment and treatment of food selectivity in natural settings. *J Appl Behav Anal, 36*: 383–386.

Patel, M. R., Piazza, C. C., Kelly, L., Ochsner, C. A., Santana, C. M. (2001). Using a fading procedure to increase fluid consumption in a child with feeding problems. *J Appl Behav Anal, 34*: 357–360.

Patel, M. R., Piazza, C. C., Layer, S. A., Coleman, R., Swartzwelder, D. M. (2005). A systematic evaluation of food textures to decrease packing and increase oral intake in children with pediatric feeding disorders. *J Appl Behav Anal, 38*: 89–100.

Patel, M. R., Piazza, C. C., Santana, C. M., Volkert, V. M. (2002). An evaluation of food type and texture in the treatment of a feeding problem. *J Appl Behav Anal, 35*: 183–186.

Patel, M. R., Reed, G. K., Piazza, C. C., Bachmeyer, M. H., Layer, S, A., Pabico, R. S. (2006). An evaluation of a high-probability instructional sequence to increase acceptance of food and decrease inappropriate behavior in children with pediatric feeding disorders. *Res Dev Disabil, 27*: 430–442.

Piazza, C. C., Fisher, W. W., Brown, K.A., et al. (2003). Functional analysis of inappropriate mealtime behaviors. *J Appl Behav Anal, 36*:187–204.

Piazza, C. C., Patel, M. R., Gulotta, C. S., Sevin, B. M., Layer, S. A. On the relative contributions of positive reinforcement and escape extinction in the treatment of food refusal. *J Appl Behav Anal, 36*: 309–324.

Piazza, C. C., Patel, M. R., Santana, C. M., Goh, H. L., Delia, M. D., Lancaster, B. M. (2002). An evaluation of simultaneous and sequential presentation of preferred and nonpreferred food to treat food selectivity. *J Appl Behav Anal, 35*: 259–270.

Reed, G. K., Piazza, C. C., Patel, M. R., et al. (2004). On the relative contributions of noncontingent reinforcement and escape extinction in the treatment of food refusal. *J Appl Behav Anal, 37*:27–42.

Rommel, N., De Meyer, A. M., Feenstra, L., & Veereman-Wauters, G. (2003). The complexity of feeding problems in 700 infants and young children presenting to a tertiary care institution. *Journal of Pediatric Gastroenterology and Nutrition, 37*: 75–82.

Sevin, B.M., Gulotta, C.S., Sierp, B. J., Rosica, L. A., Miller, L. J. (2002). Analysis of response covariation among multiple topographies of food refusal. *J Appl Behav Anal, 35*: 65–68.

Twachtman-Reilly, J., Amaral, S. C., Zebrowski, P. P. (2008). Addressing feeding disorders in children on the autism spectrum in school-based settings: Physiological and behavioral issues. *Language, Speech, and Hearing Services in Schools, 39*: 261–272.

Volkert, V. M., Piazza, C. C. (in press). Empirically supported treatments for pediatric feeding disorders. In P. Sturmey and M. Herson (Eds.), *Handbook of Evidence-Based Practice in Clinical Psychology*. Honoken, NJ: Wiley.

Werle, M. A., Murphy, T.B., Budd, K. S. (2002). Treating chronic food refusal in young children: Home-based parent training. *J Appl Behav Anal, 26*: 421–433.

Chapter 26. Gastrointestinal Disease: Emerging Concensus, by Dr. Arthur Krigsman

Afzal N, Murch S, Thirrupathy K, Berger L, Fagbemi A, Heuschkel R. Constipation with acquired megarectum in children with autism. Pediatrics. 2003 Oct;112(4):939–42.

Ashwood P, Wakefield AJ. Immune activation of peripheral blood and mucosal CD3+ lymphocyte cytokine profiles in children with autism and gastrointestinal symptoms. J Neuroimmunol. 2006 Apr;173(1-2):126–34.

Balzola F, Barbon V, Repici A, Rizzetto M. Panenteric IBD-like disease in a patient with regressive autism shown for the first time by the wireless capsule enteroscopy: another piece in the jigsaw of this gut-brain syndrome? Am J Gastro. 2005; 979–981.

Balzola F, Daniela C, Repici A, Barbon V, Sapino A, Barbera C, Calvo PL, Gandione M, Rigardetto R, Rizzetto M. Autistic enterocolitis: confirmation of a new inflammatory bowel disease in an Italian cohort of patients. Gastroenterology. 2005;128:Suppl.2;A–303.

Bolte ER. Autism and Clostridium tetani. Med Hypotheses. 1998 Aug;51(2):133–44.

Buie T, Campbell D, Fuchs G, Furuta G, Levy J, VandeWater J, Whitaker A, Atkins D, Bauman M, Beaudet A, Carr E, Gershon M, Hyman S, Jirapinyo P, Jyonouchi H, Kooros K, Kushak R, Levitt P, Levy S, Lewis J, Murray K, Natowicz M, Sabra A, Wershil B, Weston S, Zeltzer L, Winter H. Evaluation, Diagnosis, and Treatment of Gastrointestinal Disorders in Individuals With ASDs: A Consensus Report Pediatrics, Jan 2010; 125: S1 - S18.

Buie T, Fuchs G, Furuta G, Kooros K, Levy J, Lewis J, Wershil B, Winter H. Recommendations for Evaluation and Treatment of Common Gastrointestinal Problems in Children With ASDs Pediatrics, Jan 2010; 125: S19 - S29.

D'Eufemia P, Celli M, Finocchiaro R, Pacifico L, Viozzi L, Zaccagnini M, Cardi E, Giardini O. Abnormal intestinal permeability in children with autism. Acta Paediatr. 1996 Sep;85(9):1076–9.

Finegold SM, Molitoris D, Song Y, Liu C, Vaisanen ML, Bolte E, McTeague M, Sandler R, Wexler H, Marlowe EM, Collins MD, Lawson PA, Summanen P, Baysallar M, Tomzynski TJ, Read E, Johnson E, Rolfe R, Nasir P, Shah H, Haake DA, Manning P, Kaul A. Gastrointestinal microflora studies in late onset autism. Clin Infect Dis. 2002 Sep 1;35(Suppl 1):S6–S16.

Furlano RI, Anthony A, Day R, Brown A, McGavery L, Thomson MA, Davies SE, Berelowitz M, Forbes A, Wakefield AJ, Walker-Smith JA, Murch SH. Colonic CD8 and gamma delta T-cell infiltration with epithelial damage in children with autism. Pediatrics 2001;138:366–72.

Gonzalez L, Lopez K, Navarro D, Negron L, Flores L, Rodriguez R, Martinez M, Sabra A. Endoscopic and Histological Characteristics of the digestive mucosa in autistic children with gastrointestinal symptoms. Arch Venez Pueric Pediatr 69;1:19–25.

Horvath K, Papadimitriou JC, Rabazlan A. Gastrointestinal abnormalities in children with autistic disorder. J Pediatr 1999, 135:559–563.

Horvath K, Perman JA. Autistic disorder and gastrointestinal disease. Curr Opin Pediatr. 2002 Oct;14(5):583–7.

Jyonouchi, H, Geng, L, Ruby, A and Zimmerman-Bier, B. Dysregulated innate immune responses in young children with autism spectrum disorders: their relationship to gastrointestinal symptoms and dietary intervention. Neuropsychobiology, 2005;51(2):77-85.

Jyonouchi, H, Sun, S and Le, H. Proinflammatory and regulatory cytokine production associated with innate and adaptive immune responses in children with autism spectrum disorders and developmental regression. Journal of Neuroimmunology, 2001;120(1-2):170-179.

Knivsberg AM, Reichelt KL, Hoien T, Nodland M. A randomised, controlled study of dietary intervention in autistic syndromes. Nutr Neurosci. 2002 Sep;5(4): 251–61.

Knivsberg AM, Reichelt KL, Nodland M, Hoein T: Autistic Syndromes and Diet: a follow-up study. Scandinavian Journal of Educational Research 1995; 39: 223–236.

Knivsberg AM, Reichelt KL, Nodland M. Reports on dietary intervention in autistic disorders. Nutr Neurosci. 2001;4(1): 25–37.

Krigsman A, Boris M, Goldblatt A, Stott C. Clinical Presentation and Histologic Findings at Ileocolonoscopy in Children with Autistic Spectrum Disorder and Chronic gastrointestinal Symptoms. Autism Insights 2010:2 1–11.

Kuddo T, Nelson KB. How common are gastrointestinal disorders in children with autism. Curr Opin Pediatr 2003: 15(3); 339–343.

Kushak R, Winter H, Farber N, Buie T. Gastrointestinal symptoms and intestinal disaccharidase activities in children with autism. Abstract of presentation to the North American Society of Pediatric Gastroenterology, Hepatology, and Nutrition, Annual Meeting, October 20-22, 2005, Salt Lake City, Utah.

Melmed RD, Schneider CK, Fabes RA. Metabolic markers and gastrointestinal symptoms in children with autism and related disorders. J Pediatr Gastroenterol Nutr 2000:31(suppl 2)S31–32.

Parracho HM, Bingham MO, Gibson GR, McCartney AL. Differences between the gut microflora of children with autistic spectrum disorders and that of healthy children. J Med Microbiol. 2005 Oct;54(Pt 10):987–91.

Sandler RH, Finegold SM, Bolte ER, Buchanan CP, Maxwell AP, Vaisanen ML, Nelson MN, Wexler HM. Short-term benefit from oral vancomycin treatment of regressive-onset autism. J Child Neurol. 2000 Jul;15(7):429–35.

Song Y, Liu C, Finegold SM. Real-time PCR quantitation of clostridia in feces of autistic children. Appl Environ Microbiol. 2004 Nov;70(11):6459–65.

Torrente F, Machado N, Perez-Machado M, Furlano R, Thomson M, Davies S, Wakefield AJ, Walker-Smith JA, Murch SH. Enteropathy with T cell infiltration and epithelial IgG deposition in autism. Mol Psychiatry. 2002;7:375–382.

Torrente F, Anthony A. Heuschkel, RB, Thomson, M, Ashwood, P, Murch S. Focal-enhanced gastritis in regressive autism with features distinct from Crohn's disease and helicobacter Pylori gastritis. Am J Gastroenterol 2004 Apr;99(4):598–605.

Valicenti-McDermott M, McVicar K, Rapin I, Wershil BK, Cohen H, Shinnar S. Frequency of gastrointestinal symptoms in children with autistic spectrum disorders and association with family history of autoimmune disease. J Dev Behav Pediatr. 2006 Apr;27(2 Suppl):S128–36.

Wakefield AJ, Murch SH, Anthony A et al. Ileal-lymphoid nodular hyperplasia non-specific colitis and pervasive developmental disorder in children. Lancet. 1998;351:637–41.

Wakefield, AJ, Anthony, A, Murch, S, et al. Enterocolitis in Children with Developmental Disorders. American Journal of Gastroenterology, 2000;95(9):2285-2295.

Chapter 27. Helminthic Therapy, by Judith Chinitz

Ashwood, P., Anthony, A., Torrente, F., Wakefield, A. J. (2004). Spontaneous mucosal lymphocyte cytokine profiles in children with autism and gastrointestinal symptoms: mucosal immune activation and reduced counter regulatory interleukin-10. *Journal of Clinical Immunology,* 24(6): 664–673.

Ashwood, P., Wakefield, A. J. (2006). Immune activation of peripheral blood and mucosal CD3+ lymphocyte cytokine profiles in children with autism and gastrointestinal symptoms. *Journal of Neuroimmunology, 173*(1-2):126–134.

Bashir, M. E. H., Andersen, P., Fuss, I., Shi, H. N., Nagler-Anderson, C. (2002). An enteric helminth infection protects against an allergic response to dietary antigen. *The Journal of Immunlogy, 169*: 3284–3292.

Becker, K. (2007). Autism, asthma, inflammation, and the hygiene hypothesis. *Medical Hypothesis,* doi:10.1016/j.mehy.2007.02.019.

Correale, J., Farez, M. (2007). Association between parasite infection and immune responses in multiple sclerosis. *Annals of Neurology, 61*: 97–108.

Croonenberghs, J., Bosmans, E., Deboutte, D., Kenis, G., Maes, M. (2002). Activation of the inflammatory response system in autism. *Neuropsychobiology, 45*(1):1–6.

Croese, J., O'Neil, J., Masson, J., Cooke, S., Melrose, W., Pritchard, D. Speare, R., (2006). A proof of concept study establishing Necator americanus in Crohn's patients and reservoir donors. *Gut, 55*: 136–137.

Elliott, D. E., Summers, R. W., Weinstock, J. V. (2007). Helminths as governors of immune-mediated inflammation. *International Journal of Parasitology, 37*(5): 457–464.

Elliott, D. E., Summers, R. W., Weinstock, J. V. (2005). Helminths and the modulation of mucosal inflammation. *Current Opinion in Gastroenterology, 21*: 51–58.

Feillet, H., Bach, J.F. (2004). Increased incidence of inflammatory bowel disease: the price of the decline of infectious burden? Current Opinion in Gastroenterology:20(6):560–4.

Fumagalli, M., Pozzoli, U., Cagliani, R., Comi, G.P., Stefania, R., Clerici, M., Bresolin, N., Sironi, M. (2009). Parasites represent a major selective force for interleukin genes and shape the genetic predisposition to autoimmune conditions. *Journal of Experimental Medicine, 206*(6): 1395–1408.

Gupta, S., Aggarwal, S., Rashanravan, B., Lee, T. (1998). Th1- and Th2-like cytokines in CD4+ and CD8+ cells in autism. *Journal of Neuroimmunlogy, 85*(1): 106–109.

Hamilton, G. (2008). Why we need germs. The Ecologist Report. Retrieved August 4, 2008 from www.mindfullly.org/Health/We-Need-Germs.htm.

Jyonouchi, H., Sun, S., Le H. (2001). Proinflammatory and regulatory cytokine production associated with innate and adaptive immune responses in children with autism spectrum disorders and developmental regression. *Journal of Neuroimmunology: 120*(1-2):170–179.

Li, X., Chauhan, A., Sheikh, A.M., Patil, S., Chauhan, V., Li, X.M., Ji L., Brown, T., Malik, M. (2009). Elevated immune response in the brain of autistic patients. *Journal of Neuroimmunology, 207*(1-2):111–116.

Maizels, R. M., Yazdanbakhsh, M. (2003). Immune regulation by helminth parasites: cellular and molecular mechanisms. *Nature Reviews/Immunlogy,* volume 3.

Mangan, N.E., Fallon, R.E., Smith, P., van Rooijen, N., McKenzie, A.N., Fallon, P.G. (2004). Helminth infection protects mice from anaphylaxis via IL-10-producing B cells. *Journal of Immunology, 173*: 6346–6356.

Molloy, C. A., Morrow, A. L., Meinzen-Derr, J., Schleifer, K., Dienger, K., Manning-Courtney, P., Altaye, M., Wills-Karp, M. (2006). Elevated cytokine levels in ch ildren with autism spectrum disorders. *Journal of Neuroimmunlogy, 172*(1-2):198–205.

Newman, A.(1999). In pursuit of autoimmune worm cure. *The New York Times* on the Web. Retrieved March, 25, 2008 from http://query.nytimes.com/gst/fullpage.html?res=9A0DE6DB113BF932A0575BC0A96F958260&scp=1&sq=in%20pursuit%20of%20an%20autoimmune%20cure&st=cse.

Reddy, A., Fried, B. (2007). The use of Trichuris suis and other helminth therapies to treat Crohn's disease. *Parasitology Research, 100:* 921–927.

Rook, G. (2007). The hygiene hypothesis and the increasing prevalence of chronic inflammatory disorders. *Transactions of the Royal Society of Tropical Medicine and Hygiene, 101:* 1072–1074.

Rook, G., Lowry, C. A. (2008). The hygiene hypothesis and psychiatric disorders. *Trends in Immunology, 29*(4): 150–158.

Schnoeller, C., Rausch, S., Pillai, S., Avagyan, A., Wittig, B. M., Loddenkemper, C., Hamann, A., Hamelmann, E., Lucius, R., Hartmann, S. (2008). A helminth immunomodulator reduces allergic and inflammatory responses by induction of IL-10-producing macrophages. *The Journal of Immunology, 180:* 4265–4272.

Summers, R. W., Elliott, D. E., Qadir, K., Urban, J. F. Jr, Thompson, R., Weinstock, J. V. (2003). Trichuris suis seems to be safe and possibly effective in the treatment of inflammatory bowel disease. *American Journal of Gastroenterology Sep;98*(9):2034–2041.

Summers, R. W., Elliott, D. E., Urban, J. F. Jr, Thompson, R., Weinstock, J. V. (2005) Trichuris suis therapy in Crohn's disease. *Gut, 54:* 87–90.

Turner, J. D., Jackson, J. A., Faulkner, H., Behnke, J., Else, K. J., Kamgno, J., Boussinesq, M., Bradley, J. E. (2008). Intensity of intestinal infection with multiple worm species is related to regulatory cytokine output and immune hyporesponsiveness. *Journal of Infectious Diseases, 197:* 1204–1212.

Warren, R. P., Margaretten, N. C., Pace, N. C., Foster, A. (1986). Immune abnormalities in patients with autism. *Journal of Autism and Developmental Disorders, 16*(2):189–197.

Weinstock, J. V., Elliott, D. E. (2009). Helminths and the IBD Hygiene Hypothesis. *Inflammatory Bowel Disease, 15*(1):128–133.

Zaccone, P., Fehervari, Z., Phillips, J. M., Dunne, D. W., Cooke, A. (2006). Parasitic worms and inflammatory diseases. *Parasite Immunology, 28:* 515–523.

Chapter 29. Hyperbaric Oxygen Therapy: Let's put the Pressure on Autism for Recovery, by Dr. James Neubrander

Hyperbaric Medicine Team Training, Conducted at Nix Medical Center, San Antonio, Texas, June 4-8, 2007.

Neuro-HBOT Certification Course, IHA with ICIM, October 1-2, 2008, Pittsburg, PA.

Akin, M. L., B. M. Gulluoglu, et al. (2002). "Hyperbaric oxygen improves healing in experimental rat colitis." Undersea Hyperb Med 29(4): 279–85.

Alex, J., G. Laden, et al. (2005). "Pretreatment with hyperbaric oxygen and its effect on neuropsychometric dysfunction and systemic inflammatory response after cardiopulmonary bypass: a prospective randomized double-blind trial." J Thorac Cardiovasc Surg 130(6): 1623–30.

Allen, K. D., J. S. Danforth, et al. (1989). "Videotaped modeling and film distraction for fear reduction in adults undergoing hyperbaric oxygen therapy." J Consult Clin Psychol 57(4): 554–8.

Alleva, R., E. Nasole, et al. (2005). "alpha-Lipoic acid supplementation inhibits oxidative damage, accelerating chronic wound healing in patients undergoing hyperbaric oxygen therapy." Biochem Biophys Res Commun 333(2): 404–10.

Al-Waili, N. S. and G. J. Butler (2006). "Effects of hyperbaric oxygen on inflammatory response to wound and trauma: possible mechanism of action." ScientificWorldJournal 6: 425–41.

Al-Waili, N. S., G. J. Butler, et al. (2005). "Hyperbaric oxygen in the treatment of patients with cerebral stroke, brain trauma, and neurologic disease." Adv Ther 22(6): 659–78.

Al-Waili, N. S., G. J. Butler, et al. (2006). "Hyperbaric oxygen and lymphoid system function: a review supporting possible intervention in tissue transplantation." Technol Health Care 14(6): 489–98.

Anderson, B., Jr. and J. C. Farmer, Jr. (1978). "Hyperoxic myopia." Trans Am Ophthalmol Soc 76: 116–24.

Anderson, D. C., A. G. Bottini, et al. (1991). "A pilot study of hyperbaric oxygen in the treatment of human stroke." Stroke 22(9): 1137–42.

Ansari, K. A., M. Wilson, et al. (1986). "Hyperbaric oxygenation and erythrocyte antioxidant enzymes in multiple sclerosis patients." Acta Neurol Scand 74(2): 156–60.

Ashamalla, H. L., S. R. Thom, et al. (1996). "Hyperbaric oxygen therapy for the treatment of radiation-induced sequelae in children. The University of Pennsylvania experience." Cancer 77(11): 2407–12.

Atochin, D. N., D. Fisher, et al. (2000). "Neutrophil sequestration and the effect of hyperbaric oxygen in a rat model of temporary middle cerebral artery occlusion." Undersea Hyperb Med 27(4): 185–90.

Atochin, D. N., D. Fisher, et al. (2001). "[Hyperbaric oxygen inhibits neutrophil infiltration and reduces postischemic brain injury in rats]." Ross Fiziol Zh Im I M Sechenova 87(8): 1118–25.

Atug, O., H. Hamzaoglu, et al. (2008). "Hyperbaric oxygen therapy is as effective as dexamethasone in the treatment of TNBS-E-induced experimental colitis." Dig Dis Sci 53(2): 481–5.

Bader, N., A. Bosy-Westphal, et al. (2006). "Influence of vitamin C and E supplementation on oxidative stress induced by hyperbaric oxygen in healthy men." Ann Nutr Metab 50(3): 173–6.

Bader, N., A. Bosy-Westphal, et al. (2007). "Effect of hyperbaric oxygen and vitamin C and E supplementation on biomarkers of oxidative stress in healthy men." Br J Nutr 98(4): 826–33.

Baugh, M. A. (2000). "HIV: reactive oxygen species, enveloped viruses and hyperbaric oxygen." Med Hypotheses 55(3): 232–8.

Benedetti, S., A. Lamorgese, et al. (2004). "Oxidative stress and antioxidant status in patients undergoing prolonged exposure to hyperbaric oxygen." Clin Biochem 37(4): 312–7.

Bennett, M. and H. Newton (2007). "Hyperbaric oxygen therapy and cerebral palsy--where to now?" Undersea Hyperb Med 34(2): 69–74.

Bennett, M. H., J. Wasiak, et al. (2005). "Hyperbaric oxygen therapy for acute ischaemic stroke." Cochrane Database Syst Rev(3): CD004954.

Bitterman, H. (2007). "Hyperbaric oxygen for invasive fungal infections." Isr Med Assoc J 9(5): 387–8.

Boadi, W. Y., L. Thaire, et al. (1991). "Effects of dietary factors on antioxidant enzymes in rats exposed to hyperbaric oxygen." Vet Hum Toxicol 33(2): 105–9.

Bornside, G. H., L. M. Pakman, et al. (1975). "Inhibition of pathogenic enteric bacteria by hyperbaric oxygen: enhanced antibacterial activity in the absence of carbon dioxide." Antimicrob Agents Chemother 7(5): 682–7.

Bouachour, G., P. Cronier, et al. (1996). "Hyperbaric oxygen therapy in the management of crush injuries: a randomized double-blind placebo-controlled clinical trial." J Trauma 41(2): 333–9.

Brady, C. E., 3rd, B. J. Cooley, et al. (1989). "Healing of severe perineal and cutaneous Crohn's disease with hyperbaric oxygen." Gastroenterology 97(3): 756–60.

Buchman, A. L., C. Fife, et al. (2001). "Hyperbaric oxygen therapy for severe ulcerative colitis." J Clin Gastroenterol 33(4): 337–9.

Buras, J. A., D. Holt, et al. (2006). "Hyperbaric oxygen protects from sepsis mortality via an interleukin-10-dependent mechanism." Crit Care Med 34(10): 2624–9.

Calvert, J. W., J. Cahill, et al. (2007). "Hyperbaric oxygen and cerebral physiology." Neurol Res 29(2): 132–41.

Calvert, J. W., W. Yin, et al. (2002). "Hyperbaric oxygenation prevented brain injury induced by hypoxia-ischemia in a neonatal rat model." Brain Res 951(1): 1–8.

Calvert, J. W. and J. H. Zhang (2007). "Oxygen treatment restores energy status following experimental neonatal hypoxia-ischemia." Pediatr Crit Care Med 8(2): 165–73.

Chungpaibulpatana, J., T. Sumpatanarax, et al. (2008). "Hyperbaric oxygen therapy in Thai autistic children." J Med Assoc Thai 91(8): 1232–8.

Clark, J. M. and L. M. Pakman (1971). "Inhibition of Pseudomonas aeruginosa by hyperbaric oxygen. II. Ultrastructural changes." Infect Immun 4(4): 488–91.

Collet, J. P., M. Vanasse, et al. (2001). "Hyperbaric oxygen for children with cerebral palsy: a randomised multicentre trial. HBO-CP Research Group." Lancet 357(9256): 582–6.

Colombel, J. F., D. Mathieu, et al. (1995). "Hyperbaric oxygenation in severe perineal Crohn's disease." Dis Colon Rectum 38(6): 609–14.

Connor, D. J. and M. Bennett (2002). "Response to article by Buchman et al. Use of hyperbaric oxygenation in the treatment of ulcerative colitis." J Clin Gastroenterol 35(1): 98; author reply 98.

Daugherty, W. P., J. E. Levasseur, et al. (2004). "Effects of hyperbaric oxygen therapy on cerebral oxygenation and mitochondrial function following moderate lateral fluid-percussion injury in rats." J Neurosurg 101(3): 499–504.

Dave, K. R., R. Prado, et al. (2003). "Hyperbaric oxygen therapy protects against mito-chondrial dysfunction and delays onset of motor neuron disease in Wobbler mice." Neuroscience 120(1): 113–20.

Demchenko, I. T., A. E. Boso, et al. (2000). "Hyperbaric oxygen reduces cerebral blood flow by inactivating nitric oxide." Nitric Oxide 4(6): 597–608.

Demchenko, I. T., T. D. Oury, et al. (2002). "Regulation of the brain's vascular responses to oxygen." Circ Res 91(11): 1031–7.

Demirturk, L., M. Ozel, et al. (2002). "Therapeutic efficacy of hyperbaric oxygenation in ulcerative colitis refractory to medical treatment." J Clin Gastroenterol 35(3): 286-7; author reply 287–8.

Dennog, C., A. Hartmann, et al. (1996). "Detection of DNA damage after hyperbaric oxygen (HBO) therapy." Mutagenesis 11(6): 605–9.

Dennog, C., P. Radermacher, et al. (1999). "Antioxidant status in humans after exposure to hyperbaric oxygen." Mutat Res 428(1-2): 83–9.

Dole, M., F. R. Wilson, et al. (1975). "Hyperbaric hydrogen therapy: a possible treatment for cancer." Science 190(4210): 152–4.

Efrati, S., J. Bergan, et al. (2007). "Hyperbaric oxygen therapy for nonhealing vasculitic ulcers." Clin Exp Dermatol 32(1): 12–7.

Eftedal, O. S., S. Lydersen, et al. (2004). "A randomized, double blind study of the prophylactic effect of hyperbaric oxygen therapy on migraine." Cephalalgia 24(8): 639–44.

Feldmeier, J. J., Chairman and Editor (2003). Hyperbaric oxygen 2003: indications and results: the hyperbaric oxygen therapy committee report. Kensington, MD, Undersea and Hyperbaric Medicine Society.

Feldmeier, J. J., N. B. Hampson, et al. (2005). "In response to the negative randomized controlled hyperbaric trial by Annane et al in the treatment of mandibular ORN." Undersea Hyperb Med 32(3): 141–3.

Ferrer, M. D., A. Sureda, et al. (2007). "Scuba diving enhances endogenous antioxidant defenses in lymphocytes and neutrophils." Free Radic Res 41(3): 274–81.

Fry, D. E. (2005). "The story of hyperbaric oxygen continues." Am J Surg 189(4): 467–8.

Gill, A. L. and C. N. Bell (2004). "Hyperbaric oxygen: its uses, mechanisms of action and outcomes." QJM 97(7): 385–95.

Girnius, S., N. Cersonsky, et al. (2006). "Treatment of refractory radiation-induced hemorrhagic proctitis with hyperbaric oxygen therapy." Am J Clin Oncol 29(6): 588–92.

Golden, Z., C. J. Golden, et al. (2006). "Improving neuropsychological function after chronic brain injury with hyperbaric oxygen." Disabil Rehabil 28(22): 1379–86.

Golden, Z. L., R. Neubauer, et al. (2002). "Improvement in cerebral metabolism in chronic brain injury after hyperbaric oxygen therapy." Int J Neurosci 112(2): 119–31.

Gorgulu, S., G. Yagci, et al. (2006). "Hyperbaric oxygen enhances the efficiency of 5-aminosalicylic acid in acetic acid-induced colitis in rats." Dig Dis Sci 51(3): 480–7.

Gosalvez, M., J. Castillo Olivares, et al. (1973). "Mitochondrial respiration and oxidative phosphorylation during hypothermic hyperbaric hepatic preservation." J Surg Res 15(5): 313–8.

Gottlieb, S. F. (1971). "Effect of hyperbaric oxygen on microorganisms." Annu Rev Microbiol 25: 111–52.

Granowitz, E. V., E. J. Skulsky, et al. (2002). "Exposure to increased pressure or hyperbaric oxygen suppresses interferon-gamma secretion in whole blood cultures of healthy humans." Undersea Hyperb Med 29(3): 216–25.

Gregorevic, P., G. S. Lynch, et al. (2001). "Hyperbaric oxygen modulates antioxidant enzyme activity in rat skeletal muscles." Eur J Appl Physiol 86(1): 24–7.

Gulec, B., M. Yasar, et al. (2004). "Effect of hyperbaric oxygen on experimental acute distal colitis." Physiol Res 53(5): 493–9.

Gurbuz, A. K., E. Elbuken, et al. (2003). "A different therapeutic approach in patients with severe ulcerative colitis: hyperbaric oxygen treatment." South Med J 96(6): 632–3.

Gurbuz, A. K., E. Elbuken, et al. (2003). "A different therapeutic approach in severe ulcerative hyperbaric oxygen treatment." Rom J Gastroenterol 12(2): 170–1.

Gutsaeva, D. R., H. B. Suliman, et al. (2006). "Oxygen-induced mitochondrial biogenesis in the rat hippocampus." Neuroscience 137(2): 493–504.

Hammarlund, C. and T. Sundberg (1994). "Hyperbaric oxygen reduced size of chronic leg ulcers: a randomized double-blind study." Plast Reconstr Surg 93(4): 829-33; discussion 834.

Harabin, A. L., J. C. Braisted, et al. (1990). "Response of antioxidant enzymes to intermittent and continuous hyperbaric oxygen." J Appl Physiol 69(1): 328–35.

Harch, P. G. (2006). "Medicine that overlooks the evidence." Arch Phys Med Rehabil 87(4): 592-3; author reply 593.

Harch, P. G., C. Kriedt, et al. (2007). "Hyperbaric oxygen therapy improves spatial learning and memory in a rat model of chronic traumatic brain injury." Brain Res 1174: 120–9.

Hardy, P., J. P. Collet, et al. (2002). "Neuropsychological effects of hyperbaric oxygen therapy in cerebral palsy." Dev Med Child Neurol 44(7): 436–46.

Hardy, P., K. M. Johnston, et al. (2007). "Pilot case study of the therapeutic potential of hyperbaric oxygen therapy on chronic brain injury." J Neurol Sci 253(1-2): 94–105.

Harrison, D. K., N. C. Abbot, et al. (1994). "Protective regulation of oxygen uptake as a result of reduced oxygen extraction during chronic inflammation." Adv Exp Med Biol 345: 789–96.

Helms, A. K., H. T. Whelan, et al. (2007). "Hyperbaric oxygen therapy of acute ischemic stroke." Stroke 38(4): 1137; author reply 1138–9.

Henninger, N., L. Kuppers-Tiedt, et al. (2006). "Neuroprotective effect of hyperbaric oxygen therapy monitored by MR-imaging after embolic stroke in rats." Exp Neurol 201(2): 316–23.

Heuser, G., S. A. Heuser, et al. (2002). "Treatment of neurologically impaired adults and children with "mild" hyperbaric oxygenation (1.3 atm and 24% oxygen). In Hyperbaric oxygenation for cerebral palsy and the brain-injured child. Edited by Joiner JT. Flagstaff, Arizona: Best Publications."

Hollis, A. L., W. I. Butcher, et al. (1992). "Structural alterations in retinal tissues from rats deficient in vitamin E and selenium and treated with hyperbaric oxygen." Exp Eye Res 54(5): 671–84.

Hu, Z. Y., X. F. Shi, et al. (1991). "The protective effect of hyperbaric oxygen on hearing during chronic noise exposure." Aviat Space Environ Med 62(5): 403–6.

Inamoto, Y., F. Okuno, et al. (1991). "Effect of hyperbaric oxygenation on macrophage function in mice." Biochem Biophys Res Commun 179(2): 886–91.

Jacobs, E. A., P. M. Winter, et al. (1969). "Hyperoxygenation effect on cognitive functioning in the aged." N Engl J Med 281(14): 753–7.

Kiralp, M. Z., S. Yildiz, et al. (2004). "Effectiveness of hyperbaric oxygen therapy in the treatment of complex regional pain syndrome." J Int Med Res 32(3): 258–62.

Kudchodkar, B. J., A. Pierce, et al. (2007). "Chronic hyperbaric oxygen treatment elicits an anti-oxidant response and attenuates atherosclerosis in apoE knockout mice." Atherosclerosis 193(1): 28–35.

Lavy, A., G. Weisz, et al. (1994). "Hyperbaric oxygen for perianal Crohn's disease." J Clin Gastroenterol 19(3): 202–5.

Leach, R. M., P. J. Rees, et al. (1998). "Hyperbaric oxygen therapy." BMJ 317(7166): 1140–3.

Lee, A. K., R. B. Hester, et al. (1993). "Increased oxygen tensions modulate the cellular composition of the adaptive immune system in BALB/c mice." Cancer Biother 8(3): 241–52.

Lee, A. K., R. B. Hester, et al. (1994). "Increased oxygen tensions influence subset composition of the cellular immune system in aged mice." Cancer Biother 9(1): 39–54.

Lou, M., Y. Chen, et al. (2006). "Involvement of the mitochondrial ATP-sensitive potassium channel in the neuroprotective effect of hyperbaric oxygenation after cerebral ischemia." Brain Res Bull 69(2): 109–16.

Lou, M., J. H. Wang, et al. (2008). "[Effect of hyperbaric oxygen treatment on mitochondrial free radicals after transient focal cerebral ischemia in rats]." Zhejiang Da Xue Xue Bao Yi Xue Ban 37(5): 437–43.

Marois, P. and M. Vanasse (2003). "Hyperbaric oxygen therapy and cerebral palsy." Dev Med Child Neurol 45(9): 646-7; author reply 647–8.

Miljkovic-Lolic, M., R. Silbergleit, et al. (2003). "Neuroprotective effects of hyperbaric oxygen treatment in experimental focal cerebral ischemia are associated with reduced brain leukocyte myeloperoxidase activity." Brain Res 971(1): 90–4.

Moon, R. E. and J. J. Feldmeier (2002). "Hyperbaric oxygen: an evidence based approach to its application." Undersea Hyperb Med 29(1): 1–3.

Neubauer, R. A. (2001). "Hyperbaric oxygenation for cerebral palsy." Lancet 357(9273): 2052; author reply 2053.

Neubauer, R. A. and E. End (1980). "Hyperbaric oxygenation as an adjunct therapy in strokes due to thrombosis. A review of 122 patients." Stroke 11(3): 297–300.

Neubauer, R. A. and S. F. Gottlieb (1993). "Hyperbaric oxygen for brain injury." J Neurosurg 78(4): 687–8.

Neubauer, R. A., S. F. Gottlieb, et al. (1992). "Identification of hypometabolic areas in the brain using brain imaging and hyperbaric oxygen." Clin Nucl Med 17(6): 477–81.

Neubauer, R. A., S. F. Gottlieb, et al. (1994). "Hyperbaric oxygen for treatment of closed head injury." South Med J 87(9): 933–6.

Neubauer, R. A. and P. James (1998). "Cerebral oxygenation and the recoverable brain." Neurol Res 20 Suppl 1: S33–6.

Nie, H., L. Xiong, et al. (2006). "Hyperbaric oxygen preconditioning induces tolerance against spinal cord ischemia by upregulation of antioxidant enzymes in rabbits." J Cereb Blood Flow Metab 26(5): 666–74.

Pelaia, P., P. Volturo, et al. (1990). "[Mechanical ventilation in hyperbaric environment: experimental evaluation of the Drager Hyperlog]." Minerva Anestesiol 56(10): 1371.

Poliakova, L. V., V. L. Lukich, et al. (1991). "[Hyperbaric oxygenation and drug therapy in treatment of nonspecific ulcerative colitis and Crohn's disease]." Fiziol Zh 37(5): 120–3.

Qibiao, W., W. Hongjun, et al. (1995). "Treatment of children's epilepsy by hyperbaric oxygenation: analysis of 100 cases." Proceedings of the Eleventh International Congress on Hyperbaric Medicine. Flagstaff, AZ: Best Publishing: 79–81.

Rachmilewitz, D., F. Karmeli, et al. (1998). "Hyperbaric oxygen: a novel modality to ameliorate experimental colitis." Gut 43(4): 512–8.

Reillo, M., R. Altieri, et al. (1994). "Hyperbaric oxygen therapy to relieve chronic fatigue associated with HIV/AIDS [letter]." AIDS Patient Care 8(3): 106–7.

Reillo, M. R. and R. J. Altieri (1996). "HIV antiviral effects of hyperbaric oxygen therapy." J Assoc Nurses AIDS Care 7(1): 43–5.

Rocco, M., M. Antonelli, et al. (2001). "Lipid peroxidation, circulating cytokine and endothelin 1 levels in healthy volunteers undergoing hyperbaric oxygenation." Minerva Anestesiol 67(5): 393–400.

Rockswold, G. L. and S. E. Ford (1985). "Preliminary results of a prospective randomized trial for treatment of severely brain-injured patients with hyperbaric oxygen." Minn Med 68(7): 533–5.

Rockswold, S. B., G. L. Rockswold, et al. (2001). "Effects of hyperbaric oxygenation therapy on cerebral metabolism and intracranial pressure in severely brain injured patients." J Neurosurg 94(3): 403–11.

Rossignol, D. A. (2007). "Hyperbaric oxygen therapy might improve certain pathophysiological findings in autism." Med Hypotheses 68(6): 1208–27.

Rossignol, D. A. (2008). The use of hyperbaric oxygen therapy in autism. Hyperbaric oxygen for neurological disorders. J. H. Zhang. Flagstaff, AZ, Best Publishing Company: 209–258.

Rossignol, D. A. and J. J. Bradstreet (2008). "Evidence of mitochondrial dysfunction in autism and implications for treatment." American Journal of Biochemistry and Biotechnology 4(2): 208–217.

Rossignol, D. A. and L. W. Rossignol (2006). "Hyperbaric oxygen therapy may improve symptoms in autistic children." Med Hypotheses 67(2): 216–28.

Rossignol, D. A., L. W. Rossignol, et al. (2007). "The effects of hyperbaric oxygen therapy on oxidative stress, inflammation, and symptoms in children with autism: an open-label pilot study." BMC Pediatr 7(1): 36.

Rothfuss, A., C. Dennog, et al. (1998). "Adaptive protection against the induction of oxidative DNA damage after hyperbaric oxygen treatment." Carcinogenesis 19(11): 1913–7.

Rothfuss, A., P. Radermacher, et al. (2001). "Involvement of heme oxygenase-1 (HO-1) in the adaptive protection of human lymphocytes after hyperbaric oxygen (HBO) treatment." Carcinogenesis 22(12): 1979–85.

Saito, K., Y. Tanaka, et al. (1991). "Suppressive effect of hyperbaric oxygenation on immune responses of normal and autoimmune mice." Clin Exp Immunol 86(2): 322–7.

Sénéchal, C., S. Larivée, et al. (2007). "Hyperbaric Oxygenation Therapy in the Treatment of Cerebral Palsy: A Review and Comparison to Currently Accepted Therapies." Journal of American Physicians and Surgeons 12(4): 109–113.

Sethi, A. and A. Mukherjee (2003). "To see the efficacy of hyperbaric oxygen therapy in gross motor abilities of cerebral palsy children of 2-5 years, given initially as an adjunct to occupational therapy. ." The Indian Journal of Occupational Therapy 25(1): 7–11.

Sheffield, P. J. and D. A. Desautels (1997). "Hyperbaric and hypobaric chamber fires: a 73-year analysis." Undersea Hyperb Med 24(3): 153–64.

Shi, X. Y., Z. Q. Tang, et al. (2006). "Evaluation of hyperbaric oxygen treatment of neuropsychiatric disorders following traumatic brain injury." Chin Med J (Engl) 119(23): 1978–82.

Shi, X. Y., Z. Q. Tang, et al. (2003). "Cerebral perfusion SPECT imaging for assessment of the effect of hyperbaric oxygen therapy on patients with postbrain injury neural status." Chin J Traumatol 6(6): 346–9.

Stoller, K. P. (2005). "Quantification of neurocognitive changes before, during, and after hyperbaric oxygen therapy in a case of fetal alcohol syndrome." Pediatrics 116(4): e586–91.

Sumen, G., M. Cimsit, et al. (2001). "Hyperbaric oxygen treatment reduces carrageenan-induced acute inflammation in rats." Eur J Pharmacol 431(2): 265–8.

Sumen-Secgin, G., M. Cimsit, et al. (2005). "Antidepressant-like effect of hyperbaric oxygen treatment in forced-swimming test in rats." Methods Find Exp Clin Pharmacol 27(7): 471–4.

Takeshima, F., K. Makiyama, et al. (1999). "Hyperbaric oxygen as adjunct therapy for Crohn's intractable enteric ulcer." Am J Gastroenterol 94(11): 3374–5.

Thom, S. (1993). "A role for hyperbaric oxygen in clostridial myonecrosis." Clin Infect Dis 17(2): 238.

Thom, S. R., V. M. Bhopale, et al. (2006). "Stem cell mobilization by hyperbaric oxygen." Am J Physiol Heart Circ Physiol 290(4): H1378–86.

Tomaszewski, C. A. and S. R. Thom (1994). "Use of hyperbaric oxygen in toxicology." Emerg Med Clin North Am 12(2): 437–59.

Vitullo, V., P. Pelaia, et al. (1990). "[The role of hyperbaric oxygenation in treatment of retinal occlusive pathology]." Minerva Anestesiol 56(10): 1379.

Vlodavsky, E., E. Palzur, et al. (2006). "Hyperbaric oxygen therapy reduces neuroinflammation and expression of matrix metalloproteinase-9 in the rat model of traumatic brain injury." Neuropathol Appl Neurobiol 32(1): 40–50.

Wada, K., T. Miyazawa, et al. (2001). "Preferential conditions for and possible mechanisms of induction of ischemic tolerance by repeated hyperbaric oxygenation in gerbil hippocampus." Neurosurgery 49(1): 160-6; discussion 166–7.

Wada, K., T. Miyazawa, et al. (2000). "Mn-SOD and Bcl-2 expression after repeated hyperbaric oxygenation." Acta Neurochir Suppl 76: 285–90.

Weber, C. A., C. A. Duncan, et al. (1990). "Depletion of tissue glutathione with diethyl maleate enhances hyperbaric oxygen toxicity." Am J Physiol 258(6 Pt 1): L308–12.

Weisz, G., A. Lavy, et al. (1997). "Modification of in vivo and in vitro TNF-alpha, IL-1, and IL-6 secretion by circulating monocytes during hyperbaric oxygen treatment in patients with perianal Crohn's disease." J Clin Immunol 17(2): 154–9.

Wilson, H. D., J. R. Wilson, et al. (2006). "Hyperbaric oxygen treatment decreases inflammation and mechanical hypersensitivity in an animal model of inflammatory pain." Brain Res 1098(1): 126–8.

Xu, X., H. Yi, et al. (1997). "Differential sensitivities to hyperbaric oxygen of lymphocyte subpopulations of normal and autoimmune mice." Immunol Lett 59(2): 79–84.

Yang, Z., J. Nandi, et al. (2006). "Hyperbaric oxygenation ameliorates indomethacin-induced enteropathy in rats by modulating TNF-alpha and IL-1beta production." Dig Dis Sci 51(8): 1426–33.

Yang, Z. J., G. Bosco, et al. (2001). "Hyperbaric O2 reduces intestinal ischemia-reperfusion-induced TNF-alpha production and lung neutrophil sequestration." Eur J Appl Physiol 85(1-2): 96–103.

Yang, Z. J., C. Camporesi, et al. (2002). "Hyperbaric oxygenation mitigates focal cerebral injury and reduces striatal dopamine release in a rat model of transient middle cerebral artery occlusion." Eur J Appl Physiol 87(2): 101–7.

Yatsuzuka, H. (1991). "[Effects of hyperbaric oxygen therapy on ischemic brain injury in dogs]." Masui 40(2): 208–23.

Yildiz, S., G. Uzun, et al. (2006). "Hyperbaric oxygen therapy in chronic pain management." Curr Pain Headache Rep 10(2): 95–100.

Yin, W., A. E. Badr, et al. (2002). "Down regulation of COX-2 is involved in hyperbaric oxygen treatment in a rat transient focal cerebral ischemia model." Brain Res 926(1-2): 165–71.

Chapter 30. Integrated Play Groups (IPG) Model, by Dr. Pamela Wolfberg

Bottema, K. (2008) *Integrated teen social groups: A qualitative analysis of peer socialization in teens with Autism Spectrum Disorder*. Unpublished position paper. University of California, Berkeley with SFSU.

California Department of Education. (1997) *Best practices for designing and delivering effective programs for individuals with Autistic Spectrum Disorders*. RiSE, Resources in Special Education, Sacramento, CA.

Fuge, G & Berry, R. (2004) *Pathways to Play! Combining Sensory Integration and Integrated Play Groups. Theme-based activities for children with Autism Spectrum and Other Sensory Processing Disorders*. Shawnee Mission, KS: Autism Asperger Publishing Company

Gonsier-Gerdin, J. (1992). *Elementary school children's perspectives on peers with disabilities in the context of Integrated Play Groups: "They're not really disabled, they're like plain kids."* (unpublished study) UC Berkeley-San Francisco State University.

Iovannone, R. Dunlop, G, Huber, H. & Kincaid, D. (2003). Effective educational practices for students with ASD. *Focus on Autism and Other Developmental Disabilities,* 18 (3), 150–165.

Julius, H. & Wolfberg, P. (2009) *Integrated Play and Drama Groups for Children and Adolescents on the Autism Spectrum. Alexander von Humboldt Foundation TransCoop Program: Transatlantic Cooperation in the Humanities, Social Sciences, Law, and Economics (2009–2012).*

Lantz, J. F., Nelson, J. M. & Loftin, R. L. (2004) Guiding Children with Autism in Play: Applying the Integrated Play Group Model in School Settings. *Exceptional Children,* 37(2), 8–14.

Mikaelan, B. (2003) *Increasing language through sibling and peer support play.* Unpublished Master Thesis, San Francisco State University, CA. National Research Council (2001) *Educating Children with Autism.* Committee on Educational Interventions for Children with Autism: Division of Behavioral and Social Sciences and Education, National Academy Press: Washington, D.C. National Autism Center (2009) *National standards project report- findings and conclusions: Addressing the need for evidence-based practice guidelines for Autism Spectrum Disorder.* Integrated Play Groups™ (IPG) model identified as "Established" practice within category of "Peer Intervention Package" based on studies reviewed; cited on p. 14, 30, & 50.

Neufeld, D. & Wolfberg, P.J. (2010) From novice to expert: Guiding children on the autism spectrum in Integrated Play Groups. In Schaefer, C. (Ed.) *Play therapy for preschool children.* Washington, D.C: American Psychological Association.

O'Connor, T. (1999). *Teacher perspectives of facilitated play in Integrated Play Groups.* Unpublished Master Thesis, San Francisco State University, CA.

Richard, V, & Goupil, G. (2005). Application des groupes de jeux integres aupres d'eleves ayant un trouble envahissant du development (Implementation of Integrated Play Groups with PDD Students). *Revue quebecoise de psychologie, 26(3),* 79–103

Vygotsky, L. (1966). Play and its role in the mental development of the child. *Soviet Psychology, 12,* 6–18 (Original work published in 1933).

Vygotsky, L. S. (1978). *Mind in society: The development of higher psychological processes.* Cambridge, MA: Harvard University Press.

Wolfberg, P. J. (1988). *Integrated play groups for children with autism and related disorders.* Unpublished master's field study, San Francisco State University.

Wolfberg, P.J. (1994). *Case illustrations of emerging social relations and symbolic activity in children with autism through supported peer play* (Doctoral dissertation, University of California at Berkeley with San Francisco State University). *Dissertation Abstracts International,* #9505068.

Wolfberg, P. J., & Schuler, A. L. (1992). *Integrated play groups project: Final evaluation report* (Contract # HO86D90016). Washington, DC: Department of Education, OSERS.

Wolfberg, P.J. (2009). *Play and imagination in children with autism.* (second edition) New York: Teachers College Press, Columbia University.

Wolfberg, P., Turiel., E., & DeWitt, M., (2008). *Integrated Play Groups: Promoting symbolic play, social engagement and communication with peers across settings in children with autism.* Autism Speaks Treatment Grant (2008–2011).

Wolfberg, P.J. (2003) *Peer play and the autism spectrum: The art of guiding children's socialization and imagination.* Shawnee, KS: Autism Asperger Publishing Company.

Wolfberg, P.J., & Schuler, A.L. (1992). *Integrated play groups project: Final evaluation report* (Contract # HO86D90016). Washington, DC: U.S.Department of Education, OSERS.

Wolfberg, P. J. (1988). *Integrated play groups for children with autism and related disorders.* Unpublished master's field study, San Francisco State University.

Wolfberg, P. (2010).

Wolfberg, P. J., & Schuler, A. L. (1993). Integrated Play Groups: A model for promoting the social and cognitive dimensions of play in children with autism. *Journal of Autism and Developmental Disorders, 23*(3), 467–489.

Yang, T., Wolfberg, P. J., Wu, S, Hwu, P. (2003) Supporting children on the autism spectrum in peer play at home and school: Piloting the Integrated Play Groups model in Taiwan. *Autism: The International Journal of Research and Practice, 7*(4) 437–453.

Zercher, C., Hunt, P., Schuler, A. L., & Webster, J. (2001). Increasing joint attention, play and language through peer supported play. *Autism: The International Journal of Research and Practice, 5,* 374–398.

Chapter 31. Intestine, Leaky Gut, Autism, and Probiotics, by Dr. Alessio Fasano

Fasano A. Pathological and therapeutical implications of macromolecule passage through the tight junction. *In* Tight Junctions. Boca Raton, FL: CRC Press, Inc., 2001, p. 697–722.

Fasano A. Physiological, pathological, and therapeutic implications of zonulin-mediated intestinal barrier modulation: living life on the edge of the wall. *Am J Pathol.* 173:1243–52, 2008.

White JF. Intestinal pathophysiology in Autism. *Exp Biol Med* 228:639–649, 2003.Prevalence of autism spectrum disorders - Autism and Developmental Disabilities Monitoring Network, United States, 2006. Autism and Developmental Disabilities Monitoring Network Surveillance Year 2006 Principal Investigators; Centers for Disease Control and Prevention (CDC). *MMWR Surveill Summ.* 2009; 58:1–20.

Buie T, Campbell DB, Fuchs GJ, III, et al Evaluation, Diagnosis, and Treatment of Gastrointestinal Disorders in Individuals With ASDs: A Consensus Report. *Pediatrics* 2010;125;S1–S18.

Buie T, Fuchs GJ, III, Furuta GT, Kooros K, Levy J, Lewis JD, Wershil BK, Winter H. Recommendations for Evaluation and Treatment of Common Gastrointestinal Problems in Children With ASDs. *Pediatrics* 2010;125;S19–S29

Guarner F Prebiotics, probiotics and helminths: the 'natural' solution? *Dig Dis.* 2009;27: 412–417. www.usprobiotics.org

Golnik AE, Ireland M., Complementary alternative medicine for children with autism: a physician survey. *J Autism Dev Disord.* 2009; 39: 996–1005.

Chapter 32. Intravenous Immunoglobulin (IVIG), by Dr. Michael Elice

Gupta, S, Aggarwal S., Heads, C. Dysregulated immune system in children with autism: beneficial effects of intravenous gamma globulin on autistic characteristics. J autism Dev disord 1996;26: 439–452.

Plioplys A V. Intravenous gamma globulin in children with autism. J Child Neurol 1998;13:79–82

Delgiudice-Asch G, Simon L, Schmeidler J, Cunningham-Rundles C, Hollander E. A pilot clinical triial of intravenous gamma globulin in childhood autism. *J Autism Dev Disord* 1999 199;29:157–160.

Boris M, goldblatt A, Galanko j, James J. Association of MTHFR gene variants with autism. *J Phys Surg* 2004;29:157–160.

National Institutes of Health. Intravenous immunoglobulin: prevention and treatment of disease. NIH consensus Statement 1990;8(2):1–23.

Latov N, Chaudhry V, Koski CL, Lisak RP Apatoff BR, Hahn AF, Howard AF. Use of intravenous gamma globulins in neuroimmunologic diseases. *J Allerg Clin Immunol* 2001;108:S126–132.

Comi AM, Zimmmerman AW, Frye VH, Law PA, Peeden JN. Familial Clustering of autoimmune disorders and evaluation of medical risk factors in autism. *J Child Neurol* 1999;14:388–394.

Swedo, SE. Sydenham's chorea: a model for childhood autoimmune neuropsychiatric disorders. *JAMA* 1994;272(22): 1788–1791.

Swedo SE, Rapoport JL, Cheslow DL, et al. High prevalence of obsessive-compulsive symptoms in patients with sydenham's chorea. *Am J Psychiatry*. 1989;46:335–341.

Swedo SE, Leonard HL, Garvey M, et al. Pediatric autoimmune neuropsychiatric disorders associated with streptococcal infections (PANDAS): a clinical description of the first fifty cases. Am J Psychiatry. 1998;155:264–271.

Giedd JN, Rapoport JL, Leonard HL, etal. Case study, acute basal ganglia enlargement and obsessive-compusive symptoms in an adolescent boy. J Am Acad Child Adolsc Pshychiatry. 1996,35(7):913–915

Garvey MA, Perlmutter SJ, Allen AJ, etal. A pilot study of penicillin prophylaxis for neuropsychiatric exacerbations triggered by streptococcal infections. Biol Psychiatry. 1999,45:1564–1571

Barron KS, Sher MR, Silverman ED. Intravenous immunoglobulin therapy: magic or black magic. J Theumatol. 1992; 19:94–97

Perlmutter SJ, Leitman SF, Garvey MA etal. Therapeutic plasma exchange and intravenous immunoglobulin for obsessive-compulsive disorder and tic disorders in childhood. Lancet. 1999;50(6):429–439

Martino D, Defazio G, Giovannoni G. The PANDAS subgroup of tic disorders and childhood-onset obsessive-compulsive disorder. J Psychosom Res. 2009/Nov30;170(1):3–6

Gilbert DL, Kurlan R. PANDAS horse or zebra? Neurology. 2009 Oct 20;73(16):1252–3

Shulman ST. Pediatric autoimmune neuropsychiatric disorders associated with streptococci (PANDAS) update. Cuyrr Opin Pediatr. 2009 Feb;21(1): 127–30

Pavone P. Parano E, Rizzo R, Trifiletti RR.Autoimmune neuropsychiatric disorders associated with streptococcal infection: Sydenham chorea. PANDAS and PANDAS variants. J Child Neurol. 2006.Aug.21(8):678–689

Swedo SE, Grant PJ. Annotation: PANDAS: a model for human autoimmune disease. J child Psychol Psychiatry. 2005 Mar; 46(3): 227–34

Chapter 33. Linwood Method, by Bill Moss

Koegel, R. L., & Koegel, L. K. (2006). *Pivotal Response Treatments for Autism*. Baltimore: Brooks Publishing Company.

Chapter 36. Melatonin Therapy for Sleep Disorders, by Dr. James Jan

1. JE Jan and RD Freeman. Melatonin therapy for circadian rhythm sleep disorders in children with multiple disabilities: what have we learned in the last decade? Developmental Medicine and Child Neurology. 2004, 46:776–782.
2. JE Jan, MB Wasdell, MD Weiss, RD Freeman. What is the correct dose of melatonin in sleep therapy? Biological Rhythm Research. 2007, 38:85–86.
3. JE Jan, MD Wasdell, RJ Reiter, MD Weiss, KP Johnson, A.Ivanenko, RD Freeman. Melatonin therapy of pediatric sleep disorders:recent advances,why it works,who are the candidates and how to treat. Current Pediatric Reviews.2007,3:214–324.
4. R Carr, MB Wasdell, D Hamilton, MD Weiss, RD Freeman, J Tai,WJ Rietveld, JE Jan. Long-term effectiveness outcome of melatonin therapy in children with treatment-resistant circadian rhythm sleep disorders. Journal of Pineal Research. 2007, 43:351–359.

Chapter 37. MERIT Approach: Integrating ABA with Developmental Models, by Jenifer Clark

Fonagy, P., Gergely, G., Jurist, E. & Target, M. (2002). Affect regulation, mentalization, and the development of the self. New York: Other Press

Chapter 38. Methyl-B$_{12}$: Myth or Masterpiece, by Dr. James Neubrander

1. Akesson B, Fehling C, Jagerstad M. Lipid composition and metabolism in liver and brain of vitamin B12-deficient rat sucklings. Br J Nutr. 1979 Mar;41(2):263-74.
2. Allen RH, Stabler SP, Lindenbaum J. Relevance of vitamins, homocysteine and other metabolites in neuropsychiatric disorders. Eur J Pediatr. 1998 Apr;157 Suppl 2:S122-6.
3. Allen RH, Seetharam B, Allen NC, Podell ER, Alpers DH. Correction of cobalamin malabsorption in pancreatic insufficiency with a cobalamin analogue that binds with high affinity to R protein but not to intrinsic factor. In vivo evidence that a failure to partially degrade R protein is responsible for cobalamin malabsorption in pancreatic insufficiency. J Clin Invest. 1978 Jun;61(6):1628-34.
4. Arnold GL, Hyman SL, Mooney RA, Kirby. RS.Plasma amino acids profiles in children with autism: potential risk of nutritional deficiencies. J Lab Clin Med. 1973 Apr;81(4):557-67.
5. Bachli E, Fehr J. [Diagnosis of vitamin B12 deficiency: only apparently child's play] Schweiz Med Wochenschr. 1999 Jun 12;129(23):861-72.
6. Banerjee R, Ragsdale SW. The many faces of vitamin B12: catalysis by cobalamin-dependent enzymes. Annu Rev Biochem. 2003;72:209-47.
7. Banerjee R. The Yin-Yang of cobalamin biochemistry. Chem Biol. 1997 Mar;4(3):175-86.

8. Berliner N, Rosenberg LE. Uptake and metabolism of free cyanocobalamin by cultured human fibroblasts from controls and a patient with transcobalamin II deficiency. Metabolism. 1981 Mar;30(3):230-6.

9. Berentsen S, Talstad I. [Homocysteine and methylmalonic acid. New tests--for what benefit?] Tidsskr Nor Laegeforen. 1996 Sep 20;116(22):2677-9.

10. Bhatt HR, Linnell JC. Vitamin B12 homoeostasis after haemorrhage in the rat: the importance of skeletal muscle. Clin Sci (Lond). 1987 Dec;73(6):581-7.

11. Bohr KC . [Effect of vitamin B12 on sleep quality and performance of shift workers] Wien Med Wochenschr. 1996;146(13-14):289-91.

12. Bolann BJ, Solli JD, Schneede J, Grottum KA, Loraas A, Stokkeland M, Stallemo A, Schjoth A, Bie RB, Refsum H, Ueland PM. Evaluation of indicators of cobalamin deficiency defined as cobalamin-induced reduction in increased serum methylmalonic acid. Clin Chem. 2000 Nov;46(11):1744-50.

13. Brandt LJ, Bernstein LH, Wagle A. Production of vitamin B 12 analogues in patients with small-bowel bacterial overgrowth. Ann Intern Med. 1977 Nov;87(5):546-51.

14. Burger RL, Schneider RJ, Mehlman CS, Allen RH. Human plasma R-type vitamin B12-binding proteins. II. The role of transcobalamin I, transcobalamin III, and the normal granulocyte vitamin B12-binding protein in the plasma transport of vitamin B12. J Biol Chem. 1975 Oct 10;250(19):7707-13.

15. Choi SW. Vitamin B12 deficiency: a new risk factor for breast cancer? Nutr Rev. 1999 Aug;57(8):250-3.

16. Csanaky I, Gregus Z. Effect of phosphate transporter and methylation inhibitor drugs on the disposition of arsenate and arsenite in rats. Toxicol Sci. 2001 Sep;63(1):29-36.

17. Culley, D.J., Raghavan, S.V., Waly, M., Baxter, M.G., Yukhananov, R., Deth, R.C. and Crosby, G. : Nitrous oxide decreases cortical methionine synthase transiently but produces lasting memory impairment in aged rats. Anesthesia and Analgesia 105: 83-88 (2007).

18. Delva MD. Vitamin B12 replacement. To B12 or not to B12? Can Fam Physician. 1997 May;43:917-22.

19. Deth, R., Muratore, C., Benzecry, J., Power-Charnitsky, V., and Waly, M. How environmental and genetic factors combine to cause autism: A Redox/Methylation Hypothesis. Neurotoxicology (Under Review).

20. Deth, R.C., Kuznetsova, A. and Waly, M.: Attention-related signaling activities of the D4 dopamine receptor in *Cognitive Neuroscience of Attention*, Michael Posner Ed., Guilford Publications Inc., New York (2004). p 269-282.

21. Deth RC., Ph.D., Molecular Aspects of Thimerosal-induced Autism; Congressional Testimony; October 6, 2003.

22. Deth, R.C. Molecular Origins of Attention: The Dopamine-Folate Connection Kluwer Academic Publishers (April, 2003)

23. Deth, R.C., Sharma, A. and Waly, M.: Dopamine-stimulated solid-state signaling: A novel role for single-carbon folates in human attention. In: Proc. 12th Int. Symp. Chem. Pteridines and Folates. Kluwer Academic Press (2002).

24. Donaldson, RM Jr: Intrinsic factor and the transport of cobalamin, in Johnson LR (ed): *Physiology of the Gastrointestinal Tract*, New York, Raven, 1981.

25. el Kholty S, Gueant JL, Bressler L, Djalali M, Boissel P, Gerard P, Nicolas JP. Portal and biliary phases of enterohepatic circulation of corrinoids in humans. Gastroenterology. 1991 Nov;101(5):1399-408

26. Ertel R, Brot N, Taylor R, Weissbach H. Studies on the nature of the bound cobamide in E. coli N5-methyltetrahydrofolate-homocysteine transmethylase. Arch Biochem Biophys. 1968 Jul;126(1):353-7.

27. Flippo TS, Holder WD Jr. Neurologic degeneration associated with nitrous oxide anesthesia in patients with vitamin B12 deficiency. Arch Surg. 1993 Dec;128(12):1391-5.

28. Fowler B. Genetic defects of folate and cobalamin metabolism. Eur J Pediatr. 1998 Apr;157 Suppl 2:S60-6.

29. Frenkel EP, Kitchens RL. Intracellular localization of hepatic propionyl-CoA carboxylase and methylmalonyl-CoA mutase in humans and normal and vitamin B12 deficient rats. Br J Haematol. 1975 Dec;31(4):501-13.

30. Funada U, Wada M, Kawata T, Mori K, Tamai H, Kawanishi T, Kunou A, Tanaka N, Tadokoro T, Maekawa A. Changes in CD4+CD8-/CD4-CD8+ ratio and humoral immune functions in vitamin B12-deficient rats. Int J Vitam Nutr Res. 2000 Jul;70(4):167-71.

31. Giannella RA, Broitman SA, Zamcheck N. Competition between bacteria and intrinsic factor for vitamin B 12 : implications for vitamin B 12 malabsorption in intestinal bacterial overgrowth. Gastroenterology. 1972 Feb;62(2):255-60.

32. Golenko OD, Ryzhova NI. [Transplacental effect of methylcobalamine on the growth of embryonic mouse kidney tissue in organotypic cultivation] Biull Eksp Biol Med. 1986 Apr;101(4):471-4.

33. Goto I, Nagara H, Tateishi J, Kuroiwa Y. Effects of methylcobalamin on vitamin B1- and B-deficient encephalopathy in rats. J Neurol Sci. 1987 Jan;77(1):97-102.

34. Hall CA, Begley JA, Chu RC. Methionine synthetase activity of human lymphocytes both replete in and depleted of vitamin B12. J Lab Clin Med. 1986 Oct;108(4):325-31.

35. Hall LL, George SE, Kohan MJ, Styblo M, Thomas DJ. In vitro methylation of inorganic arsenic in mouse intestinal cecum. Toxicol Appl Pharmacol. 1997 Nov;147(1):101-9.

36. Herbert V. Detection of malabsorption of vitamin B12 due to gastric or intestinal dysfunction. Semin Nucl Med. 1972 Jul;2(3):220-34.

37. Hogenkamp HP, Bratt GT, Sun SZ. Methyl transfer from methylcobalamin to thiols. A reinvestigation. Biochemistry. 1985 Nov 5;24(23):6428-32.

38. Honma K, Kohsaka M, Fukuda N, Morita N, Honma S. Effects of vitamin B12 on plasma melatonin rhythm in humans: increased light sensitivity phase-advances the circadian clock? Experientia. 1992 Aug 15;48(8):716-20.

39. Hvas AM, Ellegaard J, Nexo E. [Diagnosis of vitamin B12 deficiency--time for reflection] Ugeskr Laeger. 2003 May 5;165(19):1971-6.

40. Hvas AM, Ellegaard J, Nexo E. Vitamin B12 treatment normalizes metabolic markers but has limited clinical effect: a randomized placebo-controlled study. Clin Chem. 2001 Aug;47(8):1396-404.

41. Goto I, Nagara H, Tateishi J, Kuroiwa Y. Effects of methylcobalmin on vitamin B1- and B-deficient encephalopathy in rats. J Neurol Sci. 1987 Jan;77(1):97-102.

42. Ide H, Fujiya S, Asanuma Y, Tsuji M, Sakai H, Agishi Y. Clinical usefulness of intrathecal injection of methylcobalamin in patients with diabetic neuropathy. Clin Ther. 1987;9(2):183-92.

43. Imamura N, Dake Y, Amemiya T. Circadian rhythm in the retinal pigment epithelium related to vitamin B12. Life Sci. 1995;57(13):1317-23.

44. Isoyama R, Baba Y, Harada H, Kawai S, Shimizu Y, Fujii M, Fujisawa S, Takihara H, Koshido Y, Sakatoku J. [Clinical experience of methylcobalamin (CH3-B12)/ clomiphene citrate combined treatment in male infertility] Hinyokika Kiyo. 1986 Aug;32(8):1177-83.

45. Jalaludin MA. Methylcobalamin treatment of Bell's palsy. Methods Find Exp Clin Pharmacol. 1995 Oct;17(8):539-44.

46. James SJ, Melnyk S, Jernigan S, Cleves MA, Halsted CH, Wong DH, Cutler P, Bock K, Boris M, Bradstreet JJ, Baker SM, Gaylor DW. Metabolic endophenotype and related genotypes are associated with oxidative stress in children with autism. Am J Med Genet B Neuropsychiatr Genet. 2006 Dec 5;141(8):947-56.

47. James SJ, Slikker W 3rd, Melnyk S, New E, Pogribna M, Jernigan S. Thimerosal neurotoxicity is associated with glutathione depletion: protection with glutathione precursors. Neurotoxicology. 2005 Jan;26(1):1-8.

48. James SJ, Cutler P, Melnyk S, Jernigan S, Janak L, Gaylor DW, Neubrander JA. Metabolic biomarkers of increased oxidative stress and impaired methylation capacity in children with autism. Am. J. Clinical Nutrition, Dec 2004; 80: 1611–1617.

49. Jin X, Jin X, Sheng X. Methylcobalamin as antagonist to transient ototoxic action of gentamicin. Acta Otolaryngol. 2001 Apr;121(3):351-4.

50. Kaji R, Kodama M, Imamura A, Hashida T, Kohara N, Ishizu M, Inui K, Kimura J. Effect of ultrahigh-dose methylcobalamin on compound muscle action potentials in amyotrophic lateral sclerosis: a double-blind controlled study. Muscle Nerve. 1998 Dec;21(12):1775-8.

51. Kal'nev VR, Rachkus IuA, Kanopkaite SI. [Cobalamins and tRNA methyltrans-ferase activity in E. coli cells] Biokhimiia. 1981 Oct;46(10):1773-9.

52. Kapadia CR. Vitamin B12 in health and disease: part I--inherited disorders of func-tion, absorption, and transport. Gastroenterologist. 1995 Dec;3(4):329-44.

53. Kasuya M. The effect of methylcobalamin on the toxicity of methylmercury and mercuric chloride on nervous tissue in culture. Toxicol Lett. 1980 Nov;7(1):87-93.

54. Kawata T, Tashiro A, Tamiki A, Suga K, Kamioka S, Yamada K, Wada M, Tadokoro T, Maekawa A. Utilization of dietary protein in the vitamin B12-deficient rats. Int J Vitam Nutr Res. 1995;65(4):248-54.

55. Kelly GS. Folates: supplemental forms and therapeutic applications. Altern Med Rev. 1998 Jun;3(3):208-20.

56. Kosonen T, Pihko H. [Development regression in a child caused by vitamin B12 deficiency] Duodecim. 1994;110(6):588-91.

57. Kiuchi T, Sei H, Seno H, Sano A, Morita Y. Effect of vitamin B12 on the sleep-wake rhythm following an 8-hour advance of the light-dark cycle in the rat. Physiol Behav. 1997 Apr;61(4):551-4.

58. Kolhouse JF, Allen RH. Recognition of two intracellular cobalamin binding proteins and their identification as methylmalonyl-CoA mutase and methionine synthetase. Proc Natl Acad Sci U S A. 1977 Mar;74(3):921-5

59. Kubota K, Kurabayashi H, Kawada E, Okamoto K, Shirakura T. Restoration of abnormally high CD4/CD8 ratio and low natural killer cell activity by vitamin B12 therapy in a patient with post-gastrectomy megaloblastic anemia. Intern Med. 1992 Jan;31(1):125-6.

60. Kurimoto S, Iwasaki T, Nomura T, Noro K, Yamamoto S. Influence of VDT (visual display terminals) work on eye accommodation. J UOEH. 1983 Mar 1;5(1):101-10

61. Kuwabara S, Nakazawa R, Azuma N, Suzuki M, Miyajima K, Fukutake T, Hattori T. Intravenous methylcobalamin treatment for uremic and diabetic neuropathy in chronic hemodialysis patients. Intern Med. 1999 Jun;38(6):472-5.

62. Kuznetsova, A.Y., and Deth, R.C.: A model for gamma oscillations induced by D4 dopamine receptor-mediated phospholipid methylation. J. Computational Neuroscience (Under Review).

63. Lindstedt G. [Nitrous oxide can cause cobalamin deficiency. Vitamin B12 is a simple and cheap remedy] Lakartidningen. 1999 Nov 3;96(44):4801-5.

64. Linnell JC, Wilson MJ, Mikol YB, Poirier LA. Tissue distribution of methylcobalamin in rats fed amino acid-defined, methyl-deficient diets. J Nutr. 1983 Jan;113(1):124-30.

65. Linnel JC: The fate of cobalamin in vivo, in Babior BM (ed): *Cobalamin Biochemistry and Pathophysiology,* New York, Wiley, 1975, p287.

66. Maltin CA, Duncan L, Wilson AB. Mitochondrial abnormalities in muscle from vitamin B12-deficient sheep. J Comp Pathol. 1983 Jul;93(3):429-35.

67. Marsh EN. Coenzyme B12 (cobalamin)-dependent enzymes. Essays Biochem. 1999;34:139-54.

68. Masson C. [Combined sclerosis of the spinal cord «revisited»] Presse Med. 1999 Nov 27;28(37):2048-9.

69. Matthews RG. Cobalamin-dependent methyltransferases. Acc Chem Res. 2001 Aug;34(8):681-9.

70. McCaddon A, Regland B, Hudson P, Davies G. Functional vitamin B(12) deficiency and Alzheimer disease. Neurology. 2002 May 14;58(9):1395-9.

71. Mellman IS, Youngdahl-Turner P, Willard HF, Rosenberg LE. Intracellular binding of radioactive hydroxocobalamin to cobalamin-dependent apoenzymes in rat liver. Proc Natl Acad Sci U S A. 1977 Mar;74(3):916-20.

72. Metz J. Cobalamin deficiency and the pathogenesis of nervous system disease. Annu Rev Nutr. 1992;12:59-79.

73. Mikhailov VV, Rusanova AG, Chikina NA, Avakumov VM. [Effect of methylcobalamine on the processes of posttraumatic regeneration of the salivary glands] Biull Eksp Biol Med. 1984 Jul;98(7):95-7.

74. Mori K, Kaido M, Fujishiro K, Inoue N, Ide Y, Koide O. Preventive effects of methylcobalamin on the testicular damage induced by ethylene oxide. Arch Toxicol. 1991;65(5):396-401.

75. Moriyama H, Nakamura K, Sanda N, Fujiwara E, Seko S, Yamazaki A, Mizutani M, Sagami K, Kitano T. [Studies on the usefulness of a long-term, high-dose treatment of methylcobalamin in patients with oligozoospermia] Hinyokika Kiyo. 1987 Jan;33(1):151-6.

76. Nishizawa Y, Goto HG, Tanigaki Y, Fushiki S, Nishizawa Y. Induction of apoptosis in an androgen-dependent mouse mammary carcinoma cell line by methylcobalamin. Anticancer Res. 2001 Mar-Apr;21(2A):1107-10.

77. Nishizawa Y, Yamamoto T, Tanigaki Y, Kasugai T, Mano M, Ishiguro S, Fushiki S, Poirier LA, Nishizawa Y. Methylcobalamin decreases mRNA levels of androgen-induced growth factor in androgen-dependent Shionogi carcinoma 115 cells. Nutr Cancer. 1999;35(2):195-201.

78. [No authors listed] Vitamin B12, cognitive impairment, survival and HHV-6A. Posit Health News. 1998 Spring;(No 16):12-3.

79. [No authors listed] Methylcobalamin. Altern Med Rev. 1998 Dec;3(6):461-3.

80. Ohta T, Iwata T, Kayukawa Y, Okada T. Daily activity and persistent sleep-wake schedule disorders. Prog Neuropsychopharmacol Biol Psychiatry. 1992 Jul;16(4):529-37.

81. Okawa M, Mishima K, Nanami T, Shimizu T, Iijima S, Hishikawa Y, Takahashi K. Vitamin B12 treatment for sleep-wake rhythm disorders. Sleep. 1990 Feb;13(1):15-23.

82. Okuda K, Yashima K, Kitazaki T, Takara I. Intestinal absorption and concurrent chemical changes of methylcobalamin. J Lab Clin Med. 1973 Apr;81(4):557-67.

83. Pan-Hou HS, Imura N. Involvement of mercury methylation in microbial mercury detoxication. Arch Microbiol. 1982 Mar;131(2):176-7.

84. Pema PJ, Horak HA, Wyatt RH. Myelopathy caused by nitrous oxide toxicity. AJNR Am J Neuroradiol. 1998 May;19(5):894-6.

85. Peracchi M, Bamonti Catena F, Pomati M, De Franceschi M, Scalabrino G. Human cobalamin deficiency: alterations in serum tumour necrosis factor-alpha and epidermal growth factor. Eur J Haematol. 2001 Aug;67(2):123-7.

86. Pfohl-Leszkowicz A, Keith G, Dirheimer G. Effect of cobalamin derivatives on in vitro enzymatic DNA methylation: methylcobalamin can act as a methyl donor. Biochemistry. 1991 Aug 13;30(32):8045-51.

87. Raux E, Schubert HL, Warren MJ. Biosynthesis of cobalamin (vitamin B12): a bacterial conundrum. Cell Mol Life Sci. 2000 Dec;57(13-14):1880-93.

88. Ray JG, Cole DE, Boss SC. An Ontario-wide study of vitamin B12, serum folate, and red cell folate levels in relation to plasma homocysteine: is a preventable public health issue on the rise?. Clin Biochem. 2000 Jul;33(5):337-43.

89. Reynolds EH, Bottiglieri T, Laundy M, Stern J, Payan J, Linnell J, Faludy J. Subacute combined degeneration with high serum vitamin B12 level and abnormal vitamin B12 binding protein. New cause of an old syndrome. Arch Neurol. 1993 Jul;50(7):739-42.

90. Rosenblatt DS, Fenton WA: Inborn errors of cobalamin metabolism, in Banerjee R (ed): *Chemistry and Biology of B12*: New York, John Wiley, 1999, p. 367.

91. Scalabrino G, Buccellato FR, Veber D, Mutti E. New basis of the neurotrophic action of vitamin B12. Clin Chem Lab Med. 2003 Nov;41(11):1435-7.

92. Scalabrino G, Tredici G, Buccellato FR, Manfridi A. Further evidence for the involvement of epidermal growth factor in the signaling pathway of vitamin B12 (cobalamin) in the rat central nervous system. J Neuropathol Exp Neurol. 2000 Sep;59(9):808-14.

93. Scriver, Charles R., et. al, 2001. The Metabolic and Molecular Bases of Inherited Disease, 8th Edition, McGraw Hill Medical Publishing Division: New York, St. Louis, San Francisco. pp. 2164-2193; pp. 3896-3933.

94. Seetharam B: Gastrointestinal absorption and transport of cobalamin (vitamin B12) in Johnson LR (ed): *Physiology of the Gastrointestinal Tract*, New York, Raven, 1997.

95. Sennett C, Rosenberg LE, Mellman IS. Transmembrane transport of cobalamin in prokaryotic and eukaryotic cells. Annu Rev Biochem. 1981;50:1053-86.

96. Sharma, A. and Deth, R.C.: Protein kinase C regulates basal and D4 dopamine receptor-mediated phospholipid methylation in neuroblastoma cells. Eur. J. Pharmacol. 427: 83-90 (2001).

97. Sharma, A., Kramer, M., Wick, P.F., Liu, D., Chari, S., Shim, S., Tan, W.-B., Ouellette, D., Nagata, M., DuRand, C., Kotb, M. and Deth, R.C.: Dopamine D4 receptor-

mediated methylation of membrane phospholipids and its implications for mental illnesses such as schizophrenia. Molecular Psychiatry 4: 235-246 (1999).

98. Shimizu N, Hamazoe R, Kanayama H, Maeta M, Koga S. Experimental study of antitumor effect of methyl-B12. Oncology. 1987;44(3):169-73

99. Small DH, Carnegie PR, Anderson RM. Cycloleucine-induced vacuolation of myelin is associated with inhibition of protein methylation. Neurosci Lett. 1981 Feb 6;21(3):287-92.

100. Sponne IE, Gaire D, Stabler SP, Droesch S, Barbe FM, Allen RH, Lambert DA, Nicolas JP. Inhibition of vitamin B12 metabolism by OH-cobalamin c-lactam in rat oligodendrocytes in culture: a model for studying neuropathy due to vitamin B12 deficiency. Neurosci Lett. 2000 Jul 21;288(3):191-4.

101. Takahashi K, Okawa M, Matsumoto M, Mishima K, Yamadera H, Sasaki M, Ishizuka Y, Yamada K, Higuchi T, Okamoto N, Furuta H, Nakagawa H, Ohta T, Kuroda K, Sugita Y, Inoue Y, Uchimura N, Nagayama H, Miike T, Kamei K. Double-blind test on the efficacy of methylcobalamin on sleep-wake rhythm disorders. Psychiatry Clin Neurosci. 1999 Apr;53(2):211-3.

102. Takase M, Taira M, Sasaki H. Sleep-wake rhythm of autistic children. Psychiatry Clin Neurosci. 1998 Apr;52(2):181-2.

103. Taniguchi H, Ejiri K, Baba S. Improvement of autonomic neuropathy after mecobalamin treatment in uremic patients on hemodialysis. Clin Ther. 1987;9(6):607-14

104. Tashiro S, Sudou K, Imoh A, Koide M, Akazawa Y. Phosphatidylethanolamine methyltransferase activity in developing, demyelinating, and diabetic mouse brain. Tohoku J Exp Med. 1983 Dec;141 Suppl:485-90.

105. Taylor RT, Weissbach H. Escherichia coli B N5-methyltetrahydrofolate-homocysteine methyltransferase: sequential formation of bound methylcobalamin with S-adenosyl-L-methionine and N5-methyltetrahydrofolate. Arch Biochem Biophys. 1969 Feb;129(2):728-44.

106. Taylor RT, Weissbach H. Escherichia coli B N5-methyltetrahydrofolate-homocysteine vitamin-B12 transmethylase: formation and photolability of a methylcobalamin enzyme. Arch Biochem Biophys. 1968 Jan;123(1):109-26.

107. Taylor RT, Weissbach H. Enzymic synthesis of methionine: formation of a radioactive cobamide enzyme with N5-methyl-14C-tetrahydrofolate. Arch Biochem Biophys. 1967 Mar;119(1):572-9.

108. Tefferi A, Pruthi RK. The biochemical basis of cobalamin deficiency. Mayo Clin Proc. 1994 Feb;69(2):181-6.

109. Tomczyk A, Helewski K, Glowacka M, Konecki J, Stepien M. [Neurological picture and selected diagnostic indices of vitamin b12 malabsorption syndrome]

110. [Neurological picture and selected diagnostic indices of vitamin b12 malabsorption syndrome] Wiad Lek. 2001;54(5-6):305-10.

111. Tomoda A, Miike T, Matsukura M. Circadian rhythm abnormalities in adrenoleukodystrophy and methyl B12 treatment. Brain Dev. 1995 Nov-Dec;17(6):428-31.

112. Toskes PP, Hansell J, Cerda J, Deren JJ. Vitamin B 12 malabsorption in chronic pancreatic insufficiency. N Engl J Med. 1971 Mar 25;284(12):627-32.

113. Tsao CS, Miyashita K, Young M. Cytotoxic activity of cobalamin in cultured malignant and nonmalignant cells. Pathobiology. 1990;58(5):292-6.

114. Tsao CS, Myashita K. Influence of cobalamin on the survival of mice bearing ascites tumor. Pathobiology. 1993;61(2):104-8

115. Turley CP, Brewster MA. Alpha-tocopherol protects against a reduction in adenosyl-cobalamin in oxidatively stressed human cells. J Nutr. 1993 Jul;123(7):1305-12.

116. Tsukerman ES, Korsova TL, Poznanskaia AA. [Cobalamins in normal and pathological states (review)] Vopr Med Khim. 1985 Sep-Oct;31(5):7-17.

117. Uchiyama M, Mayer G, Okawa M, Meier-Ewert K. Effects of vitamin B12 on human circadian body temperature rhythm. Neurosci Lett. 1995 Jun 2;192(1):1-4.

118. Van Hove JL, Van Damme-Lombaerts R, Grunewald S, Peters H, Van Damme B, Fryns JP, Arnout J, Wevers R, Baumgartner ER, Fowler B. Cobalamin disorder Cbl-C presenting with late-onset thrombotic microangiopathy. Am J Med Genet. 2002 Aug 1;111(2):195-201.

119. Vieira-Makings E, van der Westhuyzen J, Metz J. Both valine and isoleucine supplementation delay the development of neurological impairment in vitamin B12 deficient bats. Int J Vitam Nutr Res. 1990;60(1):41-6.

120. Vitols E, Walker GA, Huennekens FM. Enzymatic conversion of vitamin B-12s to a cobamide coenzyme, alpha-(5,6-dimethylbenzimidazolyl)deoxyadenosylcobamide (adenosyl-B-12). J Biol Chem. 1966 Apr 10;241(7):1455-61.

121. Wada M, Kawata T, Yamada K, Funada U, Kuwamori M, Endo M, Tanaka N, Tadokoro T, Maekawa A. Serum C3 content in vitamin B(12)-deficient rats. Int J Vitam Nutr Res. 1998;68(2):94-7.

122. Walker GA, Murphy S, Huennekens FM. Enzymatic conversion of vitamin B 12a to adenosyl-B 12: evidence for the existence of two separate reducing systems. Arch Biochem Biophys. 1969 Oct;134(1):95-102.

123. Waly, M, and Deth, R.C.: Glutathione and methylcobalamin-dependent methionine synthase activity in neuronal cells: Implications for neurodevelopmental and neurodegenerative disorders. (In Preparation). 124. Waly, M., Power-Charnitsky, V., Deth, R.C.: Reduced activation of phospholipid methylation by the seven-repeat variant of the D4 dopamine receptor. Eur. J. Pharmacol. (Submitted).

125. Waly, M., Banerjee, R., Choi, S.W., Mason, J., Benzecry, J., Power-Charnitsky, V.A, Deth, R.C. PI3-kinase regulates methionine synthase: Activation by IGF-1 or dopamine and inhibition by heavy metals and thimerosal Molecular Psychiatry 9: 358-370 (2004).

126. Waly M, Olteanu H, Banerjee R, Choi SW, Mason JB, Parker BS, Sukumar S, Shim S, Sharma A, Benzecry JM, Power-Charnitsky VA, Deth RC. Activation of methionine synthase by insulin-like growth factor-1 and dopamine: a target for neurodevelopmental toxins and thimerosal. Mol Psychiatry. 2004 Jan 27 [Epub ahead of print]

127. Wang FK, Koch J, Stokstad EL. Folate coenzyme pattern, folate linked enzymes and methionine biosynthesis in rat liver mitochondria. Biochem Z. 1967 Jan 27;346(5):458-66.

128. Watanabe F, Nakano Y. [Vitamin B_{12}] Nippon Rinsho. 1999 Oct;57(10):2205-10.

129. Weinberg JB, Shugars DC, Sherman PA, Sauls DL, Fyfe JA. Cobalamin inhibition of HIV-1 integrase and integration of HIV-1 DNA into cellular DNA. Biochem Biophys Res Commun. 1998 May 19;246(2):393-7.

130. Weir DG, Scott JM. The biochemical basis of the neuropathy in cobalamin deficiency. Baillieres Clin Haematol. 1995 Sep;8(3): 479-97.

131. Weissbach H, Taylor R. Role of vitamin B12 in methionine synthesis. Fed Proc. 1966 Nov-Dec;25(6):1649-56.

132. Yagihashi S, Tokui A, Kashiwamura H, Takagi S, Imamura K. In vivo effect of methylcobalamin on the peripheral nerve structure in streptozotocin diabetic rats. Horm Metab Res. 1982 Jan;14(1):10-3.

133. Yamadera H, Takahashi K, Okawa M. A multicenter study of sleep-wake rhythm disorders: therapeutic effects of vitamin B12, bright light therapy, chronotherapy and hypnotics. Psychiatry Clin Neurosci. 1996 Aug;50(4):203-9.

134. Yamashiki M, Nishimura A, Kosaka Y. Effects of methylcobalamin (vitamin B12) on in vitro cytokine production of peripheral blood mononuclear cells. J Clin Lab Immunol. 1992;37(4):173-82

135. Yaqub BA, Siddique A, Sulimani R. Effects of methylcobalamin on diabetic neuropathy. Clin Neurol Neurosurg. 1992;94(2):105-11.

136. Yeomans ND, St John DJ. Small intestinal malabsorption of vitamin B(12) in iron-deficient rats. Pathology. 1975 Jan;7(1):35-44.

137. Youngdahl-Turner P, Mellman IS, Allen RH, Rosenberg LE. Protein mediated vitamin uptake. Adsorptive endocytosis of the transcobalamin II-cobalamin complex by cultured human fibroblasts. Exp Cell Res. 1979 Jan;118(1):127-34.

138. Youngdahl-Turner P, Rosenberg LE, Allen RH. Binding and uptake of transcobalamin II by human fibroblasts. J Clin Invest. 1978 Jan;61(1):133-41.

139. Zakharyan RA, Aposhian HV. Arsenite methylation by methylvitamin B12 and glutathione does not require an enzyme. Toxicol Appl Pharmacol. 1999 Feb 1;154(3):287-91.

140. Zhao W, Mosley BS, Cleves MA, Melnyk S, James SJ, Hobbs CA. Neural tube defects and maternal biomarkers of folate, homocysteine, and glutathione metabolism. Birth Defects Res A Clin Mol Teratol. 2006 Apr;76(4):230-6.

141. Zhao, R., Chen, Y., Tan, W., Waly, M., Malewicz, B., Stover, P., Rosowsky, A. and Deth, R.C.: Influence of single-carbon folate and *de novo* purine synthesis pathways on D4 dopamine receptor-mediated phospholipid methylation. J. Neurochem. 78: 788-796 (2001).

Chapter 40. Music Therapy, by the American Music Therapy Association

1. Gold, C., & Wigram, T. (2006). Music therapy for autistic spectrum disorder. *Cochrane Database of Systematic Reviews, 1.*

2. Reitman, M. R. (2005). Effectiveness of music therapy interventions on joint attention in children diagnosed with autism: A pilot study (Doctoral dissertation, Carlos Albizu University, 2005). *Dissertation Abstracts International, B66*(11). (AAT 3195248)

3. Umbarger, G.T. (2007). State of the evidence regarding complementary and alternative medical treatments for autism spectrum disorders. *Education and Training in Developmental Disabilities*, 42(4): 437–447.

4. Wigram, T. (2002). Indications in music therapy. *British Journal of Music Therapy, 16*(1), 11–28.

5. Standley, J. M. (1996). A meta-analysis on the effects of music as reinforcement for education/therapy objectives. *Journal of Research in Music Education, 44*(2), 105–133.

6. Whipple, J. (2004). *Music in intervention for children and adolescents with autism: A meta-analysis.* Journal of Music Therapy, 41*(2), 90–106. (Listed in* Database of Abstracts of Reviews of Effects *produced by the Centre for Reviews and Dissemination, 2007.)*

7.   Kaplan, R. S., & Steele, A. L. (2005). An analysis of music therapy program goals and outcomes for clients with diagnoses on the autism spectrum. *Journal of Music Therapy, 42*(1), 2–19.

Chapter 41. Neurofeedback (Neurotherapy or EEG Biofeedback), by Dr. Betty Jarusiewicz

1.   www.eegspectrum.com/FAQ/
2.   Jarusiewicz, B. Diagram of Dysregulated vs. Typical Brain Behavior Steinberg, M & Othmer, S. (2004). *ADD: The 20-Hour Solution. Training minds to concentrate and self-regulate naturally without medication*. 35.
3.   www.eegspectrum.com/FAQ/
4.   Sichel, A.G., Fehmi, L.G., & Goldstein, D.M. (1995). Positive outcome with Neurofeedback treatment in a case of mild autism. *Journal of Neurotherapy, 1* (1), 60–64.
5.   Hauri, P.J. (1981). Treating psychophysiologic insomnia with biofeedback. *Archives of General Psychiatry, 38*(7), 752–758.
6.   Kaiser, D.A. & Othmer, S. (1995). Efficacy of smr-beta Neurofeedback on attentional processes. *Affiliate Package Section IV, Publication/Research*. Encino, CA: EEG Spectrum Inc.
7.   Lantz, D. & Sterman, M.B. (1992). Neuropsychological prediction and outcome measure in relation to EEG feedback training for the treatment of epilepsy. In T.L. Bennet (Ed.), *Critical issues in neuropsychology* (pp 21–231). New York: Plenum Press.
8.   Linden, M., Habib, T., & Radojevic, V. (1996). A controlled study of the effects of EEG biofeedback on cognition and behavior of children with attention deficit disorders and learning disability. *Biofeedback and Self-Regulation, 21*, 35–50.
9.   Lubar, J.F., & Shouse, M.N. (1976). Use of biofeedback in the treatment of seizure disorders and hyperactivity. *Advances in Clinical Child Psychology, 1*, 203–265.
10.   Swingle, P.G. (1996). Subthreshold 10-Hz sound suppresses EEG theta: Clinical application for the potentiation of Neurofeedback treatment of ADD/ADHD. *Journal of Neurotherapy, 2* (1), 1–11.
11.   Tansey, M.A. (1990), Righting the rhythms of reason. EEG biofeedback training as a therapeutic modality in a clinical office setting. *Medical Psychotherapy, 3,* 57–68.
12.   Thomas. .E., & Sattlberger, E. (1997). Treatment of chronic anxiety disorder with neurotherapy: A Case Study. *Journal of Neurotherapy, 2* (3), 1–8.
13.   Jarusiewicz, B. (2002). Efficacy of Neurofeedback for children in the autistic spectrum: A pilot study. *Journal of Neurotherapy, 6* (4), 39–49.
14.   J.R. Evans, Ed. (2007). Jarusiewicz, B.: Use of Neurofeedback with Autistic Spectrum Disorders. *Handbook of Neurofeedback*, The Haworth Medical Press. 321–340.
15.   Coben, R. & Padolsky, I. (2007). Assessment-Guided Neurofeedback for Autistic Spectrum Disorder. *Journal of Neurotherapy, 11*(1), 5–23.
16.   www.biocompresearch.org/biofeedback-institute-research.html.
17.   www.amenclinics.com.
18.   www.brainmapping.org.
19.   www.ucsd.tv/search-details.aspx?showID=14663.
20.   www.irlen.com.
21.   Jarusiewicz, B. (2002). Efficacy of Neurofeedback for children in the autistic spectrum: A pilot study. *Journal of Neurotherapy, 6* (4), 39–49.
22.   www.ari-atec.com.

23. Coben, R. & Padolsky, I. (2007). Assessment-Guided Neurofeedback for Autistic Spectrum Disorder. *Journal of Neurotherapy, 11*(1), 5–23.
24. www.umaccweb.com/diagnostic_tools/index.html.
25. Hirshberg, L. personal communication
26. Jarusiewicz, B. Hints for All Parents.

Chapter 43. NeuroProtek, Flavonoids, and Allergies, by Dr. Theoharis Theoharides

Theoharides TC, Spanos C, Pang X, Alferes L, Ligris K, Letourneau R, Rozniecki JJ, Webster E, Chrousos GP. Stress-induced intracranial mast cell degranulation: a corticotropin-releasing hormone-mediated effect. **Endocrinology.** 1995 Dec;136(12):5745-50.

Esposito P, Gheorghe D, Kandere K, Pang X, Connolly R, Jacobson S, Theoharides TC. Acute stress increases permeability of the blood-brain-barrier through activation of brain mast cells. **Brain Res.** 2001 Jan 5;888(1):117-127.

Theoharides TC, Konstantinidou AD. Corticotropin-releasing hormone and the blood-brain-barrier. **Front Biosci.** 2007 Jan 1;12:1615-28.

Theoharides TC, Doyle R. Autism, gut-blood-brain barrier, and mast cells. **J Clin Psychopharmacol.** 2008 Oct;28(5):479-83.

Theoharides TC, Francis K, Vasiadi M, Sideri K, Chliva K, Christoni Z, Kempuraj K, Theoharides A, Kalogeromitros D. Increased serum neurotensin, IL-6 and IL-17 in young children with autism. **J Neuroimmunol,** 2010, in press.

Theoharides, TC. Autistic spectrum diseases and mastocytosis. **Intl J Immunopathol Pharmacol.** 2009 Oct-Dec;22(4):859-65.

Theoharides TC, Doyle R, Francis K, Conti P, Kalogeromitros D. Novel therapeutic targets for autism. **Trends Pharmacol Sci.** 2008 Aug;29(8):375-82.

Theoharides TC, Kempuraj D, Redwood L. Autism: an emerging 'neuroimmune disorder' in search of therapy. **Expert Opin Pharmacother.** 2009 Sep;10(13):2127-43.

Theoharides TC, Angelidou A, Alysandratos K-D. Neonatal mast cell activation and autism. **Brain Behavior Immunity,** in press, 2010.

Theoharides TC, Kalogeromitros D. The critical role of mast cells in allergy and inflammation. *Ann N Y Acad Sci.* 2006 Nov;1088:78-99.

Theoharides TC, Kempuraj D, Tagen M, Conti P, Kalogeromitros D. Differential release of mast cell mediators and the pathogenesis of inflammation. *Immunol Rev.* 2007 Jun;217:65-78.

Kempuraj D, Asadi S, Zhang B, Manola A, Hogan J, Peterson E, Theoharides Mercury induces inflammatory mediator release from human mast cells. **J Neuroinflamm,** in press, 2010.

Middleton E Jr, Kandaswami C, Theoharides TC. The effects of plant flavonoids on mammalian cells: implications for inflammation, heart disease, and cancer. **Pharmacol Rev.** 2000 Dec;52(4):673-751.

Kempuraj D, Madhappan B, Christodoulou S, Boucher W, Cao J, Papadopoulou N, Cetrulo CL, Theoharides TC. Flavonols inhibit proinflammatory mediator release, intracellular calcium ion levels and protein kinase C theta phosphorylation in human mast cells. **Br J Pharmacol.** 2005 Aug;145(7):934-44.

Kandere-Grzybowska K, Kempuraj D, Cao J, Cetrulo CL, Theoharides TC. Regulation of IL-1-induced selective IL-6 release from human mast cells and inhibition by quercetin. **Br J Pharmacol.** 2006 May;148(2):208-15.

Kempuraj D, Tagen M, Iliopoulou BP, Clemons A, Vasiadi M, Boucher W, House M, Wolfberg A, Theoharides TC. Luteolin inhibits myelin basic protein-induced human mast cell activation and mast cell-dependent stimulation of Jurkat T cells. **Br J Pharmacol**. 2008 Dec;155(7):1076-84.

Harwood M, Danielewska-Nikiel B, Borzelleca JF, Flamm GW, Williams GM, Lines TC. A critical review of the data related to the safety of quercetin and lack of evidence of in vivo toxicity, including lack of genotoxic/carcinogenic properties. **Food Chem Toxicol**. 2007 Nov;45(11):2179-205.

Chapter 45. Parent Support, by Dr. Lauren Tobing-Puente

1. Tobing, L., & Glenwick, D. S. (2002). Relation of the Childhood Autism Rating Scale-Parent Version to diagnosis, stress, and age. *Research in Developmental Disabilities, 23,* 211–223.

2. Brobst, J.B., Clopton, J. R., & Hendrick, S.H. (2009). Parenting children with autism spectrum disorders: The couple's relationship. *Focus on Autism and Other Developmental Disabilities, 24,* 38–49.

3. Konstantareas, M. M., Homatidis, S., & Plowright, C. M. S. (1992). Assessing resources and stress in parents of severely dysfunctional children through the Clarke modification of Holroyd's Questionnaire on Resources and Stress. *Journal of Autism and Developmental Disorders, 22,* 217–234.

4. Fisman, S., & Wolf, L. (1991). The handicapped child: Psychological effects on parental, marital and sibling relationships. *Psychiatric Clinics of North America, 14,* 199–217.

5. Tobing, L. E., & Glenwick, D. S. (2006). Predictors and moderators of psychological distress in mothers of children with pervasive developmental disorders. *Journal of Family Social Work, 10,* 1–22.

6. Rodrigue, J. R., Morgan, S. B., & Geffken, G. (1990). Families of autistic children: Psychological functioning of mothers. *Journal of Clinical Child Psychology, 19,* 371–379.

7. Greenspan, S. I., & Wieder, S. (2006). *Engaging autism: Using the floortime approach to help children relate, communicate and think.* Cambridge, MA: Da Capo Press

Chapter 48. Physical Therapy, by Meghan Collins

1. Description of Physical Therapy—The World Confederation for Physical Therapy (WCPT) www.wcpt.org/description_of_physical_therapy

2. Bly, L (1983). The Components of Normal Development During the First Year of Life. Neuro-Developmental Treatment Association, Inc.

3. Schmidt, R.A. (1988). *Motor Control and Learning: A Behavioral Emphasis.* 2nd ed. Champaign, IL: Human Kinetics.

4. Campbell, SK Physical Therapy for Children Second Edition. WB Saunders, 2000 Cohen S *Targering Autism: What we Know, Don't Know, and Can do to Help Young Children with Autism and Related Disorders.* California: University of California Press. 1998

Chapter 49. PPAR Agonists (Actos), by Dr. Michael Elice

1. Stubbs EG, Autistic children exhibit undetectable hem agglutination-inhibition antibody titers despite previous rubella vaccination, J> Autism child Schizophrenia. 1976; 6:269–274

2. Stubbs, EG and Crawford ML, Depressed lymphocyte responsiveness in autistic children, J.Autism Child Schizophr. 1977;749–55

3. Molloy CA, Morrow AL, etal. Elevated cytokine levels in children with autism spectrum disorder. J. Neuroimmunology. 2005 Dec 14

4. Pershadsingh HA, Peroxisome proliferators-activated receptor-g: therapeutic target for diseases beyond diabetes:quo vadis? Expert Opinion on Investigational Drugs. 2004;13:3

5. Mrak, RE and Landreth, GE. PPAR-g, neuroinflammation, and disease. J. of Neuroinflammation. 2004,1:5

6. Roberts-Thomson SJ. Peroxisome proliferator-activated receptors in tumorigenesis: targets of tumour promotion and treatment: Immunol Cell Biol 2000; 78:436–41

7. Gelman, L, Fruchart JC, Auwerx J. an update on the mechanisms of action of the peroxisome proliferators-activated receptors (PPARs) and their roles in inflammation and cancer. Cell Mol Life Sci 1999;55:932–43

8. Baba, S, Pioglitazone: a review of Japanese clinical studies. Curr Med Res Opin, 2001. 17(3): 166–89

9. Diagnostic and Statistical Manual of the American Psychiatric Association 4th ed. (DSM-IV) American Psychiatric Association, 1994

Chapter 52. Respen-A, by Dr. Fred Starr

1. World Health Organization (2006). "F84. Pervasive developmental disorders". *International Statistical Classification of Diseases and Related Health Problems* (10th ed. (ICD-10) ed.).

2. Catherine R. Prevalence of Autism Spectrum Disorders - Autism and Developmental Disabilities Monitoring Network, 14 Sites, United States, 2002. Surveillance summaries. February 9, 2007 MMWR 56(SS01);12–28.

3. Gardener H, Spiegelman D, Buka SL (2009). "Prenatal risk factors for autism: comprehensive meta-analysis". *Br J Psychiatry* 195 (1): 7–14

4. Taylor B (2006). "Vaccines and the changing epidemiology of autism". *Child Care Health Dev* 32 (5): 511–9.

5. Posey DJ, Stigler KA, Erickson CA, McDougle CJ (2008). "Antipsychotics in the treatment of autism". *J Clin Invest* 118 (1): 6–14.

6. Eikeseth S (2009). "Outcome of comprehensive psycho-educational interventions for young children with autism". *Res Dev Disabil* 30 (1): 158–78.

7. Myers SM, Johnson CP, Council on Children with Disabilities (2007). "Management of children with autism spectrum disorders". *Pediatrics* 120 (5): 1162–82.

8. Oswald DP, Sonenklar NA (2007). "Medication use among children with autism spectrum disorders". *J Child Adolesc Psychopharmacol* 17 (3): 348–55.

9. Chavez B, Chavez-Brown M, Sopko MA Jr, Rey JA (2007). "Atypical antipsychotics in children with pervasive developmental disorders". *Pediatr Drugs* 9 (4): 249–66.

10. Angley M, Semple S, Hewton C, Paterson F, McKinnon R (2007). "Children and autism—part 2—management with complementary medicines and dietary interventions". *Aust Fam Physician* 36 (10): 827–30.

11. Levy SE, Hyman SL (2005). "Novel treatments for autistic spectrum disorders". *Ment Retard Dev Disabil Res Rev* 11 (2): 131–42.

12. Millward C, Ferriter M, Calver S, Connell-Jones G (2008). "Gluten- and casein-free diets for autistic spectrum disorder". *Cochrane Database Syst Rev* (2): CD003498.

13. Bartz JA, Hollander E (2008). "Oxytocin and experimental therapeutics in autism spectrum disorders". *Prog Brain Res* 170 (451–62): 451.

14. Andersen IM, Kaczmarska J, McGrew SG, Malow BA (2008). "Melatonin for insomnia in children with autism spectrum disorders". *J Child Neurol* 23 (5): 482–5.

15. Rossignol DA, Rossignol LW, Smith S *et al.* (2009). "Hyperbaric treatment for children with autism: a multicenter, randomized, double-blind, controlled trial" (PDF). *BMC Pediatrics* 9: 21

16. Vijayalakshmi V, Lele JV, Daginawala HF (1978). "Effect of reserpine on the monoamine oxidase (MAO) activity in rat liver and brain". *Biochemical Pharmacology* 27(15): 1985–1986.

Chapter 54. Sensory-Based Antecedent Interventions, by Ginny Van Rie and Dr. L.Juane Heflin

Alberto, P. A., & Troutman, A. C. (2009). *Applied behavior analysis for teachers* (8th ed.). Upper Saddle River, NJ: Pearson Merrill Prentice–Hall.

Ben-Sasson, A., Cermak, S. A., Orsmond, G. I., Tager-Flusberg, H., Carter, A. S., Kadlec, M. B., & Dunn, W. (2007). Extreme sensory modulation behaviors in toddlers with autism spectrum disorders. *The American Journal of Occupational Therapy, 61,* 584–592.

Banda, D., & Kubina Jr., R. (2006). The effects of a high-probability request sequencing technique in enhancing transition behaviors. *Education & Treatment of Children*, *29*, 507–516.

Crane, L., Goddard, L., & Pring, L. (2009). Sensory processing in adults with autism spectrum disorders. *Autism: The International Journal of Research & Practice*, *13*, 215–228.

Ermer, J., & Dunn, W. (1998). The sensory profile: a discriminate analysis of children with and without disabilities. *American Journal of Occupational Therapy, 52,* 283–289.

Dunn, W. (1997). The impact of sensory processing abilities on the daily lives of young children and their families: A conceptual model. *Infants and Young Children, 9(4),* 23–35.

Dunn, W. (1999). *Sensory profile.* San Antonio, TX: Pearson.

Dunn, W. (2001). The sensations of everyday life: Empirical, theoretical, and pragmatic considerations, 2001 Eleanor Clarke Slagle lecture. *American Journal of Occupational Therapy, 55,* 608–620.

Harrison, J., & Hare, D. J. (2004). Brief report: Assessment of sensory abnormalities in people with autistic spectrum disorders. *Journal of Autism and Developmental Disabilities, 34,* 727–730.

Heflin, L. J., & Alaimo, D. F. (2007). *Students with autism spectrum disorders: Effective instructional practices.* Upper Saddle River, NJ: Pearson Merrill Prentice Hall.

Hess, K., Morrier, M., Heflin, L., & Ivey, M. (2008). Autism Treatment Survey: Services received by children with autism spectrum disorders in public school classrooms. *Journal of Autism & Developmental Disorders, 38,* 961–971.

Leuba, C. (1955). Toward some integration of learning theories: The concept of optimal stimulation. *Psychological Reports, 1,* 27–32.

Keeling, K., Myles, B., Gagnon, E., & Simpson, R. (2003). Using the power card strategy to teach sportsmanship skills to a child with autism. *Focus on Autism & Other Developmental Disabilities, 18,* 103.

McIntosh, D. N., Miller, L. J., Shyu, V., & Dunn, W. (1999). Overview of the Short Sensory Profile (SSP). In W. Dunn, *Sensory Profile: User's Manual* (59–73). San Antonio, TX: Pearson.

Myles, B. S. Cook, K. T., Miller, N. E., Rinner, L. & Robbins, L. A. (2000). *Asperger syndrome and sensory issues: Practical solutions for making sense of the world.* Shawnee, KS: AAPC.

Napolitano, D., Tessing, J., McAdam, D., Dunleavy, I., & Cifuni, N. (2006). The influence of idiosyncratic antecedent variables on problem behavior displayed by a person with PDD. *Journal of Developmental & Physical Disabilities, 18,* 295–305.

National Autism Center. (2009a). *National standards report: The national standards project addressing the need for evidence-based practice guidelines for autism spectrum disorders.* Randolph, MA: Author.

National Autism Center. (2009b). *Evidence-based practice and autism in the schools: A guide to providing appropriate interventions to students with autism spectrum disorders.* Randolph, MA: Author.

Parker, R. I., & Vannest, K. J. (in press). Pairwise data overlap for single case research. *School Psychology Review.*

Reinhartsen, D., Garfinkle, A., & Wolery, M. (2002). Engagement with toys in two-year-old children with autism: Teacher selection versus child choice. *Journal of the Association for Persons with Severe Handicaps, 27,* 175–87.

Rogers, S. J., Hepburn, S., & Wehner, E. (2003). Parent reports of sensory symptoms in toddlers with autism and those with other developmental disorders. *Journal of Autism and Developmental Disorders, 33,* 631–642.

Schilling, D., & Schwartz, I. (2004). Alternative seating for young children with autism spectrum disorder: Effects on classroom behavior. *Journal of Autism & Developmental Disorders, 34,* 423–432.

Sweeney, H., & LeBlanc, J. (1995). Effects of task size on work-related and aberrant behaviors of youths with autism and mental retardation. *Research in Developmental Disabilities, 16,* 97–115.

Taber, T., Seltzer, A., Heflin, L., & Alberto, P. (1999). Use of self-operated auditory prompts to decrease off-task behavior for a student with autism and moderate mental retardation. *Focus on Autism and Other Developmental Disabilities, 14,* 159–66, 90.

Tomcheck, S. D., & Dunn, W. (2007). Sensory processing in children with and without autism: A comparative study using the Short Sensory Profile. *The American Journal of Occupational Therapy, 61,* 190–200.

Van Rie, G. L., & Heflin, L. J. (2009). The effect of sensory activities on correct responding for children with autism spectrum disorders. *Research in Autism Spectrum Disorders, 3,* 783–796.

Yack, E., Aquilla, P., & Sutton, S. (2002). *Building bridges through sensory integration* (2nd ed.). Las Vegas, NV: Sensory Solutions.

Zentall, S. S., & Zentall, T. R. (1983). Optimal stimulation: A model of disordered activity and performance in normal and deviant children. *Psychological Bulletin, 94,* 446–471.

Chapter 60. Speech-Language Therapy, by Lavinia Pereira and Michelle Solomon

Buschbacher, Pamelazita W., and Fox, Lise (2003). Understanding and Intervening with the Challenging Behavior of Young Children with Autism Spectrum Disorder. *Language, Speech, and Hearing Services in Schools, 34,* 217–227.Bibby, P., Eikeseth, S., Martin, N., Mudford, O., & Reeves, D. (2001). Progress and Outcomes for Children With Autism Receiving Parent-Managed Intensive Interventions. *Research in Developmental Disabilities*, 22, 425–447. Hegde, M.N., (1999). *PocketGuide to Assessment in Speech-Language Pathology.* San Diego, Singular Publishing Group, Inc.

Kashinath, Shubha; Woods, Juliann.; and Goldstein, Howard. (2006). Enhancing Generalized Teaching Strategy Use in Daily Routines by Parents of Children with Autism. *Journal of Speech, Language and Hearing Research*, 49, 466–485.

Kaufman, Nancy, and Tamara Kasper. "Shaping Verbal Language for Children on the Spectrum of Autism Who Also Exhibit Apraxia of Speech. Apraxia-KIDS." www.apraxia-kids.org.

Peppe, Susan; McCann, Joanne, Gibboa, Fiona; O'Hare, Anne; Rutherford, Marion. (2007) Receptive and Expressive Prosodic Ability in Children With High-Functioning Autism. *Journal of Speech, Language and Hearing Research*, 50, 1015–1028.

Prelock, Patricia PhD. "Treatment Efficacy Summary." www.asha.org.

Ruddell.R.B. (2002).*Teaching Children to Read and Write: Becoming an Effective Literacy Teacher.* Boston: Allyn & Bacon.

Schlosser, Ralf, W., and Wendt, Oliver. (2008). Effects of Augmentative and Alternative Communication Intervention on Speech Production in Children With Autism: A Systematic Review. *American Journal of Speech-Language Pathology*, 17, 221–230.

Schwartz, Heatherann and Drager, Kathryn, D.R. (2008). Training and Knowledge in Autism Among Speech-Language Pathologists: A Survey. *Language, Speech and Hearing Services in Schools*, 39, 66–77.

Siegel, Bryna. (1996). *The World of the Autistic Child.* New York, Oxford University Press, Inc.

Sweeney-Kerwin, E., Zecchin-Tirri, G., Carbone, V.J.; Janeckey, M.; Murrary, D. & McCarthy, K. (2005). Improving the Speech Production of Children with Autism. *Proceedings of the 31st Annual International Convention Association for Behavior Analysis.* Atlanta, Georgia.

Chapter 64. Transcranial Magnetic Stimulation, by Joshua Baruth, Dr. Estate Sokhadze, Dr. Ayman El-Baz, Dr. Grace Mathai, Dr. Lonnie Sears, and Dr. Manuel Casanova.

American Psychiatric Association. (2000). Diagnostic and statistical manual of mental disorders (DSM-IV TR) (4th ed.). Washington, DC: American Psychiatric Association. (text revised).

Barker, A.T., Jalinous, R., Freeston, I.L. (1985). Non-invasive magnetic stimulation of the human motor cortex. *Lancet*, 1,1106–1107.

Belmonte, M.K., and Yurgelun-Todd, D.A. (2003). Functional anatomy of impaired selective attention and compensatory processing in autism. Cognitive Brain Research, 17, 651–664.

Bodfish, J.W., Symons, F.J., and Lewis, M.H. (1999). Repetitive Behavior Scale. Western Carolina Center Research Reports.

Boroojerdi, B., Prager, A., Muellbacher, W., et al. (2000). Reduction of human visual cortex excitability using 1-Hz transcranial magnetic stimulation. *Neurology*, 54, 1529–1531.

Brown, C., Gruber, T., Boucher, J., Rippon, G., Brock, J. (2005). Gamma abnormalities during perception of illusory figures in autism. *Cortex*, 41, 364-76.

Casanova, M. F., Buxhoeveden, D. P., Switala, A. E., & Roy, E. (2002a). Minicolumnar pathology in autism. *Neurology*, 58, 428–432.

Casanova, M. F., Buxhoeveden, D. P., Switala, A. E., & Roy, E. (2002b). Neuronal density and architecture (gray level index) in the brains of autistic patients. *Journal of Child Neurology*, 17, 515–521.

Casanova, M. F., van Kooten, I., Switala, A. E., van England, H., Heinsen, H., Steinbuch, H. W. M., et al. (2006a). Abnormalities of cortical minicolumnar organization in the prefrontal lobes of autistic patients. *Clinical Neuroscience Research*, 6, 127–133.

Casanova, M. F., van Kooten, I., van Engeland, H., Heinsen, H., Steinbursch, H. W. M., Hof, P. R., et al. (2006b). Minicolumnar abnormalities in autism. *Acta Neuropathologica*, 112, 287–303.

Casanova, M.F. (2007). The neuropathology of autism. *Brain Pathology*, 17, 422–33.

Charman T. (2008). Autism spectrum disorders. *Psychiatry*, 7, 331–334.

Farady M: Effects on the production of electricity from magnetism (1831), in Michael Faraday. Edited by Williams LP. New York, Basic Books, 1965, p 531.

George and Belmaker (2007) *Transcrainial Magenetic Stimulation in Clinical Psychiatry.* Arlington, VA: American Psychiatric Publishing, Inc.

George, M.S., Wassermann, E.M., Williams, W.A., Callahan, A., Ketter, T.A., Basser, P., Hallett, M., Post, R.M. (1995). Daily repetitive transcranial magnetic stimulation (rTMS) improves mood in depression. *Neuroreport*, 6, 1853–6.

Gillberg, C., Billstedt, E. (2000). Autism and Asperger syndrome: coexistence with other clinical disorders. *Acta Psychiatrica Scandinavica*,102, 321–30.

Hoffman, R. E., & Cavus, I. (2002). Slow transcranial magnetic stimulation, long-term depotentiation, and brain hyperexcitability disorders. *American Journal of Psychiatry*, 159, 1093–1102.

Mountcastle, V.B. (2003). Introduction.Computation in cortical columns. *Cerebral Cortex*, 13, 2–4.

Pascual-Leone, A., Valls-Sole, J., Wasserman, E.M., et al. (1994). Responses to rapid-rate transcranial magnetic stimulation of the human cortex. *Brain*, 117, 847–858.

Pascual-Leone, A., Walsh, V., Rothwell, J. (2000). Transcranial magnetic stimulation in cognitive neuroscience—virtual lesion, chronometry, and functional connectivity. *Current Opinion in Neurobiology*, 10, 232–7.

Quintana, H. (2005). Transcranial magnetic stimulation in persons younger than the age of 18. *The Journal of ECT*, 21:88–95.

Rippon, G., Brock, J., Brown, C., & Boucher, J. (2007). Disordered connectivity in the autistic brain: Challenges for the 'new psychophysiology'. *International Journal of Psychophysiology*, 63, 164–172.

Rubenstein, J.L.R., Merzenich, M.M. (2003). Model of autism: increased ratio of excitation/inhibition in key neural systems. *Genes, Brain, and Behavior*, 2, 255–267.

Sokhadze, E., Baruth, J., Tasman, A., Sears, L., Mathai, G., El-Baz, A., Casanova, M. (2009a). Event-related potential study of novelty processing abnormalities in autism. *Applied Psychophysiology and Biofeedback*, 34, 37–51.

Sokhadze, E., El-Baz, A., Baruth, J., Mathai, G., Sears, L., Casanova, M. (2009b). Effects of low frequency repetitive transcranial magnetic stimulation (rTMS) on gamma frequency oscillations and event-related potentials during processing of illusory figures in autism. *Journal of Autism and Developmental Disorders*, 39, 619–34.

Sokhadze, E., Baruth, J., Tasman, A., Mansoor, M., Ramaswamy, R., Sears, L., Mathai, G., El-Baz, A., Casanova, M.F. (2009c). Low-Frequency Repetitive Transcranial Magnetic Stimulation (rTMS) Affects Event-Related Potential Measures of Novelty Processing in Autism. *Applied Psychophysiology and Biofeedback*, Nov 26. [Epub ahead of print]

Wassermann, E.M. (1996). Risk and safety of repetitive transcranial magnetic stimulation: report and suggested guidelines from the International Workshop on the Safety of Repetitive

Transcranial Magnetic Stimulation, June 5–7. *Electroencephalography and Clinical Neurophysiology*, 108:1–16.

Whittington, M.A., Traub, R.D., Kopell, N., Ermentrout, B., Buhl, E.H. (2000). Inhibition-based rhythms: experimental and mathematical observations on network dynamics. *International Journal of Psychophysiology*, 38, 315–336.

Wu, A.D., Fregni, F., Simon, D.K., Deblieck, C., Pascual-Leone, A. (2008). Noninvasive Brain Stimulation for Parkinson's Disease and Dystonia. *Neurotherapeutics*, 5:345–61.

Chapter 65. Viruses and Autism, by Dr. Mary Megson

1. Libbey, J. E., Sweeton, T. L., McMahon, W. M., Fujinami, R. S. Autistic disorder and viral infections. *J. Neurovirol.* 2005. Feb; 11(1) 1-10.

2. Jyonouchi H., Geng L., Ruby A., Zimmerman-Bier. Dipregulated innate immune responses in young children with autism spectrum disorders. *Neuropsychobiology.* 2005. May; 146(5): 605-610.

3. Sporn M., Roberts A., Goodman D. *The Retinoids: Biology, Chemistry, and Medicine.* New York: Raven Press, 1994, 536-537.

4. Vojdani A., Campbell A. W., Anyanwa E., Kashanian A., Boch K., Vojdani E. Antibodies to neuron-specific antigens in children with autism. J. Musoimmurd. 2002 Aug; 129(1-2): 168-177.

5. McCandless J. Low-*dose naltrexone for mood and immune system modulation in autism.* DAN! Conference, Oct. 6-9, 2006.

6. Vargas D., Zimmerman A., Pardo C. Neurological Activation and Neuroinflammation in the Brain of Patients with Autism. *Ann. Neur.* 2005. Jan. 57(1): 67-81.

Chapter 66. Vision Therapy, by Dr. Jeffrey Becker

Becker, J. (2009). Vision Therapy Can Help Spectrum Children With Visual Dysfunctions. *The Autism File USA* 33, 76–81

Cohen, A. H., Lowe, S.E., Steele, G.T., Suchoff, I.B., Gottlieb, D.D., & Trevorrow, T.L. (1988). The efficacy of optometric vision therapy, *Journal Of The American Optometric Association, 59*(2), 95–105.

Holmes, J., Rice, M., Karlsson, V., Nielsen, B., Sease, J., & Shevlin, T. (2008). The best treatment determined for childhood eye problem. *Archives of Ophthalmology, 126*(10) 1336–1349. HTS Inc. (2009). 6788 S. Kings Ranch Rd., Gold Canyon, AZ 85118. NeuroSensory Centers of America. (2009). 300 Beardsley Road, Austin, TX 78746

Taub, M.B., & Russell, R. (2007). Autism spectrum disorders: A primer for the optometrist. *Review of Optometry. 144*(5). 82–91

Trachtman, J.N. (2008). Background and history of autism in relation to vision care, *Optometry*, *79*(7), 391–396.

THERAPIES OF THE FUTURE

Chapter 67. Anti-allergic, anti-inflammatory and other future treatments, by Dr. Theoharis Theoharides

Theoharides TC, Spanos C, Pang X, Alferes L, Ligris K, Letourneau R, Rozniecki JJ, Webster E, Chrousos GP. Stress-induced intracranial mast cell degranulation: a corticotropin-releasing hormone-mediated effect. **Endocrinology.** 1995 Dec;136(12):5745-50.

Esposito P, Gheorghe D, Kandere K, Pang X, Connolly R, Jacobson S, Theoharides TC. Acute stress increases permeability of the blood-brain-barrier through activation of brain mast cells. **Brain Res.** 2001 Jan 5;888(1):117-127.

Theoharides TC, Konstantinidou AD. Corticotropin-releasing hormone and the blood-brain-barrier. **Front Biosci.** 2007 Jan 1;12:1615-28.

Theoharides TC, Doyle R. Autism, gut-blood-brain barrier, and mast cells. **J Clin Psychopharmacol.** 2008 Oct;28(5):479-83.

Theoharides TC, Francis K, Vasiadi M, Sideri K, Chliva K, Christoni Z, Kempuraj K, Theoharides A, Kalogeromitros D. Increased serum neurotensin, IL-6 and IL-17 in young children with autism. **J Neuroimmunol,** 2010, in press.

Theoharides, TC. Autistic spectrum diseases and mastocytosis. **Intl J Immunopathol Pharmacol.** 2009 Oct-Dec;22(4):859-65.

Theoharides TC, Doyle R, Francis K, Conti P, Kalogeromitros D. Novel therapeutic targets for autism. **Trends Pharmacol Sci.** 2008 Aug;29(8):375-82.

Theoharides TC, Kempuraj D, Redwood L. Autism: an emerging 'neuroimmune disorder' in search of therapy. **Expert Opin Pharmacother.** 2009 Sep;10(13):2127-43.

Theoharides TC, Angelidou A, Alysandratos K-D. Neonatal mast cell activation and autism. **Brain Behavior Immunity,** in press, 2010.

Theoharides TC, Kalogeromitros D. The critical role of mast cells in allergy and inflammation. *Ann N Y Acad Sci.* 2006 Nov;1088:78-99.Theoharides TC, Kempuraj D, Tagen M, Conti P, Kalogeromitros D. Differential release of mast cell mediators and the pathogenesis of inflammation. *Immunol Rev.* 2007 Jun;217:65-78.

Kempuraj D, Asadi S, Zhang B, Manola A, Hogan J, Peterson E, Theoharides Mercury induces inflammatory mediator release from human mast cells. **J Neuroinflamm,** in press, 2010.

Middleton E Jr, Kandaswami C, Theoharides TC. The effects of plant flavonoids on mammalian cells: implications for inflammation, heart disease, and cancer. **Pharmacol Rev.** 2000 Dec;52(4):673-751.

Kempuraj D, Madhappan B, Christodoulou S, Boucher W, Cao J, Papadopoulou N, Cetrulo CL, Theoharides TC. Flavonols inhibit proinflammatory mediator release, intracellular calcium ion levels and protein kinase C theta phosphorylation in human mast cells. **Br J Pharmacol.** 2005 Aug;145(7):934-44.

Kandere-Grzybowska K, Kempuraj D, Cao J, Cetrulo CL, Theoharides TC. Regulation of IL-1-induced selective IL-6 release from human mast cells and inhibition by quercetin. **Br J Pharmacol**. 2006 May;148(2):208-15.

Kempuraj D, Tagen M, Iliopoulou BP, Clemons A, Vasiadi M, Boucher W, House M, Wolfberg A, Theoharides TC. Luteolin inhibits myelin basic protein-induced human mast cell activation and mast cell-dependent stimulation of Jurkat T cells. **Br J Pharmacol**. 2008 Dec;155(7):1076-84.

Harwood M, Danielewska-Nikiel B, Borzelleca JF, Flamm GW, Williams GM, Lines TC. A critical review of the data related to the safety of quercetin and lack of evidence of in vivo toxicity, including lack of genotoxic/carcinogenic properties. **Food Chem Toxicol**. 2007 Nov;45(11):2179-205.

Chapter 68. Research at the University of Louisville Autism Center, by Dr. Manuel Casanova, Dr. Estate Sokhadze, Dr. Ayman El-Baz, Joshua Baruth, Dr. Grace Mathai, and Dr. Lonnie Sears

Sokhadze EM, El-Baz A, Baruth J, Mathai G, Sears L, Casanova MF: Effects of low frequency transcranial magnetic stimulation (rTMS) on gamma frequency oscillations and event-related potentials during processing of illusory figures in autism. *Journal of Autism and Developmental Disorders*, 39:619–634, 2009.

Chapter 69. Research being conducted at the Seaver Autism Center, by Dr. David Grodberg, et al.

1. Prevalence of autism spectrum disorders - Autism and Developmental Disabilities Monitoring Network, United States, 2006. MMWR Surveill Summ, 2009. **58**(10): p. 1–20.

2. Szatmari, P., et al., Mapping autism risk loci using genetic linkage and chromosomal rearrangements. Nat Genet, 2007. **39**(3): p. 319–28.

3. Wang, K., et al., Common genetic variants on 5p14.1 associate with autism spectrum disorders. Nature, 2009. **459**(7246): p. 528–33.

4. Buxbaum, J.D., Multiple rare variants in the etiology of autism spectrum disorders. Dialogues Clin Neurosci, 2009. **11**(1): p. 35–43.

5. Buxbaum, J.D., et al., Mutation screening of the PTEN gene in patients with autism spectrum disorders and macrocephaly. Am J Med Genet B Neuropsychiatr Genet, 2007. **144B**(4): p. 484–91.

6. Bear, M.F., K.M. Huber, and S.T. Warren, The mGluR theory of fragile X mental retardation. Trends Neurosci, 2004. **27**(7): p. 370–7.

7. Cai, G., et al., Multiplex ligation-dependent probe amplification for genetic screening in autism spectrum disorders: efficient identification of known microduplications and identification of a novel microduplication in ASMT. BMC Med Genomics, 2008. **1**: p. 50.

8. Silverman, J.M., et al., Autism-related routines and rituals associated with a mitochondrial aspartate/glutamate carrier SLC25A12 polymorphism. Am J Med Genet B Neuropsychiatr Genet, 2008. **147**(3): p. 408–10.

9. Bartz, J.A. and E. Hollander, Oxytocin and experimental therapeutics in autism spectrum disorders. Prog Brain Res, 2008. **170**: p. 451–62.

LIST OF AUTISM ORGANIZATIONS

NATIONAL

ACT Today!
Autism Care & Treatment Today!
19019 Ventura Blvd. Suite 200
Tarzana, CA 91356
818-705-1625
Info@act-today.org

ACT Today! is a nonprofit organization whose mission is to provide funding and support to families that cannot afford the treatments their autistic children need to achieve their full potential.

Advancing Futures for Adults with Autism (AFAA)
(917) 475-5059
AFAA@autismspeaks.org
www.afaa-us.org

AFAA was created to inform adolescents and adults with autism about living options and new developments, and promote active community involvement from adults with autism.

Autism Collaboration
4182 Adams Avenue
San Diego, CA 92116
(619) 281-7165
www.autism.org

The Autism Collaboration brings together the most experienced autism advocacy organizations in an effort dedicated to advancing autism research in the interest of all individuals living with autism today and their families.

The Autism Hope Alliance
752 Tamiami Trail
Port Charlotte, FL 33953
888.918.1118
info@autismhopealliance.org

Dedicated to the recovery of children and adults from autism, the Autism Hope Alliance ignites hope for families facing the diagnosis through education and funding to promote progress in the present moment.

AutismOne
1816 W. Houston Avenue
Fullerton, CA 92833
(714) 680-0792
earranga@autismone.org
www.autismone.org

AutismOne is a nonprofit, charity organization educating more than 100,000 families every year about prevention, recovery, safety, and change.

Autism Research Institute
4182 Adams Avenue
San Diego, CA 92116
(619) 281-7165
Media Contact: Matt Kabler
matt@autism.com
www.autism.com

ARI is devoted to conducting research and to disseminating the results of research on the triggers of autism and on methods of diagnosing and treating autism.

Autism Society
4340 East-West Hwy, Suite 350
Bethesda, MD 20814
www.autism-society.org

(301) 657-0881, (800)-3AUTISM x 150
info@autism-society.org

The Autism Society exists to improve the lives of all affected by autism by increasing public awareness about the day-to-day issues faced by people on the spectrum, advocating for appropriate services for individuals across the lifespan, and providing the latest information regarding treatment, education, research and advocacy.

Autism Speaks
2 Park Avenue, 11th Floor
New York, NY 10016
(212) 252-8584
contactus@autismspeaks.org
www.autismspeaks.org

Autism Speaks is dedicated to funding autism research, disseminating information, and providing a voice for autistic people's needs.

Generation Rescue
19528 Ventura Blvd. #117
Tarzana, CA 91356
1 (877) 98-AUTISM
www.generationrescue.org

Generation Rescue is Jenny McCarthy and Jim Carrey's autism organization dedicated to informing and assisting families touched by autism; it provides programs and services for personalized support, and Generation Rescue volunteers are researching causes and treatment for autism.

Helping Hand
1330 W. Schatz Lane
Nixa, MO 65714
(877) NAA-AUTISM (877-622-2884)
naa@nationalautism.org
www.nationalautismassociation.org/
helpinghand.php

Helping Hand is a program from the National Autism Association that provides financial assistance for autism families.

National Autism Association
1330 W. Schatz Lane
Nixa, MO 65714
(877) 622-2884
naa@nationalautism.org
www.nationalautism.org

NAA raises funds for autism research and support and also provides programs, such as Helping Hand, Family First, and FOUND, designed to aid specific needs for families dealing with autism.

SafeMinds
16033 Bolsa Chica St. #104-142
Huntington Beach, CA 92649
404-934-0777
www.safeminds.org

SafeMinds is an organization dedicated to research and awareness of mercury's involvement in such neurological disorders as autism, attention deficit disorder, and more.

Talk About Curing Autism (TACA)
3070 Bristol Street, Suite 340
Costa Mesa CA 92626
949-640-4401
www.tacanow.org

TACA provides medical, diet, and educational information geared toward autistic children, and the organization also has support, resources, and community events.

U.S. Autism and Asperger Association
P.O. Box 532
Draper, UT 84020-0532
(888) 9AUTISM, (801) 649-5752
information@usautism.org
www.usautism.org

USAAA provides support, education, and resources for autistic individuals and those with Asperger's Syndrome.

Unlocking Autism
P.O. Box 208
Tyrone, GA 30290
(866) 366-3361
www.unlockingautism.org

Unlocking Autism was created to find information about autism and disseminate that information to families with autistic children; the organization also raises funds for research and awareness.

ONLINE

Age of Autism
www.ageofautism.com

Age of Autism is an online blog with daily news in the latest autism research, updates, and community happenings.

Foundation for Autism Information & Research, Inc.
1300 Jefferson Rd.
Hoffman Estates, IL 60169
info@autismmedia.org

F.A.I.R. Autism Media is a non-profit foundation creating original, up-to-date and comprehensive educational media (video documentaries) to inform the medical community and the public about the latest advances in research and biomedical & behavioral therapies for autism spectrum disorders.

Schafer Autism Report
9629 Old Placerville Road
Sacramento, CA 95827
edit@doitnow.com
www.sarnet.org

Schafer Autism Report is a publication to inform the public about autism-related issues; it can be found online.

STATE LEVEL

Alabama:

Autism Society of Alabama
4217 Dolly Ridge Road,
Birmingham, AL 35243
Jennifer Robertson, 1-877-4-AUTISM, info@autism-alabama.org
www.autism-alabama.org

ASA's mission is to improve the quality of life of persons with Autism Spectrum Disorders and their families through education and advocacy.

Alaska:

Alaska Autism Resource Center
3501 Denali Street, Suite 101
Anchorage, AK 99503-4039
866-301-7372
www.alaskaarc.org

AARC's mission is to increase understanding and support for Alaskans of all ages with autism spectrum disorder via collaboration with families, schools and communities throughout the state.

Arizona:

A.C.T. Today!
1620 N. 48th Street
Phoenix, AV 85008
Phone (602)275-1107
Fax (602) 275-1108
www.azacttoday.org

The ACT Today! Arizona chapter's mission is to support Arizona families impacted by autism by increasing their access to therapy and support. Our vision is that the quality of life for all Arizona children with autism has been improved through therapy and supports.

Southwest Autism Research & Resource Center (SARRC)
Vocational & Life Skills Academy
2225 N. 16th Street
Phoenix, AZ 85006
(602) 340-8717
sarrc@autismcenter.org
www.autismcenter.org

SARRC provides research and support as well as clinical and consultation programs for a widespread group of autistic individuals and their families.

Arkansas:

HEAR Helping Educate about Autism Recovery
Arkansas Autism Resource & Outreach Center
2001 Pershing Circle, Suite 300
North Little Rock, AR 72114-1841
Telephone/TDD: 800-342-2923
Telephone: 501-682-9900
Dianna D. Varady, Parent Coordinator,
Partners for Inclusive Communities, UAMS
DDVarady@uams.edu
www.arkansasautism.org

We are a parent-run organization based in Little Rock, Arkansas, whose focus is to provide information and support to empower families, educate providers, and increase community awareness about autism spectrum disorders.

California:

ACT Today!
Autism Care & Treatment Today!

19019 Ventura Blvd. Suite 200
Tarzana, CA 91356
818-705-1625
Info@act-today.org

ACT Today! is a nonprofit 501(c)(3) organization whose mission is to provide funding and support to families that cannot afford the treatments their autistic children need to achieve their full potential.

Autism One

1816 W. Houston Avenue
Fullerton, CA 92833
(714) 680-0792
earranga@autismone.org
www.autismone.org

AutismOne is a nonprofit, charity organization educating more than 100,000 families every year about prevention, recovery, safety, and change.

Autism Research Institute

4182 Adams Avenue
San Diego, CA 92116
(619) 281-7165
Media Contact: Matt Kabler
matt@autism.com
www.autism.com

ARI is devoted to conducting research and to disseminating the results of research on the triggers of autism and on methods of diagnosing and treating autism.

Canine Companions for Independence

P.O. Box 446
Santa Rosa, CA 95402-0446
1-866-224-3647
www.cci.org

CCI provides support dogs for assistance to those with disabilities.

Center for Autism & Related Disorders, Inc. (CARD)

19019 Ventura Blvd
Suite 300
Tarzana CA, 91356
818-345-2345
info@centerforautism.com
www.centerforautism.com

The Center for Autism and Related Disorders, Inc. (CARD) diligently maintains a repu-

tation as one of the world's largest and most experienced organizations effectively treating children with autism, Asperger's Syndrome, PDD-NOS, and related disorders. They follow the principles of Applied Behavior Analysis (ABA), and develop individualized treatment plans for each child.

The Coalition for SafeMinds

16033 Bolsa Chica St. #104-142
Huntington Beach, CA 92649
(404) 934-0777
www.safeminds.org

SafeMinds (Sensible Action For Ending Mercury-Induced Neurological Disorders) investigates and disseminates information on risks to children due to mercury in medical products.

For OC Kids Neurodevelopmental Center

1915 West Orangewood, Suite 200
Orange, CA 92868
(714) 939-6409
forockids@uci.edu
www.forockids.org

For OC Kids Neurodevelopmental Center provides education as well as treatment and support for children with developmental, behavioral, and learning issues ages 0–5.

Generation Rescue

19528 Ventura Blvd. #117
Tarzana, CA 91356
1 (877) 98-AUTISM
www.generationrescue.org

Generation Rescue is Jenny McCarthy and Jim Carrey's autism organization dedicated to informing and assisting families touched by autism; it provides programs and services for personalized support, and Generation Rescue volunteers are researching causes and treatment for autism.

SafeMinds

16033 Bolsa Chica St. #104-142
Huntington Beach, CA 92649
404-934-0777
www.safeminds.org

SafeMinds is an organization dedicated to research and awareness of mercury's involvement in such neurological disorders as autism, attention deficit disorder, and more.

Schafer Autism Report
9629 Old Placerville Road
Sacramento, CA 95827
edit@doitnow.com
www.sarnet.org

Schafer Autism Report is a publication to inform the public about autism-related issues; it can be found online.

Sensory Research Center
510 N. Prospect S-308
Redondo Beach, CA 90277
(310) 698-9008
Contact: Jennifer Hoffiz, Founder
Jhoffiz@sensorycenter.com
www.sensoryresearchcenter.org

Sensory Research Center researches treatments and provides services for children with sensory processing disorders and families without the means to participate in sensory therapy.

Talk About Curing Autism (TACA)
3070 Bristol Street, Suite 340
Costa Mesa CA 92626
949-640-4401
949-640-4424 FAX
www.tacanow.org

TACA provides medical, diet, and educational information geared toward autistic children, and the organization also has support, resources, and community events.

Colorado:

The SMART Foundation
PO Box 2181
Vail, Colorado 81658
(970) 476-7702
info@thesmartfoundation.org
www.thesmartfoundation.org

The SMART Foundation works to train professionals and provide a variety of resources and research for families dealing with autism.

Connecticut:

Autism Support Network
Box 1525
Fairfield, CT 06824
(203) 404-4929
info@AutismSupportNetwork.com
www.autismsupportnetwork.com

The Autism Support Network is a support community for individuals and groups who have dealt with autism.

Stamford Education 4 Autism, Inc.
1127 High Ridge Road PMB #315
Stamford, CT 06905
(203) 329-9310
stamforde4autism@aol.com
www.stamfordeducation4autism.org

Stamford Education 4 Autism is an organization to provide awareness and emotional support for autistic children and their families.

Delaware:

Autism Delaware
924 Harmony Road, Suite 201
Newark, DE 19713
(302) 224-6020
delautism@delautism.org
www.delautism.org

Autism Delaware provides support services, resources, and information for people with autism and their families.

Florida:

The Autism Hope Alliance
752 Tamiami Trail
Port Charlotte, FL 33953
888.918.1118
info@autismhopealliance.org

Dedicated to the recovery of children and adults from autism, the Autism Hope Alliance ignites hope for families facing the diagnosis through education and funding to promote progress in the present moment.

Healing Every Autistic Life
226-5 Solana Rd. #211
Ponte Vedra Beach, FL 32082
(904) 285-5651
info@healautismnow.org
www.healautismnow.org

The HEAL Foundation provides support for local autistic individuals through grants for organizations, information, and events.

Georgia:

Autism Society Of Northeast Georgia
PO Box 48366
Athens GA 30604-8366

(706) 208-0066
ga-northeastgeorgia@autismsocietyofamerica.
org
http://negac-autsoc.tripod.com

The Autism Society of Northeast Georgia is a chapter of the Autism Society of America that provides support, information, and meetings for autism families in Georgia.

North Georgia Autism Center
PO Box 38
Cumming, GA 30028
770-844-8624
northgaautismcen@bellsouth.net
www.northgeorgiaautismcenter.com

NGAC's mission is to promote and provide intensive home, school, and center-based behavioral therapy to children, youth and families affected by Autism Spectrum Disorders.

Hawaii:

Pacific Autism Center
670 Auahi Street, Suite A-6
Honolulu, HI 96813
808-523-8188
laura@pacificautismcenter.com
http://pacificautismcenter.com

The mission of Pacific Autism Center is to use ABA and be a foundation for those individuals (and their families) within the autism spectrum, and to also provide access to high quality researched based services that support the individual in all areas of their life.

Idaho:

Idaho Center for Autism, LLC
5353 Franklin Road
Boise, ID 83705
(208) 342-0374
Jackie Mathias, jmathias@
idahocenterforautism.com
www.idahocenterforautism.com

Idaho Center for Autism, LLC, is a small group of people who love the kids and families we work with and are committed to doing our best to help them understand that ASDs are complex disorders, with no easy answers and no guarantees, but we know that the lives of kids affected by autism can improve dramatically and are committed to working with

families in order to determine and administer appropriate treatment.

Illinois:

Easter Seals Headquarters
233 S. Wacker Dr., Suite 2400
Chicago, IL 60606
(800) 221-6827 or (312) 726-6200
www.easterseals.com

Easter Seals provides services and outreach for those with autism, including medical rehabilitation, employment, and recreation information.

Illinois Center for Autism
548 Ruby Lane
Fairview Heights, IL 62208
(618) 398-7500
info@illinoiscenterforautism.org
www.illinoiscenterforautism.org

The Illinois Center aims to prevent the unnecessary institutionalization of people with autism and to help people with autism achieve their highest level of independence within their home, school and community.

Indiana:

Hamilton County Autism Support Group
19215 Morrison Way
Noblesville, Indiana 46060
(317) 403-6705
Contact: Jane Grimes, President
janegrimes@hcasg.org
www.hcasg.org

Hamilton County Autism Support Group is a local support group that provides community awareness and resources for autistic individuals and families.

Iowa:

Eastern Central Iowa Autism Society
851 16th St SE
Cedar Rapids, IA 52403
319-431-9052
Sheri Grawe, Vice President: sherigrawe@aol.
com
www.eciautismsociety.org

Eastern Central Iowa Autism Society strives to be an advocate for all those affected with Autism Spectrum Disorder—to advance their quality of life through biomedicine, education, community awareness, and therapies.

Kansas:

Autism Awareness Association Inc.
PO Box 780898
Wichita, KS 67278
(316) 771-7335
Email: tralanajones@autismawareassoc.org

Heartspring
8700 East 29th Street North
Wichita, KS 67218
(316) 634-8881 , (800) 835-1043
Contact: kbaker@heartspring.org
www.heartspring.org

Heartspring is a facility that supports special-needs children through a variety of clinical and support services.

Kentucky:

Kentucky Autism Training Center
College of Education and Human Development
Dean's Office
University of Louisville
Louisville, KY 40292
800-334-8635 ext. 852-4631
katc@louisville.edu
https://louisville.edu/education/
kyautismtraining

The mission of the Kentucky Autism Training Center is to strengthen our state's systems of support for persons affected by autism by bridging research to practice and by providing training and resources to families and professionals.

Louisiana:

Unlocking Autism
PO Box 15388
Baton Rouge, LA 70895
866-366-3361
www.unlockingautism.org

UA's mission is constantly evolving to meet the ever-changing needs of families who are dealing with ASDs, and it includes bringing issues of autism from individual homes to the forefront of national dialogue, joining parents and professionals in one concerted effort to fight for these children who cannot lift their voices to the nation for help, and helping those

on the autism spectrum reach their greatest potential in leading fulfilling and productive lives in relationships, society and employment.

Maine:

Association for Science in Autism Treatment (ASAT)
PO Box 7468
Portland, ME 04112-7468
207-253-6058
info@asatonline.org
www.asatonline.org

ASAT's mission is to disseminate accurate, scientifically sound information about autism and treatments for autism and to improve access to effective, science-based treatments for all people with autism, regardless of age, severity of condition, income or place of residence.

Maryland:

Autism Society
4340 East-West Hwy, Suite 350
Bethesda, MD 20814
www.autism-society.org

The Autism Society exists to improve the lives of all affected by autism by increasing public awareness about the day-to-day issues faced by people on the spectrum, advocating for appropriate services for individuals across the lifespan, and providing the latest information regarding treatment, education, research and advocacy.

Center for Autism and Developmental Disabilities Epidemiology (CADDE)
Department of Epidemiology
Johns Hopkins Bloomberg School of Public Health
615 N. Wolfe Street, Suite E6031
Baltimore, MD 21205
1-877-868-8014
cadde@jhsph.edu
www.jhsph.edu/cadde

The Center serves to foster communication, coordination, and collaboration among a multi-disciplinary team of researchers around the epidemiology of Autism Spectrum Disorders (ASD) and Developmental Disabilities (DD). We also strive to bring epidemiologic data and research to public health and educational practitioners, as well as to interested ASD and DD public constituencies.

Massachusetts:

Advocates for Autism of Massachusetts
217 South Street
Waltham, MA 02453
(781) 891-6270
Contact: Judy Zacek
zacek@AFAMaction.org
www.afamaction.org

AFAM is an advocacy organization dedicated to promoting rights and providing support for those with Autism and Asperger's Syndrome.

The Autism Research Foundation (TARF)
c/o Moss-Rosene Lab, W701
715 Albany Street
Boston, MA 02118
(617) 414-7012
tarf@ladders.org
www.ladders.org/pages/TARF.html

TARF is collection of researchers looking into the neurobiological effects of autism and similar disorders.

The Doug Flutie Jr. Foundation for Autism
PO Box 767
Framingham, MA 01701
(508) 270-8855
info@flutiefoundation.org
http://dougflutiejrfoundation.org/

The Doug Flutie Jr. Foundation for Autism is committed to supporting families by providing information, resources, and access to the most current autism news and events.

First Signs
P.O. Box 358
Merrimac, MA 01860
(978) 346-4380
info@firstsigns.org
www.firstsigns.org

First Signs is an organization to inform adults about the first warning signs of autism in children.

FRAXA Research Foundation
45 Pleasant St.,
Newburyport, MA 01950
(978) 462-1866

Contact: Katie Clapp, Executive Director
info@fraxa.org, mbudek@fraxa.org, kclapp@fraxa.org
www.fraxa.org

FRAXA's mission is to accelerate progress toward effective treatments and ultimately a cure for Fragile X, by directly funding the most promising research. It also supports families affected by Fragile X and raises awareness of this important but virtually unknown disease.

The Friendship Network for Children
100 Otis St. #4B
Northborough, MA 01532
(508) 393-0030
Contact: Nancy Swanberg, Executive Director
nancy@networkforchildren.org
www.networkforchildren.org

The Friendship Network for Children is dedicated to helping promote the use of creative activities, such as music and art, to reach children with communication-related disabilities, such as autism.

The Gottschall Autism Center
2 Brandt Island Road
P.O. Box 979
Mattapoisett, MA 02739
For information call:
Pam Ferro, RN, President
508-941-4791
Cheryl Gaudino, Executive Director
774-282-0293
email: info@gottschallcenter.com

The Gottschall Autism Center partners with families to provide children and adults with optimal health interventions, support services, educational enrichment and employment.

Greenlock Therapeutic Riding Center
55 Summer St.
Rehoboth, MA 02769
508-252-5814
www.greenlock.org
Laurel Welch, PT, HPCS, Intake Therapist
greenlocktrc@gmail.com

GTRC is a non-profit organization that utilizes equine-related activities for the therapy of individuals with physical, developmental, and emotional differences.

Learning and Developmental Disabilities Evaluation & Rehabilitation Services
1 Maguire Road
Lexington, MA 02421-3114
(781) 860-1700
info@ladders.org
www.ladders.org

LADDERS is a program that evaluates patients with a variety of disabilities, including autism, and provides individual and comprehensive treatment plans.

Michigan:

Michigan Autism Partnership
1601 Briarwood Circle, Suite 500
Ann Arbor, MI 48108
P 734-997-9088
office@aacenter.org
www.mapautism.org

The Michigan Autism Partnership's vision is to create a state-wide network of parents and professionals that supports and promotes intensive, developmental, play-based programming for young children with autistic spectrum disorders.

Minnesota:

Minnesota Autism Center
5710 Baker Road
Minnetonka, MN 55345
952.767.4200
info@mnautism.org
www.mnautism.org

The Minnesota Autism Center's Mission is to promote and provide intensive home, school and center-based behavioral therapy to children, youth and families affected by Autism Spectrum Disorder.

Mississippi:

TEAAM Together Enhancing Autism Awareness in Mississippi
P.O. Box 37
Mize, MS 39116
(601) 733-0090
takeaction@TEAAM.org
www.teaam.org

TEAAM is a non-profit organization dedicated to improving the lives of Mississippians

with an Autism Spectrum Disorder by cultivating and enhancing family and community supports.

Missouri:

Family First
1330 W. Schatz Lane
Nixa, MO 65714
877-NAA-AUTISM (877-622-2884)
naa@nationalautism.org
www.nationalautismassociation.org/familyfirst.
php

Family First is a program by the National Autism Association that provides marital support and promotes unity in autism families.

FOUND
1330 W. Schatz Lane
Nixa, MO 65714
877-NAA-AUTISM (877-622-2884)
naa@nationalautism.org
www.nationalautismassociation.org/found.php

Found is a National Autism Association program that raises funds to counter the rise of wandering-related deaths.

Touchpoint Autism Services
1101 Olivette Executive Pkwy.
St. Louis, MO 63132
314.432.6200
info@touchpointautism.org
www.touchpointautism.org

TouchPoint directly works with hundreds of children and adults with autism spectrum disorders (ASD). They also work with families, helping them learn the special skills they need to care for a family member with autism.

Nebraska:

Autism Action Partnership
14301 FNB Parkway, Suite 115
Omaha, Nebraska 68154
(402) 496-7200
info@autismaction.org
www.autismaction.org

AAP's mission is to improve the quality of life of persons on the Autism Spectrum and their families through education, advocacy and support, thereby enabling them to be an integral part of the community.

Nevada:

Autism Coalition of Nevada
1790 Vassar St
Reno, NV 89502
(775) 329-2268
acon@aconv.org
www.aconv.org

Our mission is to support legislation for screening, diagnosis and treatment clinics, and receive appropriations.

New Hampshire:

The Birchtree Center
2064 Woodbury Avenue, Suite 204
Newington, New Hampshire, 03801
603-433-4192
www.birchtreecenter.org

The Birchtree Center's mission is to improve the quality of life for children and youth with autism and their families through nurturing relationships, therapeutic programming and specialized education.

New Jersey:

The Daniel Jordan Fiddle Foundation
P.O. Box 1149
Ridgewood, New Jersey 07451-1149
(877) 444-1149
info@djfiddlefoundation.org
www.djfiddlefoundation.org

The DJ Fiddle Foundation was created to both develop and support programs for autistic individuals, as well as spread current information.

The Devereux New Jersey Comprehensive Community Resources (DNJCCR)
286 Mantua Grove Road, Bldg. #4
West Deptford, NJ 08066
(856) 599-6400

DNJCCR serves nearly 400 children, adolescents, adults, and their families with special needs. It also has a residential/educational center that serves individuals with autism spectrum disorders.

New Horizons in Autism
600 Essex Rd.
Neptune, NJ 07753
(732) 918-0850

Contact: Michele Goodman, Executive Director
goodman@nhautism.org
www.nhautism.org/default.asp

New Horizons in Autism is an organization that operates six homes, a vocational program, and after-school, voucher stipend and behavior therapy support options.

New York:

Autism United
100 West Nicholai Street
Hicksville, NY 11801
(516) 933-4050
www.autismunited.org

Autism United is a community for families and individuals with autism that supports the professional community of autism researchers.

Foundation for Educating Children with Autism (FECA)
PO Box 813
Mount Kisco, NY 10549
(914) 941-FECA (3322)
questions@FECAinc.org
www.fecainc.org

FECA is a non-profit organization that provides educational opportunities for children with autism through the development of schools, inclusion and vocational programs, consumer advocacy and community outreach.

Special Needs Activity Center for Kids NYC (SNACK NYC)
220 E 86th Street (Lower Level)
New York, NY 10028
(212) 439-9996
info@snacknyc.com
www.snacknyc.com

SNACK is a New York-based activity center where children with special needs can socialize; it has after-school and weekend programs that include a variety of creative activities.

North Carolina:

Autism Services of Mecklenburg County, Inc.
2211-A Executive Street
Charlotte, NC 28208
704-392-9220
info@asmcinc.com

www.asmcinc.com/index.php

ASMC is a private, not-for-profit organizatio offering residential and support services for residents of North Carolina with Autism, Traumatic Brain Injuries and other developmental disabilties.

Autism Society of North Carolina
505 Oberlin Road, Suite 230
Raleigh, NC 27605
1 (800) 442-2762 (NC only), (919) 743-0204
info@autismsociety-nc.org
www.autismsociety-nc.org

The Autism Society of North Carolina provides support services and resources for individuals, professionals, and families dealing with autism in North Carolina.

North Dakota:

North Dakota Autism Center
4733 Amber Valley Parkway, Suite 200
Fargo, ND 58104
701.277.8844
info@ndautismcenter.org
www.ndautismcenter.org

North Dakota Autism Center's mission is to help children affected by autism spectrum disorders to reach their full potential through excellence in care, therapy, instruction and support

Ohio:

4 Paws for Ability
253 Dayton Ave.
Xenia, Ohio 45385
(937) 374-0385
Contact: Karen Shirk
karen4paws@aol.com
www.4pawsforability.org
4 Paws provides service dogs for disabled people, and the company specializes in dogs that are specifically trained to work with autistic people.

Ohio Center for Autism and Low Incidence (OCALI)
470 Glenmont Ave
Columbus OH 43214
(614) 410-0321, (866)-886-2254
ocali@ocali.org
www.ocali.org

OCALI's mission is to support, promote, and train individuals with autism and other low-incidence disorders to live fulfilling and successful lives.

Oklahoma:

Oklahoma Family Center for Autism
3901 Northwest 63rd St.
Oklahoma City, OK
(405) 842-9995
melinda@okautism-efca.org
www.okautism.org

The OFCA provides a way for organizations operating in the state of Oklahoma to share information and help each other advance the cause of families affected by autism. The OFCA is a resource and leadership forum for group leaders in Oklahoma who have a passion to serve their communities.

Oregon:

Autism Service Dogs of America
4248 Galewood St., Lake Oswego, Oregon 97035
info@autismservicedogsofamerica.com
http://autismservicedogsofamerica.com

Autism Service Dogs of America trains service dogs for autistic children.

Northwest Autism Foundation
519 Fifteenth Street
Oregon City , OR 97045
503-557-2111
www.autismnwaf.org

The Northwest Autism Foundation is a non-profit organization whose goal is to provide education and information for free or at a nominal cost to families, caregivers and professionals of autistic children.

Pennsylvania:

Advisory Board on Autism and Related Disorders (ABOARD)
35 Wilson Street, Suite 100
Pittsburgh, PA 15223
(412) 781-4116
support@aboard.org
www.aboard.org

ABOARD is a Pennsylvania-based support society for parents and autistic children, which provides both access to support groups and to a variety of autism information.

Autism Spectrum News
16 Cascade Drive
Effort, PA 18329
(570) 629-5960
Contact: Ira Minot, Executive Director
iraminot@mhnews.org
www.mhnews-autism.org/index.html

The Autism Spectrum News is a publication from Mental Health News Education, Inc. that informs the autism community about research, autism information, and current happenings.

Rhode Island:

About Families, CEDARR Family Center
203 Concord St., Suite 335
Pawtucket, RI 02860
401-365-6855
info@aboutfamilies.org
www.aboutfamilies.org

The About Families CEDARR Center is committed to supporting families of children who have autism spectrum disorders, mental health and substance abuse difficulties, and development, physical, and medical disabilities by providing state of the art information, evaluative, diagnostic, prescriptive, and support services that build on the strengths of the child, family, and community.

Advocates in Action
PO Box 41528
Providence, RI 02940-1528
401-785-2028
www.aina-ri.org

Together we work to help people understand information more clearly, learn about rights, participate in their communities and share their unique gifts with the rest of society.

Autism Project of RI
1516 Atwood Avenue
Johnston, RI 02919
(401) 785-2666
inquiries@riautism.org
www.riautism.org

Autism Project of RI was founded by parents intended to be a resource for other parents in the Rhode Island community who have members of their families who live with ASD.

Rhode Island Technical Assitance Project at the Department of Education
RIDE Office of Special Populations
255 Westminster St.
Providence, RI 02903
401-222-6030
Sue Constable sconstable@ritap.org
www.ritap.org

RITAP provides practitioners, parents, and policymakers the knowledge and resources necessary to increase their capacity to provide comprehensive and coordinated services to all children including those with disabilities that result in improved educational performance and enhanced life-long outcomes.

South Carolina:

Autism Advocate Foundation
PO Box 7061
Myrtle Beach, SC 29572
(843) 213-0217
www.autismadvocatefoundation.com

To provide emotional, financial and therapeutic support for individuals with Autism Spectrum Disorders throughout their lifespan, while achieving their personal goals and dreams with integrity and distinction in their least restrictive environment.

National Autism Association
PO Box 1547
Marion, SC 29571
877-622-2884
naa@nationalautism.org
www.nationalautismassociation.org

The mission of the National Autism Association is to educate and empower families affected by autism and other neurological disorders, while advocating on behalf of those who cannot fight for their own rights.

Tennessee:

The Autism Solution Center, Inc.
9282 Cordova Park Road

Cordova, TN 38018
Phone: 901-758-8288
Fax: 901-758-1806
info@autismsolutioncenter.com

The Autism Solution Center, Inc. is a non-profit organization being developed to address an unmet, ongoing need within our communities for autism therapy, support services, research and other assistance.

Faces of Hope Children's Therapy Center
301 Hancock Street
Gallatin, Tennessee 37066
(615) 206-1176
Contact: Leslie Face, Executive Director
leslie@facesofhopetn.com
www.facesofhopetn.com

Faces of Hope provides speech, occupational, and physical therapies for autistic children in Tennessee and certain areas of Kentucky.

Texas:

ATC Rehabilitation Agency – Dallas
10610 Metric Dr., Suite 101
Dallas, TX 75243
214.221.4405

ATC Rehabilitation Agency – San Antonio
10615 Perrin-Beitel, Suite 801
San Antonio, TX 78247
210.599.7733

Autism Treatment Center – Dallas
10503 Metric Dr.
Dallas, TX 75243
972.644.2076
Anna P. Hundley, CEO

The mission of the Autism Treatment Center is to assist people with autism and related disorders throughout their lives as they learn, play, work and live in the community.

Autism Treatment Center – San Antonio
16111 Nacogdoches Road
San Antonio, TX 78247
210.590.2107
Anna P. Hundley, Executive Director

Vermont:

Howard Center
208 Flynn Avenue Suite 3J
Burlington, Vermont 05401
(802) 488-6000
Contact: Todd Centybear, Executive Director
www.howardcenter.org

Howard Center provides developmental, mental health, substance abuse, and child, youth, and family services through funding, support, and community programs.

Virginia:

Autism Learning Center
7600 Leesburg Pike #410
Falls Church, VA 22043
(703) 506-1930
autismlc@aol.com
www.autismlearningcenter.org

ALC emphasizes a positive and systematic approach to teaching skills and reducing problematic behaviors, taking a creative and flexible approach and capitalizing on the resources available for each child.

Organization for Autism Research
2000 North 14th Street, Suite 710
Arlington, VA 22201
703.243.9710
info@researchautism.org
www.researchautism.org

OAR's mission is to apply practical research that examines issues and challenges that children and adults with autism and their families face everyday to the treatment of individuals living with autism.

Washington:

Families for Effective Autism Treatment (FEAT) of Washington
14434 NE 8th St., Second Floor
Bellevue, WA 98007
206.763.3373
featwa@featwa.org
www.featwa.org

FEAT's mission is to provide families with hope and guidance to help their children with autism reach their full potential.

Washington, D.C.:

Autistic Self-Advocacy Network
1025 Vermont Avenue, NW, Suite 300
Washington, DC 20005
Contact: Ari Ne'eman, Founding President
aneeman@autisticadvocacy.org
www.autisticadvocacy.org

ASAN was created to encourage autistic individuals to seek rights and promote the positive aspects of a diverse community.

West Virginia:

Autism Services Center
The Keith Albee Building
929 4th Avenue, Second Floor
Huntington, WV 25701
(304) 525-8014

ASC is a nonprofit, licensed behavioral health care agency founded in 1979 by Ruth Christ Sullivan, Ph. D. Though specializing in autism, the agency provides comprehensive, community integrated services for individuals with all developmental disabilities, throughout their lifespan.

West Virginia Autism Training Center
Marshall University
One John Marshall Drive
Huntington, WV 25755
1-800-642-3463
www.marshall.edu/coe/atc

The mission of the Autism Training Center is to provide education, training and treatment programs for West Virginians who have Autism, Pervasive Developmental Disorder (NOS) or Asperger's Disorder and have been formally registered with the Center. This is done through appropriate education, training and support for professional personnel, family members or guardians and other important in the life of a person with autism.

Wisconsin:

Chileda Habilitation Institute
1825 Victory Street
La Crosse, WI 54601
Ruth Wiseman, President/CEO
608-782-6480 Ext. 237
www.chileda.org

Chileda is a nationally recognized and respected program for students with exceptional needs and exceptional potential. They serve children and young adults from ages 6 to 21.

Good Friend, Inc.
808 Cavalier Drive
Waukesha, WI 53186
(414) 510-0385, (262) 391-1369
Contacts: Chelsea Budde and Denise Schamens, Founders
chelsea@goodfriendinc.com, denise@goodfriendinc.com
www.goodfriendinc.com

Good Friend, Inc. was created to spread awareness and understanding from regularly-developing children for autistic children; the organization offers information, events, and workshops.

Wyoming:

Casper Autism Society
750 West 58th Street
Casper, WY 82601
307-234-5838
cgarner@tribcsp.com
http://casperautismsociety.com/

The Casper Autism Society serves as a support group for all families affected by autism and for those on the Autism Spectrum (ASD). Monthly meetings are held and a free lending library is available.

INTERNATIONAL

Autism Canada Foundation
(519) 695-5858
www.autismcanada.org

The Autism Acceptance Project
P.O. Box 23030
Toronto, Ontario Canada M5N 3A8
Contact: Estée Klar-Wolfond, Founder and Executive Director
esteewolfond@mac.com
www.taaproject.com

TAAP is a site to promote public understanding and acceptance of autistic people. This site also has an online gallery with creations completely contributed by autistic artists.

The Autism File
PO Box 144
Hampton, TW12 2FF
England
020 8979 2525
info@autismfile.com
www.autismfile.com

The Autism File is a magazine covering autism spectrum disorders, providing information about biomedical research and treatments, education and therapies, advocacy issues, perspectives of individuals on the spectrum, and more.

The Autism Trust
Brackenwood
Hill View Road
Claygate
Surrey KT10 0TU
UNITED KINGDOM
020 8979 2525
info@theautismtrust.org.uk
www.autismtrust.com

The Autism Trust provides a variety of facilities and centers that assist autistic individuals by providing resources and support in health issues, residential needs, professional information, and more.

Child Early Intervention Medical Center, FZ LLC
Dubai Health Care City Al Razi Building, Block B, Suite 2010
P.O. Box 505122 ,Dubai, UAE
Tel: +971 4 423 3667
Fax:+971 4 429 8474
Mobile: +971505512319
www.childeimc.com

Curando el Autismo
www.curandoelautismo.org

EmergenzAutismo (Italy)
www.emergenzautismo.org

MINDD Foundation
PO Box 151 Vaucluse
NSW 2030 Australia
+61 2 9337 3600
info@mindd.org
www.mindd.org

MINDD was created to inform and provide research findings on new and alternative treatments for disorders like autism, such as Chiropractic care, Chinese medicine, and holistic care.

Research Autism
Westbourne House
14-16 Westbourne Grove
London, W2 5RH020 8292 8900
UK
info@researchautism.net
www.researchautism.net

Research Autism is a UK-based charity dedicated to autism research, and is designed for anyone with an interest in autism.

Treating Autism
222 Bramhall Lane South
Bramhall, Stockport
Cheshire SK7 3AA UK
treatingautismuk@aol.com
www.treatingautism.co.uk

Treating Autism has a membership society that receives resources and newsletters, groups that meet for support, and conferences in the UK to inform about biomedical and therapeutic developments for autism.

LIST OF AUTISM
SCHOOLS

Alabama:

Glenwood
The Autism and Behavioral Health Center
150 Glenwood Lane
Birmingham, Alabama 35242-5700
Main Phone: (205) 969-2880

Glenwood provides treatment and education services in a least restrictive setting, through a continuum of care, with the highest respect for individuals and families served.

Arizona:

Arizona Centers for Comprehensive Education and Life-Skills (ACCEL)
10251 North 35th Ave
Phoenix, AZ 85051
(602) 995-7366
Contact: Nancy Molder, Vice President of Educational Services.
nmolder@accel.org

ACCEL is a private, non-profit special education day school providing educational, behavioral and vocational services to students, ages 3-21, with cognitive, emotional, orthopedic, and/or behavioral challenges and Autism.

Chrysalis Academy
600 E. Baseline Rd., Ste. B6
Tempe, AZ 85283
(480) 839-6000
play.aba@gmail.com
www.play-aba.com

Chrysalis Academy is a private year-round school that serves children with autism and related disorders using ABA teaching methods.

Gateway Academy
7655 E. Gelding Drive
Suite #A-3
Scottsdale, AZ 85260
(480) 998-1071
www.gatewayacademy.us/index.htm

Gateway Academy is a private Preschool - 12th Grade day school specializing in students with Asperger's Syndrome, High Functioning Autism, and PDD-nos. It incorporates special techniques into the curriculum, such as puppy therapy, equine therapy, and music therapy.

New Way Academy
1300 North 77th Street
Scottsdale, Arizona 85257
(480) 946-9112
Contact: denise@newwayacademy.org
www.newwayacademy.org

New Way Learning Academy is Arizona's only non-profit, private K-12 day school specializing in children with learning differences.

Pieceful Solutions
6101 E. Virginia St.
Mesa, AZ 85215
(480) 309-4792
piecefulsolutions@yahoo.com
www.piecefulsolutions.com

Pieceful Solutions is an non-profit organization created specifically to offer children with autism and other developmental disabilities comprehensive schooling using innovative teaching techniques. We work cooperatively with students and parents to set, plan for and achieve goals that focus on academics, social, emotional development and life skills.

Arkansas:

The Allen School
824 N. Tyler St.
Little Rock, AR 72205
(501) 664-2961
Contact: Suzy Benham, Director
www.invitingarkansas.com/charity/allen-school.asp

Since 1958, The Allen School has enabled children birth to five, with developmental disabilities, such as cerebral palsy, autism, epilepsy, and mental retardation, to achieve their dreams, through treatment, nurturing, and education.

California:

Beacon Day School
588 N. Glassell Street
Orange, CA 92867
Dr. Mary Jo Lang
(714) 288-4200
(714) 288-4204 FAX
contactBDS@beacondayschool.com
www.beacondayschool.com

California Autism Foundation
4075 Lakeside Drive
Richmond, CA 94806
(510) 758-0433
contactcaf@calautism.org
www.calautism.org

The mission of the California Autism Foundation is to provide people with autism and other developmental disabilities the best possible opportunities for lifetime support, training and assistance in helping them reach their highest potential for independence, productivity and fulfillment.

The Help Group
13130 Burbank Blvd.
Sherman Oaks, CA 91401
(877) 994-3588

The Help Group is a large organization that offers education in seven day schools for preschool through high-school aged students with autism and similar disorders. The schools practice diagnostic teaching, therapies, and physical education.

New Vista School
23092 Mill Creek Drive
Laguna Hills, CA 92653
(949) 455-1270
office@newvistaschool.org
www.newvistaschool.org

New Vista School is a grade 6-12+ progressive educational center that provides a safe, structured educational environment serving the needs of students with Asperger Syndrome, high-functioning Autism, and language learning disabilities who may benefit from social and transitional skills development.

Orion Academy
350 Rheem Blvd
Moraga, CA 94556-1516
(925) 377-0789
office@orionacademy.org
www.orionacademy.org

Orion Academy provides a quality college-preparatory program for secondary students whose academic success is compromised by a neurocognitive disability such as Asperger's syndrome, or NLD (Non-verbal Learning Disorder).

Pacific Autism Center for Education (School and Administrative Offices)
1880 Pruneridge Ave.
Santa Clara, CA 95050
(408) 245-3400
Contact: Jack Brown, Office Manager
admin@pacificautism.org
www.pacificautism.org

PACE has a K-12 school with programs for autistic students; an adult day program; and residential homes. The school's curriculum is based on individual assessment and programs.

PACE (Early Intervention and Sunny Days Preschool)
897 Broadleaf Ln.
San Jose, CA 95128
(408) 551-0312

Contact: Gina Baldi, Early Intervention Director
ginabaldi@pacificautism.org
www.pacificautism.org/intervention.shtml

PACE's early intervention programs focus on intellectual development for children with ASD under 6 years of age through a variety of therapies and techniques.

Pioneer Day School
4764 Santa Monica Ave.
San Diego, CA 92107
(619) 758-9424
pioneeramber@sbcglobal.net
www.pioneerdayschool.org/Home.asp

Our award winning school has created a unique and innovative model to address underlying processing deficits for students with Autism Specturm Disorders (ASD) and other special needs. We also create individualized programs for privately placed students.

Pyramid Autism Center
2830 North Glassell
Orange, CA 92865
Grace Walker, Administrative Assistant
gwalker@pyramidautismcenter.com
www.pyramidautismcenter.com

The Pyramid Autism Center (PAC) is a not-for-profit organization dedicated to serving the Orange County autism community – with specific focus on children and their families. The PAC school utilizes the Pyramid Approach to Education developed by Dr. Andrew Bondy, a world-renowned leader in autism education and research.

Springstone Middle School
1035 Carol Lane
Lafayette, CA 94549
(925) 962-9660
info@thespringstoneschool.org
http://thespringstoneschool.org

The Springstone School is an independent middle school that serves students with Asperger's Syndrome, Non-verbal Learning Disability and other executive function challenges. All instruction integrates pragmatic language, occupational therapy, organizational skills and life skills in the classroom and in the community.

Colorado:

Colorado Institute of Autism
P.O. Box 50254
Colorado Springs, Colorado 80949
(719) 593-7334

Colorado Institute of Autism is a newly established private organization dedicated to children on the autism spectrum. The institution will open its doors as the first school for children with autism, utilizing Applied Behavior Analysis principles, in the State of Colorado. Available services will include a school program, outreach, assessment, workshops, and service as a resource to the community.

The Joshua School
2303 E. Dartmouth Ave.
Englewood, CO 80113
(303) 758-7171
thejoshuaschool@yahoo.com
www.joshuaschool.org

The Joshua School serves children ages 2½ to 21 years. Our programming for learners often combines many research-validated methods (within ABA) into a comprehensive but highly individualized package.

Connecticut:

Connecticut Center for Child Development, Inc.
925 Bridgeport Ave.
Milford, CT 06460
(203) 882-8810
Peggy Fitzsimmons, Private School Program
info@cccdinc.org

The Connecticut Center for Child Development Inc. is a non-profit school that is dedicated to improving the lives of children with autism, Asperger's Syndrome and other pervasive developmental disorders.

Franklin Academy
106 River Road
East Haddam, CT 06423
(860) 873-2700
admission@fa-ct.org
www.fa-ct.org

Franklin Academy is a college preparatory school for grades 9 - 12, accredited by the New England Association of Schools and Colleges, specializing in serving students with

Nonverbal Learning Differences (NLD or NVLD) and Asperger's Syndrome (AS).

The Glenholme School
81 Sabbaday Lane
Washington, CT 06793
(860) 868-7377
info@theglenholmeschool.org
www.theglenholmeschool.org/home.htm

The Glenholme School is a specialized boarding school that provides a therapeutic program and exceptional learning environment to address varying levels of academic, social and emotional development in boys and girls ages 10 to 18.

Greenwich Education and Prep
62 Main Street
New Canaan, CT 06840
(203) 594-9777
Contacts: Katja Krumpelbeck, Assistant Director; Kirsten DeConti Ziotas, Director
katja@greenwichedprep.com; kdeconti@greenwichedprep.com
www.greenwichedprep.com

K-12 school with specialized services including Applied Behavioral Analysis (ABA) methods that teaches current public– and private-school curricula for easy transitions.

Greenwich Education and Prep
49 River Road
Cos Cob, CT 06807
(203) 661-1609
Contacts: Victoria Newman, Executive Director; Meredith Hafer, Director; Stacy Smegal, Assistant Director
vnewman@greenwichedprep.com;
meredith@greenwichedprep.com; stacy@greenwichedprep.com
www.greenwichedprep.com

K-12 school with specialized services including Applied Behavioral Analysis (ABA) methods that teaches current public– and private-school curricula for easy transitions.

Delaware:

Delaware Autism Program
Brennen School
144 Brennen Drive
Newark, DE 19713

(302) 454-2202
(302) 454-5427 FAX

Florida:

The Chase Academy
700 Reed Canal Road
South Daytona, FL 32119
(386) 690-0893
Contact: Mimi Lundell, Executive Director
mtlundell@tcaofvolusia.org
www.tcaofvolusia.org

The Chase Academy, Inc., a private non-profit corporation located in Volusia County, Florida, was established in 2006 to provide educational services specifically tailored to meet the individualized needs of students with high-functioning Autism or any of the related Autism Spectrum Disorders (ASD) and to focus these services on maximizing the students' potential for inclusion into mainstream society.

Coral Rock Academy Operated By
Gersh Educational Development
11155 SW 112th Avenue
Miami, FL 33176
631.385.3342
www.coralrockacademy.org

The Gersh Academy's primary objective is to enable students to be emotionally available to learn. They provide customized educational services to students with neurobiological disorders. Coral Rock Academy educates students grades 4-12.

Florida Autism Center of Excellence
6400 E. Chelsea St.
Tampa, FL 33610
(813) 621-FACE (3223)
www.faceprogram.org

FACE serves students ages 3 to 22 with moderate to severe autism in pre-K through 12th grade and beyond. FACE is available to families in Hillsborough, Pinellas, Pasco, Polk, Manatee and Sarasota counties.

Jacksonville School for Autism
4000 Spring Park Rd.
Jacksonville, FL 32207
(904) 732-4343
info.jsa@comcast.net

JSA is a school for children on the autism spectrum, ages 3 to 18. The school uses a variety of curriculums based on each individual child.

The Jericho School
1351 Sprinkle Drive
Jacksonville, FL 32211
(904) 744-5110
jerichos@bellsouth.net
www.thejerichoschool.org

The Jericho School serves children with autism and developmental delays using ABA and verbal behavior treatments.

Palm Beach School for Autism
1199 W. Lantana Rd. #19
Lantana, Florida 33462
(561) 533-9917
contact@pbsfa.org
www.pbsfa.org

We serve children in our preschool program ages 3-5 years of age and children in our elementary program grades kindergarten through 5th grade.

Piece by Piece Learning Center
965 Pondella Rd.
North Fort Myers, FL 33903
(239) 652-4323
info@peacebypieceinc.com
www.peacebypieceinc.com/school.html

Here our mission is to employ our extensive education and experience, in combination with Applied Behavior Analysis, to provide evidence-based and compassionate services to individuals, families, schools and organizations.

Sydney's School for Autism
St. Patrick Catholic Church
4518 South Manhattan Avenue
Tampa, FL 33611
(813) 835-4591
Contacts: Kathy Swenson, Founder; Antia Maurer, Preschool Director
autisticangels@yahoo.com, anitam@ sydneyschool.com
www.sydneysschoolhouse.com

Sydney's School for Autism serves autistic children and those with similar disorders for preschool, kindergarten, and first-grade students, based on ABA teaching methods.

Victory Center for Autism and Behavioral Challenges
18900 Northeast 25th Avenue
North Miami Beach, Florida 33180
Contact: Courtney Richel, Admission
office@thevictoryschool.org
www.thevictoryschool.org

Preschool, secondary school, and after-school program that uses Applied Behavioral Analysis (ABA) methods and one-on-one teaching in the education of children with autism and related disabilities.

Georgia:

Keystone Center for Children with Autism
1675-A Hembree Road
Alpharetta, GA 30009
404-496-4673

Keystone's mission is two-fold: first, we are dedicated to the educational and social development of children with Autism Spectrum Disorders, and second, we are committed to providing support and training to families affected by autism.

The Lionheart School
180 Academy Street
Alpharetta, Georgia 30004
770-772-4555

Lionheart's mission is to provide a developmentally appropriate program for children on the autism spectrum and other disorders of relating and communicating who need a specialized learning environment, therapeutic interventions, relationship building skills and the educational tools necessary to achieve their greatest potential.

Summit Learning Center
700 Holcomb Bridge Road
Suite 400
Roswell, Georgia 30076
Contacts: Jennifer Mitchell and Shauna Courtney, Directors
jennifer@summitlearningcenter.org, shauna@ summitlearningcenter.org
www.summitlearningcenter.org/index.html

The Summit Learning Center aims to provide individualized, effective, and scientifically based treatment for children with autism and related disabilities that is not otherwise available in the state of Georgia. The Summit Learning Center provides effective treatment, based on the science of Applied Behavior Analysis (ABA).

Hawaii:

Loveland Academy Hawaii
1506 Piikoi Street
Honolulu, HI 96822
contact_information@lovelandacademyhawaii.com
808-524-4243

As a service provider in Honolulu, Oahu, Hawaii for children and young adults with autism, the mission is to provide an array of state of the art, research based, child and family centered, culturally sensitive therapeutic and educational services targeting the biological, psychological, educational, social and emotional needs of children.

Pacific Autism Center
670 Auahi St., Suite A-6
Honolulu, HI 96813
(808) 523-8188
laura@pacificautismcenter.com

The mission of Pacific Autism Center is to use ABA and be a foundation for those individuals (and their families) within the autism spectrum, and to also provide access to high quality researched based services that support the individual in all areas of their life.

Illinois:

Giant Steps Illinois
2500 Cabot Dr
Lisle, IL 60532
(630) 455-5730
Contact: Bridget O'Connor, Executive Director
boconnor@atc-gsi.org

Students in our private day school receive an intensive educational and therapeutic program based on the strengths and individual needs of the child. Using various methodologies such as ABA, repetition and practice, errorless learning, forward and backward chaining, visual supports, hands-on manipula-

tives, sensory strategies, etc. students focus on reading and language arts, vocabulary, functional mathematics, vocational life skills and more.

Illinois Center for Autism (Children's Special Day School Program)
548 Ruby Lane
Fairview Heights, IL 62208
(618) 398-7500
info@illinoiscenterforautism.org
www.illinoiscenterforautism.org/programs/dayschool.html

ICA serves students ages 3-21 who have been diagnosed as having autism, pervasive development disorder, Aspereger's Syndrome, and/or students who exhibit compatible characteristics of autism, such as severe communications disorders, severe behavioral disorders, uneven intellectual skills, and socially inappropriate behaviors.

Soaring Eagle Academy
PO Box 63
Riverside, IL 60546
312-683-5151
contact@soaringeagleacademy.org
www.soaringeagleacademy.org

Soaring Eagle's mission is to provide a social and academic learning environment for students with special needs supporting their individual strengths and learning styles while integrating learning and interaction within a Developmental Individual-Difference Relationship (DIR®) Based Approach.

Kansas:

HeartSpring School
8700 East 29th Street North
Wichita, KS 67226
(316) 634-8730 or (800) 835-1043 (calls outside Wichita area)
admissions@heartspring.org
www.heartspring.org/school/index.php

The Heartspring School, a residential and day program, provides a warm, loving environment for children with developmental disabilities such as autism, and teams of specialists discover and develop the whole child using a multidisciplinary approach.

Rainbows United, Inc.
340 S. Broadway, Wichita, KS 67202
Phone: (316) 267-KIDS
www.rainbowsunited.org/services-child_care.
php
info@rui.org

Kids' CoveSM and Kids' PointSM services include progressive plans for all children regardless of their skill levels to provide the most trusted educational opportunities for all children ages birth through 5.

Maine:

Merrymeeting Center for Child Development
2 Davenport Circle Suite 20
Bath, ME 04530
(207) 443-6200
Contact: karenz@mccdworks.org
www.mccdworks.org/index.html

Merrymeeting Center for Child Development is committed to ensuring that children with autism, Asperger's syndrome and pervasive developmental disorder (PDD) have access to education, treatment and care that is objectively and scientifically validated as effective, delivered by professionals with specific minimum methodological competencies.

Maryland:

The IvyMount School, Inc.
11614 Seven Locks Rd.
Rockville, MD 20854
(301) 469-0223
www.ivymount.org/index.cfm

Named twice by the U.S. Department of Education as a Blue Ribbon School of Excellence, Ivymount is a non-sectarian, non-public special education day school. Ivymount's integrated approach to learning includes educational programs and therapeutic services for over 200 students annually, ages 4-21.

Linwood Center
3421 Martha Bush Drive
Ellicott City, MD 21043
(410) 465-1352
admin@linwoodcenter.org
www.linwoodcenter.org

The Linwood Center serves autistic students ages 9 to 21with residential and educational programs, and uses a variety of individualized techniques.

Massachusets:

Boston Higashi School
800 North Main Street
Randolph, MA 02368
(781) 961-0800
Contact: Deborah Donovan, President
donovan@bostonhigashi.org, admissions@
bostonhigashi.org
www.bostonhigashi.org/index.php

Boston Higashi School, Inc. is the international program serving children and young adults with autism. Our philosophy is based upon the world-renowned tenets of Daily Life Therapy® developed by the late Dr. Kiyo Kitahara of Tokyo, Japan.

Eagleton School
446 Monterey Road
Great Barrington, MA 01230
(413) 528-4385
www.eagletonschool.com

Eagleton School serves boys with PDD and Asperger's, teaching and providing daily therapy with a mainly holistic approach. Students' ages range from 9 to 22.

Melmark New England
461 River Road
Andover, MA 01810
(978) 654-4300
www.melmarkne.org/index.html

Melmark New England specializes in serving those students within our clinical profiles who are currently unable to attend public school. For some children served, the goal is to return the child to the public school setting after the benefits of a Melmark New England education are achieved. For children ages 4 - 8, classroom teachers follow a theme-based curriculum into which individual goals and objectives for each student are carefully embedded

New England Center for Children
33 Turnpike Road
Southborough, Massachusetts 01772
(508) 481-1015
Contact: Cathy Welch, Director of Admissions

cwelch@neec.org
www.necc.org

NEEC provides individualized teaching methods for children with autism and related disorders, and the school provides a variety of extra-curricular activities and therapies.

Riverview School
551 Route 6A East Sandwich
Cape Cod, MA 02537
(508) 888-0489
admissions@riverviewschool.org
www.riverviewschool.org

Riverview School provides middle-school to post-secondary school education for students with learning disabilities, focusing on transitions, personal growth, and wellness.

Minnesota:

The Fraser School
2400 W. 64th St
Minneapolis, MN 55423
612-861-1688
school@fraser.org
www.fraser.org

Fraser's mission is to make a meaningful and lasting difference in the lives of children, adults and families with special needs. We accomplish this by providing education, healthcare and housing services.

Lionsgate Academy
3420 Nevada Ave N.
Crystal, MN 55427
(763) 486-5359
Contact: Elaine Campbell, Administrative
Coordinator
ecampbell@lionsgateacademy.org
www.lionsgateacademy.org

Lionsgate Academy provides a transition-oriented and personalized learning program focused on secondary (grades 7-12) higher-functioning students on the autism spectrum that supports their full potential.

Missouri:

Ozark Center for Autism
3006 McClelland Boulevard
Joplin, Missouri 64804

(417) 347-7600
Contact: Paula Baker, Ozark Center CEO
pfbaker@freemanhealth.com
www.freemanhealth.com/ozarkcenterforautism

Ozark Center for Autism impacts lives daily through the use of Applied Behavior Analysis. Students attend school six hours a day, five days a week to minimize loss of skill.

New Jersey:

The Allegro School
125 Ridgedale Avenue
Cedar Knolls, NJ 07927
973-267-8060
www.allegroschool.org

The Allegro School is a non-profit school that provides quality education, keeps autistic children with their families, and prepares them for community living. The school serves approximately 105 students ages 3-21.

Alpine Learning Group
777 Paramus Road
Paramus, NJ 07652
201-612-7800
Bridget A. Taylor, Executive Director
btaylor@alpinelearninggroup.org
alpinelearninggroup.org/default.asp

The Alpine Learning Group is a non-profit education and treatment program facility for leraners 3 to 21 years of age that utilizes the Applied Behavior Analysis (ABA) treatment for autism.

Bancroft Schools
425 Kings Highway East, P.O. BOX 20
Haddonfield, NJ 08033
(800) 774-5516
Contact: Theresa Tolatta, Director of
Admissions and Marketing
inquiry@bnh.org.
www.bancroft.org/ID_DD/IDDD_
bancroftschool_home.html

The Bancroft School offers early education through secondary education for autistic students with a variety of techniques, including ABA, community-based instruction, and incidental learning.

Bright Beginnings Learning Center

1660 Stelton Road
Piscataway, NJ 08854
(732) 339-9331
Wendy Eaton, Principal
www.mcesc.k12.nj.us/special/bright.htm

The Bright Beginnings Learning Center provides specialized, classroom based instruction, based on the principles of Applied Behavior Analysis for students with autism or autistic-like behavior, ages 3 to 12.

Celebrate the Children School

345 South Main Street
Wharton , NJ 07885
(973) 989-4033
Contact: Monica G. Osgood, Director
info@celebratethechildren.org
www.celebratethechildren.org

Celebrate the Children School uses the developmental, individual, relationship-based model to teach autistic students ages 3 to 19 with a focus on a positive and social educational experience.

The Children's Institute

One Sunset Avenue
Verona, NJ 07044
973-509-3050
Bruce Ettinger, Ed.D., Superintendent/ CEO
webmaster@tcischool.org
www.tcischool.org/default.aspx

TCI uses a model alternative program in which each student's social/emotional and cognitive learning needs are addressed in a prescriptive Individualized Educational Plan (IEP).

Douglass Developmental Disabilities Center

151 Ryders Lane
New Brunswick, NJ 08901-8557
732-932-4500
Dr. Lara Delmolino, Ph.D., BCBA, Acting Director, Adult Services
www.dddc.rutgers.edu

The Douglass Developmental Disabilities Center (DDDC) was established by the Board of Governors of Rutgers, The State University of New Jersey in 1972 to meet the needs of people with autism spectrum disorders

and their families and continues to do so by employing ABA-based therapies.

Garden Academy

P.O. Box 188
Maplewood, NJ 07040-0188
(973) 761-6140
info@gardenacademy.org
www.gardenacademy.org

Garden Academy will serve individuals with autism ages 3-21. Garden Academy uses scientific, data-based and accountable interventions to provide an individualized education to students with autism so that they may lead lives of the greatest possible independence.

The Midland School

94 Readington Road
PO Box 5026
North Branch, New Jersey 08876
(908) 722-8222
info@midlandschool.org
www.midlandschool.org/index.asp

The Midland School is a nationally recognized program approved by the New Jersey Deparment of Education that serves children with special needs.

New Beginnings

28 Dwight Place
Fairfield, NJ 07004
(973) 882-8822
www.nbnj.org

New Beginnings is dedicated to working with children ages three to 21 diagnosed on the autism spectrum. We use a variety of techniques and resources aimed at helping individuals reach their potential and live productively—increasing social, educational and employment opportunities through integration into all aspects of community life.

Reed Academy

85 Summit Ave.
Garfield, NJ 07026
(973) 772.1188
info@reedacademy.org
www.reedacademy.org

Reed Academy is a private, not-for-profit program for individuals with autism spectrum disorders ages 3-21 using ABA techniques. In addition to an individualized full day school program, we also provide family consultation services and parent training.

Somerset Hills Learning Institute
1810 Burnt Mills Road
Bedminster, NJ 07921
(908) 719-6400
info@somerset-hills.org
www.somerset-hills.org/home.html

With our reliance on education and treatment approaches derived from the science of applied behavior analysis, some of our students will graduate to traditional education settings. Others will graduate into the workforce and independent living. None will be relegated to a bleak and inhumane future.

Stepping Stone School
45 County Road 519
Bloomsbury, NJ 08804
(908) 995-1999
Frank Jiorle, Executive Director
frankji@ptd.net
www.sstoneschool.com/page1.html

Stepping Stone School serves Children and Adolescents with Emotional Disorders,Learning Disabilities, Asperger's Syndrome, ADD,ADHD. An individualized instructional and restorative counseling program is provided as an integral part of the school experience.

Y.A.L.E. School Atlantic
(Hamilton Township, NJ)
(856) 346-0007
www.yaleschool.com/schools/atlantic

This school provides year-round, full-day educational programming to children with autism or pervasive developmental disorder not otherwise specified (PDD-NOS), ages 3-7.

Y.A.L.E. School Southeast
1004 Laurel Oak Road
Voorhees, NJ 08043
(856) 346-0007
www.yaleschool.com/schools/southeast

This school provides year-round, full-day educational programming to children with autism or pervasive developmental disorder not otherwise specified (PDD-NOS). The program provides educational services to students ages 3 to 14 years.

Y.A.L.E. School Southeast II
(856) 346-0007
www.yaleschool.com/schools/southeasttwo

This school provides year-round, full-day educational programming to children with autism or pervasive developmental disorder not otherwise specified (PDD-NOS). The program provides educational services to students ages 14 to 21 within a public Jr/Sr high school in Audubon, NJ.

New York:

Anderson Center for Autism
4885 Route 9, P.O. Box 367
Staatsburg, New York 12580
(845) 889-4034
info@ACenterforAutism.org
www.andersoncenterforautism.org

The Anderson Center for Autism is a private center with residential and educational programs for both children and adults with autism, based on ABA treatment.

Ascent: A School for Individuals with Autism
819 Grand Boulevard
Deer Park NY 11729
(631) 254-6100
Nancy Shamow, PH.D., Executive Director
NShamow@aol.com
www.ascentschool.org

Ascent is a private, non-profit school for children diagnosed with autism and atypical pervasive developmental disorders. It provides a full day, 12 month academic and behavioral treatment program to preschool and school age children ranging in age from 3 to 21 years.

Brooklyn Autism Center Academy
111 Remsen Street
Brooklyn, NY 11201
718.554.1027
info@brooklynautismcenter.org
www.brooklynautismcenter.org

The BAC is a non-profit school serving children with Autism Spectrum Disorders (ASD) in Brooklyn. Their philosophy is grounded in the Applied Behavior Analysis (ABA) model, which is the educational standard and best practice for children with autism.

The Center for Developmental Disabilities
72 South Woods Road
Woodbury NY, 11797
(516) 921-7650
vprew@centerfor.com
www.centerfor.com

The Center for Developmental Disabilities has a residential program for autistic and developmentally disabled individuals ages 5 to 21, with educational programs, access to therapy, and clinical services.

Gersh Academy (multiple locations)
358 Hoffman Lane
Hauppauge, NY 11788
254-04 Union Turnpike
Glen Oaks, NY 10004
631.385.3342
www.gershacademy.org

The Gersh Academy's primary objective is to enable students to be emotionally available to learn. They provide customized educational services to individuals with neurobiological disorders, grade 3-12.

The Gersh Experience
North Tonowanda, NY 14120
Post Secondary Program
631-385-3342
www.coralrockacademy.org./index.php/
schools/the-gersh-experience

The Gersh Experience provides a customized educational program that allows students with neurobiological disorders to successfully experience college life away from the home.

The LearningSpring Elementary School
254 West 29th Street, 4th floor
New York, NY 10001
(212) 239-4926
Margaret Poggi, Head of School
mpoggi@learningspring.org
www.learningspring.org

The LearningSpring elementary school uses a Cooperative Learning Paradigm, where academics is integrated with mastery of social/ emotional, pragmatic language, organization and sensory-motor skills.

McCarton School
350 East 82nd Street
New York, New York 10028
Phone: (212) 996-9035
info@mccartonschool.org
www.mccartonschool.org

The McCarton School provides an educational program for autistic children by using an integrated one-to-one model of therapy that is grounded in Applied Behavioral Analysis (ABA) combined with speech and language therapy, motor skills training, and peer interaction.

Millwood Learning Center
12 Schumann Road
Millwood, NY 105046
(914) 941-1991
www.devereux.org

Located in Westchester County, the Center provides year-round, full-day, intensive educational and behavioral interventions to students with autism and other pervasive developmental disorders.

New York City Center for Autism Charter School
433 E. 100 Street
New York, NY 10029
(212)-860-2580
Contact: Julie Fisher, Principal
http://schools.nyc.gov/SchoolPortals/04/M337/default.htm

This school serves grades 1 through 8 and provides special services and extra-curricular activities for children with autism.

Rebecca School
40 East 30th Street
New York, NY 10016-7374
(212) 810-4120
info@rebeccaschool.org
www.rebeccaschool.org

Therapeutic day school for children 4 to 18 that uses the Developmental Individual Difference Relationship-based (DIR) model in the education of children with PDD and autism.

Shema Kolainu-Hear Our Voices
4302 New Utrecht Ave.
Brooklyn, NY 11219
718-686-9600
info@skhov.org
www.shemakolainu.org

SK-HOV's mission is to hear the voices of the children and families they serve as they strive to achieve their full potential for independence, productivity and inclusion in the community. Shema Kolainu is dedicated to the education of children with autism spectrum disorders (ASD). Their vision is to provide the best opportunity offered anywhere for children with ASD to achieve recovery.

Summit Academy
150 Stahl Rd.
Getzville, NY 14068
Phone: 716.629.3400
Fax: 716.629.3499
www.summited.org/early.asp

West Hills Montessori School (operated by Gersh Academy)
313 Round Swamp Road
Melville, NY 11747
631.385.3342
www.gershacademy.org

It is a private, co-educational day school that serves 100 students, ages 18 months to 12 years (Toddler through 6th grade), from both Nassau and Suffolk counties.

North Carolina:

Mariposa School for Children with Autism
The Mariposa School for Children with Autism
203 Gregson Drive
Cary, NC 27511
(919) 461-0600
Contact: Dr. Jacqueline Gottlieb, Head of Mariposa School
info@MariposaSchool.org
www.mariposaschool.org

The Mariposa School staff serves and teaches autistic children by reassessing their needs constantly and giving each child an individual teaching plan.

Ohio:

Autism Academy of Learning
219 Page Street
Toledo, Ohio 43620
(419) 865-7487
Anthony Gerke, Director of Education agerke@theautismacademy.org
www.theautismacademy.org/

The Autism Academy of Learning is structured to provide every student with Autism Spectrum Disorder an appropriate foundation in the areas of academics, behavior, daily living skills, vocational skills, and independence. Our goal is to promote a higher quality of life, and the realization of the full intellectual and social development of students with Autism Spectrum Disorder.

Haugland Learning Center
3400 Snouffer Rd.
Columbus, OH 43235
614-602-6473
hlccolumbus.com

Haugland Learning Center (HLC) serves the educational needs of over 120 children with Autism or Asperger syndrome throughout the state of Ohio, accepting students from preschool through twelfth grade (including those with behaviors) and is therefore an excellent alternative to public school. All students with an Autism or Asperger's diagnosis are eligible to receive the Autism Scholarship from the Ohio Department of Education, which can be used to pay for educational services at HLC.

Oakstone Academy
5747A Cleveland Avenue
Columbus, OH 43231
(614) 865-9643

The Oakstone Academy is a non-profit, fully inclusive, chartered school dedicated to serving children with autism and their families, and we are determined to use the principles of applied behavior analysis within the natural environment and implement the most effective empirically based strategies to promote language, social, behavioral, and academic competency in children with autism.

Summit Academy Schools
www.summitacademies.com

Oregon:

Building Bridges
3533 Southeast Milwaukie
Portland, OR 97202
(503) 235-3122
http://bridgespdx.wordpress.com
Beth Mishler, Board Certified Behavior
Analyst beth@bridgespdx.com

Building Bridges is pleased to offer three behavioral classrooms for children with language and social disorders including autism spectrum disorder: primary (ages 6-8), kindergarten (ages 5-6), and preschool (ages 3-4). The curriculum includes instruction in language arts, mathematics, science, social studies, language, social skills and graphomotor skills, and functional and play skills needed in the classroom are also taught.

The Child Development School of Oregon
12208 NW Cornell Road
Portland, OR 97229
(503) 646-9135
Therese Steward

Our mission is to provide state-of-the-art education for students with autism and related disabilities and to help all our students reach their full potential in school, in the community, and in life.

School of Autism
7714 N Portsmouth
Portland, OR 97203
503-283-9603
schoolofautism@yahoo.com
www.schoolofautism.com

The School of Autism is a place that families with children with autism can go to get therapy, support and education. Through play, sensory immersion and guidance by people who actually have been through the same process, families and children with autism can be treated AND educated in one place.

Pennsylvania:

Autistic Endeavors Learning Center
7340 Jackson Street

Philadelphia, PA, 19136
Barbara A. Butkiewicz Co-Founder/President
aelcinfo@yahoo.com
www.autisticendeavors.org
(215) 360-1569

The mission of Autistic Endeavors Learning Center is to promote independent functioning of children with Autistic Spectrum Disorders. The Center will provide an intensive instructional program using, but not limited to, methods of Applied Behavior Analysis to help children with Autism acquire effective communication and socialization skills.

The Comprehensive Learning Center (CLC)
150 James Way
Southampton, PA 18966
(215) 322-7852
clcschool@clcschool.net
www.clcschool.net

The Comprehensive Learning Center's primary mission is to ensure that each of its students reaches their maximum potential through an intensive, comprehensive education and treatment program based on the scientifically validated procedures of applied behavior analysis.

Devereux Kanner/Kanner CARES
390 East Boot Road
West Chester, PA 19380
610-431-8100
www.devereux.org/site/
PageServer?pagename=kan_cares

Devereux Childhood Autism Research and Education Services (CARES) is a state of the science center-based, day education program for young children with autism using contemporary strategies and methodologies consistent with Applied Behavior Analysis (ABA).

The Melmark School
2600 Wayland Road
Berwyn, Pennsylvania 19312
(610) 325-4969
admissions@melmark.org
www.melmark.org

The Melmark School offers day and residential special education services to children and adolescents ages 5 to 21 with learning difficulties and/or challenging behaviors secondary to a diagnosis of Autism Spectrum Disorder; Acquired Brain Injury; Mental Retardation, mild to profound; Cerebral Palsy; and/or Neurological Disorders.

TALK Institute and School
(formerly Magnolia)
395 Bishop Hollow Road
Newtown Square, PA 19073
610.356.5566
www.talkinc.org/about.html
New Students
phone 610.356.5566
Email mikeabramson@comcast.net
Media Inquiries
phone 610.356.5566
Email melkot@aol.com

The Vista School
1249 Cocoa Avenue
Hershey, PA 17033
(717) 835-0310
Kristen Yurich, Clinical Director kyurich@
thevistaschool.org

Vista serves children with ASD ranging in age from pre-kindergarten to secondary school age from Berks, Cumberland, Dauphin, Franklin, Juniata, Lancaster, Lebanon, and Perry Counties, who are functioning on the moderate to severe end of the autism spectrum, who often display severe delays in communication skills, engage in higher rates of problematic or challenging behaviors, require assistance for activities of daily living, have little or limited ability to appropriately occupy their leisure time, and need one-on-one instruction for learning new skills.

Tennessee:

The King's Daughters' School for Autism
900 Trotwood Avenue
Columbia, Tennessee 38401
(931) 388-3810

The mission of The King's Daughters' School is to serve the educational and training needs of children and adults with developmental disabilities. The school strives to provide a high-quality program of personal development in a wholesome residential atmosphere aimed at allowing each person to reach

his or her fullest potential as an independent and productive citizen.

Texas:

Autism Treatment Center – Dallas
10503 Metric Drive
Dallas, Texas 75243
(972) 644-2076
www.atcoftexas.org

The mission of the Autism Treatment Center is to assist people with autism and related disorders throughout their lives as they learn, play, work and live in the community.

Capitol School of Austin
2011 West Koenig Lane
Austin, Texas 78756
(512) 467-7006

The mission of Capitol School of Austin is to provide an enriched learning environment where children with speech, language, and learning differences can reach their full potential and develop skills necessary to succeed in future educational settings.

Focus On The Future Training Center
3405 Custer Rd. Suite 100
Plano, TX 75023
(972) 599-1400
Contact: Brenda M. Batts, Director
focussped@yahoo.com
www.focussped.com/index.html

Focus on the Future Training Center is a highly regarded Pre-K to Grade 12 private school for children with autism and other mental disabilities. They offer some of the best autism early intervention and other individualized curriculum featuring Speech Therapy, Occupational Therapy, and Music Therapy.

The Monarch School
1231 Wirt Rd.
Houston, TX 77055
(713) 479-0800
Contact: Sharon Duval
sduval@monarchschool.org
www.monarchschool.org
Developmental Individuarl Difference /
FloorTime based program.

Newfound School
2206 Heads Lane, Suite 110
Carrollton, TX 75006
(214) 390-1749
www.newfoundschool.com

Newfound School is a small private school for grades PreK - 12 for children with learning and/or behavior challenges. It is designed to provide meaningful instruction and learning in a caring, nurturing atmosphere. Students are provided lifelong learning strategies for academics, behavior, and social skills.

The Westview School
1900 Kersten Drive
Houston, TX 77043
713.973.1900
Jane G. Stewart, Director
www.westviewschool.org

The Westview School is a private, non-profit school which was founded in 1981 to provide a structured, nurturing, and stimulating learning environment for children with learning differences which prevent them from being successful in regular programs.

Utah:

The Carmen B. Pingree Center for Children with Autism
780 South Guardsman
UT 84108
(801) 581-0194
Contact: Pete Nicholas, Director
petern@vmh.com
www.carmenbpingree.com

The Pingree Center is a preschool and kindergarten program for children with autism that uses a unique 5-step approach for a discrete trial format method of teaching.

Spectrum Academy
575 Cutler Drive
North Salt Lake, UT 84054
(801) 936-0318
http://spectrumcharter.org/

The Spectrum Academy is the premier charter school in Utah that tailors learning environment and curriculum to accommodate the unique needs of children with Asperger's Syndrome and other high-functioning Autism Spectrum Disorders. Our mission encompasses all children, and we are pleased to be free and offer enrollment open to the public.

Vermont:

Howard Center
208 Flynn Avenue Suite 3J
Burlington, Vermont 05401
(802) 488-6000
debs@howardcenter.org
www.howardcenter.org

The Autism Spectrum Program (ASP) at Howard Center provides intensive, specialized instructional and behavioral treatment and support services year-round to individuals with Autism Spectrum Disorders, ages 2-21 years. Services are provided in home, school, and community settings and target the teaching and shaping of essential communication, social, adaptive behavior, daily living, and functional learning skills. Multiple treatment methodologies under the principles of Applied Behavior Analysis are utilized.

INSPIRE for Autism
77 Dylan Rd.
Brattleboro, VT 05301
802-251-7301
info@inspireforautism.org
http://inspire4autism.com/

I.N.S.P.I.R.E. for Autism, Inc. will strive to maximize the potential for adolescents and young adults with Autism Spectrum Disorders to lead satisfying, self-sustaining lives in connection with their communities.

Virginia:

Alternative Paths Training School--Alexandria
5632 Mt. Vernon Memorial Highway
Alexandria, VA 22309
(703) 766-8708
Renee Loebs, Curriculum Specialist
rloebs@aptschool.org
www.aptschool.org

ATPS's mission is to provide students with the knowledge and practical skills essential for their successful integration into the community Locations in Alexandria and Fredericksburg.

Blue Ridge Autism Center
312 Whitwell Drive
Roanoke, VA 24019
540-366-7399
BRAC.1@juno.com
www.blueridgeautismcenter.com

BRAC is committed to providing resources and training to families and professionals throughout the Roanoke Valley and surrounding areas.

Dominion School for Autism
4205 Ravenswood Rd.
Richmond, VA 23222
804-355-1011
wendy.brown@dominionautism.org
www.dominionautism.org

The mission and educational philosophy of The Dominion School is to provide children with autism an individualized, ABA-based educational program in a loving and supportive atmosphere.

Spiritos School
400 Coalfield Road
Midlothian, Virginia 23113
(804) 897-7440
Janet@spiritosschool.com
www.spiritosschool.com

Our mission is to create a wealth of individualized instructional and treatment experiences that provide continual educational programming in an atmosphere of love and acceptance for children with autism and developmental delay.

The Aurora School
420 Wildman St.
Leesburg, VA 20176
540-751-1414
Courtney Deal, Program Director
cdeal@aurora-school.org

At Aurora, we believe that education works best for students and families when valid research findings from the fields of education and psychology, behavior analysis in particular, are constantly applied in the classroom, so teaching practices at the school are derived primarily from applied behavior analysis (ABA).

The Faison School
1701 Byrd Avenue
Richmond, VA 23230
804-612-1947
Dr. Kathy Mathews, Director of Education
kathy@kmaba.com
www.thefaisonschool.org

The Faison School for Autism/ACV is dedicated to giving each child the best chance he or she has to improve their life's journey by employing a three-pronged approach of empirically-driven treatment, research, and training to best serve our students. Our philosophy is a holistic one, focusing on the child, their family, and all those who touch and enrich their lives.

Virginia Institute for Autism
1414 Westwood Road
Charlottesville, VA 22901-5149
(434) 923-8252
information@viaschool.org
www.viaschool.org

VIA is dedicated to providing comprehensive, outcome-based education to people with autism; supporting families coping with the challenges that come with autism; and developing and supporting primary research, advocacy and training in the education of people with autism.

Washington:

DIR®/Floortime™ Summer Camp
20310 19th Ave NE
Shoreline, WA 98155
(206) 367-5853
Contact: Rosemary White, OTR/L, DIR® Faculty
pedptot@comcast.net

Various Locations:

Lovaas Institute
Various Locations
(856) 616-9442 (East Clinical Treatment Headquarters)
(310) 410-4450 (West Clinical Treatment Headquarters)
info@lovaas.com
www.lovaas.com

Intensive Applied Behavioral Analysis (ABA) Program that uses the Lovaas Method for autistic children ages 2 to 8 (children over the age of 5 qualify for consultative services, but not clinic-based services).

May Institute (Headquarters)
41 Pacella Park Drive
Randolph, MA 02368
(781) 440-0400
info@mayinstitute.org
www.mayinstitute.org

May Institute is one of the largest providers of private schools specifically serving children with autism. Our four May Centers for Child Development offer full-day, year-round educational services to children and adolescents with autism spectrum disorders (ASD) and other developmental disabilities. Schools are located in Massachusetts and California.

CANADA:

Autism Society Canada
PO Box 65
Orangeville
ON, L9W 2ZS

Canada
1-866-874-3334
info@autismsocietycanada.ca
www.autismsocietycanada.ca

Autism Society Canada's mission is to work with our many partners to address the national priorities facing the Autism community.

St. Marcellinus School
730 Courtneypark Dr W
Mississauga, ON L5W 1L9, Canada
(905) 564-6614
Contact: Lynda Arsenault, Admissions
lynda.arsenault@dpcdsb.org
www.dpcdsb.org/MARCL

RECOMMENDED READING

Bailey, Sally, *Wings to Fly: Bringing Theatre Arts to Studentswith Special Needs* (Woodbine House, 1993), *Dreams to Sign: Bringing Together Deaf and Hearing Audiences and Actors*, and *Barrier-Free Drama*

Barbera, Mary Lynch, and Tracy Rasmussen. *The Verbal Behavior Approach: How to Teach Children with Autism and Related Disorders.* Jessica Kingsley Publishers, 2007.

Becker, Jeffrey, published in *The Autism File*

Bluestone, Judith. *The Fabric of Autism: Weaving the Threads into a Cogent Theory.* The HANDLE Institute, 2004.

Bock, Kenneth, and Cameron Stauth. *Healing the New Childhood Epidemics: Autism, ADHD, Asthma, and Allergies: The Groundbreaking Program for the 4-A Disorders.* Ballantine Books, 2008.

Buckley, Julie A. *Healing Our Autistic Children: A Medical Plan.* Palgrave Macmillan 2010.

Casanova, Manuel F. Brain and *Brain, Behavior and Evolution* magazines, *Recent Developments in Autism Research* (Nova Biomedical Books, 2005), *Asperger's Disorder* (Medical Psychiatry Series) [Informa Healthcare, 2008], *Neocortical Modularity And The Cell Minicolumn* (Nova Biomedical Books, 2005)

Chauhan, Abha, Ved Chauhan, and Ted Brown, editors. *Autism: Oxidative Stress, Inflammation, and Immune Abnormalities.* CRC Press, 2009.

Chinitz, Judith Hope, *We Band of Mothers:Autism, My Son, and the Specific Carbohydrate Diet* (Autism Research Institute, 2007)

Davis, Dorinne S., *Every Day A Miracle: Success Stories through Sound Therapy.* Kalco Publishing LLC (October 6, 2004)

Davis, Dorinne. *Sound Bodies through Sound Therapy.* Kalco Publishing LLC, 2004.

Fine, Aubrey, and Nya M. Fine, editors. *Therapeutic Recreation for Exceptional Children : Let Me In, I Want to Play.* Delta Society, 1996.

Fine and Eisen. *Afternoons with Puppy.* Purdue University Press 2008.

Fine, Aubrey. *The Handbook on Animal Assisted Therapy: Theoretical Foundations and Guidelines for Practice.* Academic Press, 1999.

Gabriels, R. "Art therapy with children who have autism and their families." *Handbook of art therapy.* Ed. C. Malchiodi. Guilford Press, 2003.

Gottschall, Elaine G. *Breaking the Vicious Cycle: Intestinal Health Through Diet.* Kirkton Press, 1994.

Grandin, Temple and Catherine Johnson. *Animals in Translation Using the Mysteries of Autism to Decode Animal Behavior.* Houghton Mifflin Harcourt, 2005.

Greenspan, Stabley and Wieder, Serena. *Engaging Autism: Using the Floortime Approach to Help Children Relate, Communicate, and Think.* Da Capo Press, 2006.

Grinspoon, Lester, *Marihuana Reconsidered* (Harvard University press 1971, 1977, and American archives press classic edition, 1994) and *Marijuana, the Forbidden Medicine* (Yale University press, 1993, 1997)

Heflin, Juane, *Spectrum Disorders: Effective Instructional Practices* (Prentice Hall,2006)

Henley, D. R. *Exceptional children, exceptional art: Teaching art to special needs.* Worcester, MA: Davis Publications,1992.

Herskowitz, Valerie. *Autism & Computers: Maximizing Independence Through Technology.* AuthorHouse, 2009.

Heflin, L. Juane. *Students with Autism Spectrum Disorders: Effective Instructional Practices,* Prentice Hall, 2007.

Hogenboom, Marga. *Living with Genetic Syndromes Associated with Intellectual Disability.* Jessica Kingsley Publishers, 2001.

Jarusiewicz, Betty, contributed to *The Handbook of Neurofeedback*

Jepson, Bryan Jepson. *Changing the Course of Autism: A Scientific Approach for Parents and Physicians.* Sentient Publications, 2007.

Kaufman, Barry Neil. *Son Rise: The Miracle Continues.* H J Kramer, 1994.

Kawar, Frick and Frick. *Astronaut Training: A Sound Activated Vestibular-Visual Protocol for Moving, Looking & Listening.* Vital Sounds LLC, 2006.

Kirby, David. *Evidence of Harm: Mercury in Vaccines and the Autism Epidemic: A Medical Controversy.* St. Martin's Press, 2005.

Lanham, Lindyl, *The Autism File* and *The Autism Perspective* magazines

Lansky, Amy L. *Impossible Cure: The Promise of Homeopathy.* R.L. Ranch Press, 2003.

Lewis, Lisa. *Special Diets For Special Kids I & II.* Future Horizons, 2001.

Levinson, B. M. *Pet-oriented Child Psychotherapy.* Springfield, IL: Charles C. Thomas. 1969.

Marohn, Stephanie. *The Natural Medicine Guide to Autism.* Hampton Roads Pub Co, 2002.

Martin, Nicole. *Art as an Early Intervention Tool for Children with Autism.* Jessica Kingsley Publishers, 2009.

Matthews, Julie. *Nourishing Hope for Autism: Nutrition Intervention for Healing Our Children, 3rd ed.* Healthful Living Media, 2008.

Maurice, Catherine. *Let Me Hear Your Voice: A Family's Triumph over Autism.* Ballantine Books, 1994.

McCandless, Jaquelyn. *Children with Starving Brains: A Medical Treatment Guide for Autism Spectrum Disorder, 4th ed.* Bramble Books, 2009.

McCarthy, Jenny and Jerry Kartzinel. *Healing and Preventing Autism: A Complete Guide.* Penguin, 2009.

McCarthy, Jenny. *Louder Than Words: A Mother's Journey in Healing Autism.* Penguin, 2007.

McCarthy, Jenny. *Mother Warriors.* Penguin, 2008.

Mehl-Madrona, Lewis, *Coyote Medicine* (Touchstone, 1998), *Coyote Healing* (Bear & Company, 2003) *Coyote Wisdom* (Bear & Company, 2005) *Narrative Medicine* (Bear & Company, 2007) and *Healing the Mind through the Power of Story: The Promise of Narrative Psychiatry* (Bear & Company (June 15, 2010)).

Noble, J. "Art as an instrument for creating social reciprocity: Social skills group for children with autism." *Group process made visible: Group art therapy.* Ed. S. Riley. Brunner-Routledge, 2001.

Pereira, Lavinia, and Solomon Michelle, *First Sound Series* by Trafford Publishing

Prizant, Barry, Amy Wetherby, Emily Rubin, Amy Laurent and P. Rydell. *The SCERTS Model: A Comprehensive Educational Approach for Children with Autism Spectrum Disorders*. Baltimore, MD: Paul H. Brookes Publishing, 2006.

Rimland, Bernard. *Infantile Autism: The Syndrome and Its Implication for a Neural Theory of Behavior*. Prentice Hall,1964.

Rimland, Bernard, Jon Pangborn, Sidney Baker. *Autism: Effective Biomedical Treatments (Have We Done Everything We Can For This Child? Individuality In An Epidemic)*. Autism Research Institute, 2005.

Rimland, Bernard, Jon Pangborn, Sidney Baker. *2007 Supplement - Autism: Effective Biomedical Treatments (Have We Done Everything We Can for This Child? Individuality In An Epidemic)*. Autism Research Institute, 2007.

Robbins, Jim. *A Symphony in the Brain: The Evolution of the New Brain Wave Biofeedback*. Grove Press, 2008.

Rogers, Sally J. and Geraldine Dawson. *Early Start Denver Model For Young Children With Autism: Promoting Language, Learning, And Engagement*. Guilford Press, 2009.

Seroussi, Karyn. *Unraveling the Mystery of Autism and Pervasive Developmental Disorders*. Simon & Schuster, 2000.

Seroussi, Karyn and Lisa Lewis. *The Encyclopedia of Dietary Interventions for the Treatment of Autism and Related Disorders*. Sarpsborg Press, 2008.

Sicile-Kira, Chantal. *Autism Spectrum Disorders: The Complete Guide to Understanding Autism, Asperger's Syndrome, Pervasive Developmental Disorder, and Other ASDs*. Penguin, 2004.

Sicile-Kira, Chantal. *Adolescents on the Autism Spectrum: A Parent's Guide to the Cognitive, Social, Physical, and Transition Needs of Teenagers with Autism Spectrum Disorders*. Penguin, 2006.

Sicile-Kira, Chantal. *Autism Life Skills: From Communication and Safety to Self-Esteem and More - 10 Essential Abilities Every Child Needs and Deserves to Learn*. Penguin, 2008.

Silva, Louisa. *Helping your Child with Autism: A Home Program from Chinese Medicine*. Guan Yin Press, 2010.

Silver, R. A. *Developing cognitive and creative skills through art: Programs for children with communication disorders or learning disabilities* (3rd ed. revised). New York: Albin Press 1989.

Siri, Kenneth, *1001 Tips for Parents of Autistic Boys* (forthcoming)

Theoharides, Theoharis C., *Pharmacology* (Essentials of Basic Science) (Little Brown and Company, 1992) *Essentials of Pharmacology* (Essentials of Basic Science) (Lippincott Williams & Wilkins, 1996)

Wiseman, Nancy D. *The First Year: Autism Spectrum Disorders: An Essential Guide for the Newly Diagnosed Child*. Da Capo Lifelong Books, 2009.

Wolfberg, Pamela J. *Play and Imagination in Children with Autism, 2nd ed*. Autism Asperger Publishing Company, 2009.

Woodward, Bob and Marga Hogenboom. *Autism: A Holistic Approach*. Floris Books, 2001.

Yasko, Amy. *Autism: Pathways to Recovery*. Neurological Research Institute, 2009.

Yasko, Amy. *Genetic Bypass: Using Nutrition to Bypass Genetic Mutations*. Neurological Research Institute, 2005.